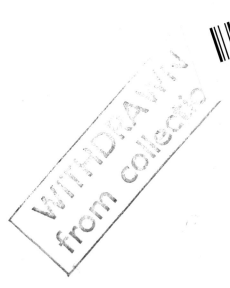

RECENT ADVANCES IN
ANIMAL NUTRITION — 2007

Recent Advances in Animal Nutrition

2007

P.C. Garnsworthy, PhD

J. Wiseman, PhD

University of Nottingham

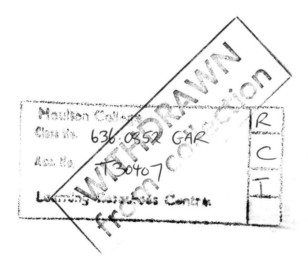

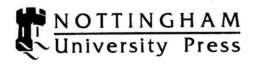

NOTTINGHAM
University Press

Nottingham University Press
Manor Farm, Main Street, Thrumpton
Nottingham, NG11 0AX, United Kingdom

NOTTINGHAM

First published 2008

British Library Cataloguing in Publication Data
Recent Advances in Animal Nutrition — 2007:
University of Nottingham Feed Manufacturers
Conference (41st, 2007, Nottingham)
I. Garnsworthy, Philip C. II. Wiseman, J.

ISBN 978-1-904761-03-7

Disclaimer

Typeset by Nottingham University Press, Nottingham
Printed and bound by Cromwell Press, Trowbridge, Wiltshire

PREFACE

The 41st University of Nottingham Feed Conference was held at the School of Biosciences, Sutton Bonington Campus, 4th – 6th September 2007. Once again, the Nottingham Cattle Fertility Conference was hosted on the preceding day so that participants had the opportunity to attend both events. With this in mind, the first seven papers of the Feed Conference are concerned with health aspects of ruminants, although mostly from a nutritional perspective to maintain relevance to the animal feed industry.

The main cause of premature culling of dairy cows is failure to conceive and poor fertility represents a significant cost to dairy industries throughout the world. Although there are genetic links with fertility, nutrition during late gestation and early lactation has a tremendous impact on health and subsequent reproductive performance of dairy cows. Therefore, the first three papers report the latest research findings from teams studying nutritional effects on health and reproductive efficiency. The first paper explains the relationship between negative energy balance and fertility, and also reviews studies where different energy sources had been used in early lactation to improve energy status and metabolism of dairy cows. The second paper outlines the findings of a large survey that identified management factors affecting fertility, including overcrowding, body condition score and milk yield as key predictors of pregnancy rate. The third paper provides a scientific approach to feeding cows during the dry period, highlights the critical role that this plays in cow health and performance, and makes practical recommendations for controlling energy intake during this period.

Lameness is another major cause of premature culling that results in significant financial losses for dairy herds. More importantly, however, lameness is also a significant welfare issue because it causes long-term pain and suffering for cows. The first of two papers on lameness looks at the impacts of practical nutritional and environmental management on lameness. The second paper looks at the basic biology of hoof structure to demonstrate how nutrition can affect the composition of the claw and its susceptibility to damage and infection.

The final two papers in the ruminant section are concerned with specific disease threats and antimicrobials respectively. The former outlines the current status of scrapie control and then considers control measures for blue tongue. The timeliness of this paper is demonstrated by the fact that, in the conference presentation, the author warned about the imminent threat of blue tongue in the UK, and then had to update the written paper to account for the first outbreak that occurred two weeks later. The second paper reports the findings of two EU projects that identified plants and their extracts with potential as antimicrobial manipulators of rumen fermentation for productivity and health benefits.

Two important issues for animal agriculture are globalisation and environmental impact. The first paper in the systems section describes the rapid growth in Indian livestock production and consumption, and discusses the tremendous implications for World markets in animal feeds and products. The second paper uses life cycle analysis to estimate the environmental burdens of animal production systems, and concludes that increases in feed efficiency in all species, and fertility in ruminant species, is the best way to reduce burdens.

Raw material issues are considered by four papers. The first looks at co-products from biodiesel production, an industry of increasing importance in Europe and elsewhere. The paper discusses glycerol, which constitutes a useful energy source for ruminants, and rapeseed meal, which constitutes a useful protein source. The second paper reports the findings of a large survey of mycotoxin contamination in feeds and raw materials, that the incidence of mycotoxins is quite high in animal feed. However, the authors could not assess the relevance of contamination levels because raw materials are diluted to varying extents and are used in a wide variety of production systems. The third paper considered the challenges faced by animal feed companies supplying the market for organic feeds; the key issues include balance of supply and demand, quality of supply, and shortages of organic feed. The fourth paper addresses the challenge of variability in feedstuff composition, which leads to uncertainty in diet formulation; allowing for variability reduces the cost of diets and improves the prediction of animal performance.

The first of the five non-ruminant papers emphasises the need for adequate water supply in pig and poultry operations, and illustrates how the simple practice of monitoring water consumption can provide a useful indication of feed intake, animal performance and health. The second paper looks at ways to manage the nutrition of outdoor pigs so as to reduce their considerable environmental impact; strategies discussed include matching diets to nutrient requirements, reducing feed wastage and excreted nutrients, and increasing vegetative capture of nutrients. The third paper provides a pig producer's perspective on salmonella control and discusses the efficacy of on-farm measures in relation to national control schemes. The fourth paper presents some novel data on the use of a commercial sports supplement to help parturition in sows and reduce perinatal mortality of piglets. The fifth paper explains the biological principles of compensatory growth in pigs and discusses how this might be used to influence the partition of nutrients between lipid and protein deposition.

We would like to take this opportunity to thank all speakers for their presentations and written papers, which have maintained the high standards and international standing of the Nottingham Feed Conference. We are grateful to all members of the Programme Committee (see the List of Participants) for their significant inputs into specifying and arranging the programme for the conference. We would also like to acknowledge the input of those who chaired sessions (Bob Webb, Mike Wilkinson, Zoë Davies, David Parker and Mike Varley) and the administrative (managed by Sue Golds), catering and support staff who ensure the smooth running of the conference. Finally we would like to thank the delegates who made significant contributions both to the discussion sessions and the general atmosphere of the meeting.

The 2008 event will be held at the University of Nottingham Sutton Bonington Campus 3rd – 4th September.

P.C. Garnsworthy
J. Wiseman

CONTENTS

Preface

1

INFLUENCES OF TRANSITION COW NUTRITION ON HEALTH AND REPRODUCTION OF DAIRY COWS

JOSÉ EDUARDO P. SANTOS
Veterinary Medicine Teaching and Research Center, School of Veterinary Medicine, University of California, Davis, USA

Introduction

Selection of dairy cattle for milk yield has linked the endocrine and metabolic controls of nutrient balance and reproductive events so that reproduction is compromised during periods of nutrient shortage such as in early lactation. Although the energy costs for ovulation, and establishment and maintenance of an early developing embryo are negligible compared with the energy needs for maintenance and lactation of the cow, the metabolic and endocrine cues associated with negative energy balance impair resumption of ovulatory cycles, oocyte and embryo quality, and establishment and maintenance of pregnancy in dairy cattle.

Nutrition during late gestation and early lactation has a tremendous impact on health and subsequent reproductive performance of dairy cows. Prevalence of periparturient diseases is high in high-producing dairy cows and these disorders tend to have negative impacts on resumption of postpartum cyclicity and fertility. Particular attention should be paid to diseases associated with energy and Ca metabolism in high-producing cows.

Inadequate energy intake after calving has a detrimental impact on reproductive performance of cows. Cows under severe negative energy balance have reduced peripheral concentrations of glucose, insulin and insulin-like growth factor-I (IGF-I), reduced peak frequency of luteinizing hormone (LH) pulses, increased concentrations of growth hormone (GH), nonesterified fatty acids (NEFA) and ß-OH-butyrate (BHBA), and impaired ovarian activity. Peripheral changes in metabolite concentrations are thought to influence granulosa cell function and oocyte quality. Slow recovery of ovarian activity during the postpartum period is a major impediment to insemination of cows immediately after the end of the voluntary waiting period. Lack of ovarian cyclicity not only influences detection of oestrus, but it also reduces conception rate, and increases the risk for pregnancy loss. Recent data indicate that cows with delayed postpartum ovulation are more likely to experience subclinical endometritis, which further reduces conception rates.

Extended postpartum anoestrus is magnified by losses of body condition (BCS) during early lactation. Cows with greater losses of BCS are more likely to experience a delay in postpartum cyclicity, and both anoestrus and low BCS negatively impact fertility. Resumption of ovulatory cycles associated with energy balance seems to be mediated by a rise in plasma insulin and IGF-I, which are linked to nutritional status. Insulin seems to be an important metabolic signal re-coupling the GH-IGF axis in the first few weeks postpartum, thereby increasing blood concentrations of IGF-I and oestradiol. Feeding diets that promote higher plasma glucose and insulin might improve the metabolic and endocrine status of cows, expedite resumption of postpartum cyclicity, and enhance fertility.

Exciting strategies have been developed to integrate nutritional and reproductive management. Feeding supplemental lipid has proven effective in enhancing reproductive performance of lactating dairy cows. Often energy status is not affected by feeding lipid and the positive impacts on fertility seem to be the result of extra-energetic effects. More specifically, some fatty acids have the ability to modulate PGF2a secretion, enhance follicle development, luteal function, fertilization rate, embryo quality, and pregnancy maintenance in dairy cows. Although lipid supplementation often improves reproduction, fertility responses to different types of fatty acids are not always consistent.

Minimizing the incidence of uterine problems and reducing the risk for subclinical and clinical ketosis are expected to improve overall cow health and reproduction. Inadequate prepartum feed intake and suppression of the immune system compromises uterine health and increases the risk for acute postpartum metritis, which reduces fertility. Proper cow management to allow adequate feeding behaviour during late gestation and early lactation is expected to minimize immune suppression and the risk for uterine diseases.

Choline is required for synthesis of lipoproteins for lipid transport. Supplementation with rumen-protected choline has consistently reduced the risk for subclinical and clinical ketosis in dairy cows, and improves milk yield, although effects on reproduction are less clear.

Nutrition and postpartum uterine health and fertility

Epidemiological studies have clearly demonstrated strong relationships between postparturient diseases and subsequent reproductive performance in dairy cattle. Cows diagnosed with clinical hypocalcaemia were 3.2 times more likely to experience retained placenta than cows that did not have clinical hypocalcaemia

(Curtis *et al.*, 1983). Whiteford and Sheldon (2005) also found that hypocalcaemia was associated with occurrence of uterine disease in lactating dairy cows. Markusfeld (1985) reported that 80% of cows with ketonuria developed metritis.

A major risk factor for uterine disease is retention of foetal membranes. Generally, cows with retained placenta have increased risk of developing metritis compared with cows not experiencing retained placenta, and both metritis and retained placenta double the risk of cows remaining with uterine inflammation at the time of first postpartum insemination (Rutigliano, 2006). In the US, a recent USDA study (NAHMS, 1996) indicated that the incidence of retained placenta in dairy cows was 7.8 ± 0.2%. A recent study in five dairy farms in Israel observed that retained placenta was diagnosed in 13.1% (9.4 to 18.1%) of multiparous cows and 9.2% (3.6 to 13.8%) of primiparous cows (Goshen and Shpiegel, 2006). In the same study, metritis affected 18.6% (15.2 to 23.5%) of multiparous cows and 30% (19.4 to 42.3%) of primiparous cows. Both retained placenta and metritis can have devastating effects on reproductive efficiency in lactating dairy cows, with reduced conception rates and extended interval to pregnancy (Goshen and Shpiegel, 2006). In fact, not only does the clinical disease negatively affect fertility of dairy cows, but subclinical endometritis, a disease characterized by increased proportion of neutrophils in uterine cytology without the presence of clinical signs of inflammation of the uterus, also has major deleterious effects on conception rates of lactating dairy cows at first postpartum insemination (Table 1).

Table 1. Subclinical endometritis and conception rate (%) at first postpartum insemination in dairy cows.

	Subclinical endometritis		
Reference	*Yes*	*No*	*P value*
Bruno *et al.* (2007)	22.5	34.3	0.02
Galvão *et al.* (2006)	28.8	41.3	0.06
Gilbert *et al.* (2005)	11.0	36.0	0.01
Kasimanickam *et al.* (2004)	18.0	32.0	0.05
Rutigliano *et al.* (2006)	18.3	35.7	0.002

There is increasing evidence to suggest that feed intake and feeding behaviour around parturition might mediate some of the increased risk for uterine diseases in dairy cattle (Hammon *et al.*, 2006; Huzzey *et al.*, 2007; Urton *et al.*, 2005). Hammon *et al.* (2006) observed that cows developing uterine disease postpartum experienced reduced dry matter intake beginning one week before calving. Similarly, cows diagnosed with severe metritis after calving were already consuming less dry matter two weeks prior to calving (Huzzey *et al.*, 2007). In the same study, even cows that subsequently developed mild metritis had reduced feed intake one week before calving compared with cows with healthy uteri. The same group (Urton *et al.*, 2005) observed that cows that developed metritis spent significantly less time eating before and after calving than cows that did not develop metritis. These data indicate that suppressed intake of nutrients or alterations in feeding behaviour prior to calving are major risk factors for development of metritis postpartum.

A potential link between nutrient intake and development of uterine diseases may be the immune status of the cow. Kimura *et al.* (2002) evaluated neutrophil function from 142 periparturient dairy cows in two herds by evaluating chemotatic and killing activity of those cells. The authors observed that 14.1% of the cows developed retained placenta, and neutrophils isolated from blood of cows with retained placenta had reduced ability to migrate to placental tissue and reduced myeloperoxidase activity, a marker for oxidative burst and killing activity of neutrophils. Interestingly, the reduced neutrophil function was observed between one and two weeks prior to calving, which suggests that the reduced innate immune function may be part of the cause of retained placenta rather than a consequence of the disease. In fact, cows that developed uterine disease, either clinical metritis or subclinical endometritis experienced reduced feed intake and neutrophil function prior to calving (Hammon *et al.*, 2006). These data suggest strongly that inadequate nutrient intake before calving might predispose cows to impaired immune function and subsequent increased risk for uterine diseases that negatively affect reproduction.

Because intake of nutrients seems to influence energy status and immune function of dairy cows, both of which seem to be related to risk of uterine diseases, it is prudent to suggest that nutritional and management strategies that optimize nutrient intake around parturition should improve uterine health and subsequent fertility of dairy cows. Perhaps, of equal or more importance than diet composition is the environment to which the preparturient cow is subjected, as inadequate cow comfort, competition for space, and hierarchical status can all influence the ability of the cow to consume nutrients (Hammon *et al.*, 2006; Huzzey *et al.*, 2007; Urton *et al.*, 2005).

Resumption of postpartum cyclicity

The onset of lactation creates an enormous drain of nutrients in high producing dairy cows which, in many cases, delays the resumption of ovulatory cycles. During early postpartum, reproduction is deferred in favour of individual survival. Therefore, in the case of the dairy cow, lactation becomes a priority to the detriment of reproductive functions.

During periods of energy restriction, oxidizable fuels consumed in the diet are prioritized toward essential processes such as cell maintenance, circulation, and neural activity (Wade and Jones, 2004). Homeorhetic controls in early lactation assure that body tissue, primarily adipose stores, will be mobilized in support of milk production. Therefore, the early lactation dairy cow that is unable to consume enough energy-yielding nutrients to meet the needs of production and maintenance will sustain high yields of milk and milk components at the expense of body tissues. This poses a problem to reproduction as delayed ovulation has been linked repeatedly with energy status (Butler, 2003). Energy deprivation reduces the frequency of pulses of LH, thereby impairing follicle maturation and ovulation. Furthermore, undernutrition inhibits oestrous behaviour by reducing responsiveness of the central nervous system to oestradiol by reducing the oestrogen receptor a content in the brain (Hileman *et al.*, 1999).

Generally, the first postpartum ovulation in dairy cattle occurs 10 to 14 days after the nadir of negative energy balance (Butler, 2003), and severe weight and BCS losses caused by inadequate feeding or illnesses are associated with anovulation and anoestrus in dairy cattle. In fact, cows with low BCS at 65 days postpartum are more likely to be anovular (Figure 1; Santos *et al.*, 2008), which compromises reproductive performance at first postpartum insemination.

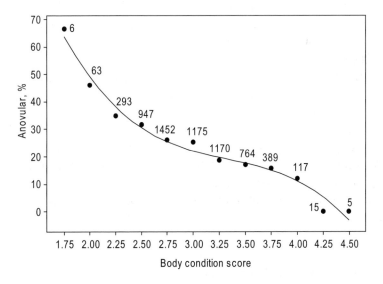

Figure 1. Relationship between frequency of lactating dairy cows classified as anovular based two sequential plasma progesterone concentrations (< 1.0 ng/mL) in the first 65 days postpartum and body condition score at 70 days postpartum. Values represent the number of cows in each body condition category (Santos *et al.*, 2008).

Prolonged postpartum anovulation or anoestrus extends the period from calving to first artificial insemination and reduces fertility during the first postpartum service

(Santos *et al.*, 2008; Stevenson *et al.*, 2001). In fact, anovular cows not only have reduced oestrous detection and conception rates, but also have compromised embryo survival (Santos *et al.*, 2004). On the other hand, an early return to cyclicity is important in regard to early conception. The timing of the first postpartum ovulation determines and limits the number of oestrous cycles occurring prior to the beginning of the insemination period. Typically, in most dairy herds, fewer than 20 % of cows should be anovular at the end of the voluntary waiting period. Oestrous expression, conception rate, and embryo survival improved when cows were cycling prior to oestrous or ovulation synchronization programs for first postpartum insemination (Santos *et al.*, 2008).

Resumption of ovarian activity in high producing dairy cows is determined by energy status of the animal. Therefore, feeding management that minimizes loss of body condition during the early postpartum period and incidence of metabolic disorders during early lactation should increase the number of cows experiencing a first ovulation during the first four to six weeks postpartum, which is critical for optimum establishment and maintenance of pregnancy following the first postpartum AI.

Energy and reproduction

Feed intake appears to have the greatest impact on energy status of lactating dairy cows. Villa-Godoy *et al.* (1988) reported that variation in energy balance in postpartum Holstein cows was influenced most strongly by dry matter intake ($r = 0.73$) and less by milk yield ($r = -0.25$). Therefore, differences among cows in the severity of energy balance are more related with how much energy they consume than with how much milk they produce.

During periods of negative energy balance, blood concentrations of glucose, insulin, and IGF-I are low, as well as the pulse frequency of GnRH and LH. Plasma progesterone concentrations are also affected by the energy balance of dairy cows. These metabolites and hormones have been shown to affect folliculogenesis, ovulation, and steroid production in vitro and in vivo. The exact mechanism by which energy affects secretion of releasing hormones and gonadotropins is not well defined, but it is clear that lower levels of blood glucose, IGF-I, and insulin may mediate this process.

It has been suggested that negative energy balance influences reproduction of dairy cows by affecting the quality and viability of the oocyte, the ovulatory follicle and the CL developing after ovulation of that follicle. Because there is substantial evidence that metabolic factors can influence early follicular development, it is conceivable that changes in metabolism during periods of negative energy balance could influence preantral follicles destined to ovulate weeks later during the breeding period. To test this hypothesis, Kendrick *et al.* (1999) randomly assigned 20 dairy cows to one of two treatments formulated so that cows consumed either 3.6 % (high energy) or 3.2 % (low energy) of their body weight. Follicles were transvaginally aspirated twice weekly and oocytes were graded based upon cumulus density and ooplasm homogeneity. Cows in better energy balance (high energy diet) had greater intrafollicular IGF-I and plasma progesterone concentrations and tended to produce more oocytes graded as good. Therefore, negative energy balance not only delays resumption of ovulatory cycles, but it might also influence the quality of oocytes ovulated at the time when cows are inseminated.

Nutritional manipulation to increase energy intake

Nutritional efforts to minimize the extent and duration of negative energy balance may improve reproductive performance. The first and most important factor that affects energy intake in dairy cows is feed availability (Grant and Albright, 1995). Therefore, dairy cows should have a high quality palatable diet available at all times to assure maximum dry matter intake (DMI). However, DMI is limited during late gestation and early lactation, which can compromise total energy intake and reproductive performance. Several nutritional management strategies have been proposed to increase energy intake during early lactation. Feeding high quality forages, increasing the concentrate:forage ratio, or adding supplemental fat to diets are some of the most common ways to improve energy intake in cows.

Intake of energy increases linearly with increasing concentrate in the diet up to 60 % of the dry matter. Diets with more than 60% concentrate and limited fibre content, particularly forage neutral detergent fibre (NDF) are associated with increased ruminal osmolarity, reduced rumen pH, increased volatile fatty acid (VFA) concentrations in the rumen and portal system, and decreased DMI. Although excessive concentrations of highly fermentable carbohydrates can be detrimental to the cow's digestive health, increased intake or ruminal digestion of dietary starch increases the proportion of propionate relative to other VFA and enhances glucose synthesis in the liver. Glucose is an insulin secretagogue, and diets with high ruminally degradable starch increase liver output of glucose (Theurer *et al.*, 1999) and plasma concentrations of glucose and insulin (Santos *et al.*, 2000).

A number of studies have demonstrated the importance of insulin as a signal mediating the effects of acute changes in nutrient intake on reproductive parameters in dairy cattle. In early postpartum dairy cattle under negative energy balance, reduced expression of hepatic GH receptor 1A (GHR-1A) is thought to be responsible for the lower concentrations of IGF-I in plasma of cows (Radcliff *et al.*, 2003). Because IGF-I is an important hormonal signal that influences reproductive events such as stimulation of cell mitogenesis, hormonal production, and embryo development, among other functions; increasing concentrations of IGF-I early postpartum are important for early resumption of cyclicity and establishment of pregnancy. It is interesting to note that insulin mediates the expression of GHR-1A in dairy cows (Butler *et al.*, 2003; Rhoads *et al.*, 2004), which results in increased concentrations of IGF-I in plasma. Because IGF-I and insulin are important for reproduction in cattle, feeding diets that promote greater insulin concentrations should benefit fertility.

Gong *et al.* (2002) fed cows of low- and high-genetic merit isoenergetic diets that differed in the ability to induce high or low insulin concentrations in plasma. The authors observed that diets that induced high insulin reduced the interval to first postpartum ovulation, increased the proportion of cows ovulating in the first 50 days postpartum, and improved conception rate at first AI (Table 2).

Table 2. Effect of diets designed to alter plasma insulin concentrations on reproductive parameters of high- and low-genetic merit postpartum dairy cows (adapted from Gong *et al.*, 2002).

| | *Diet* | | | |
| | *Low insulin* | | *High insulin* | |
Genetic merit	*Low*	*High*	*Low*	*High*
Plasma insulin,1 ng/mL	0.34	0.21	0.48	0.32
Ovulation in first 50 d postpartum,1 %	60	50	100	80
Days to first ovulation	43	54	28	41
Conception rate to first AI, %	62.5	37.5	66.7	44.4

[1] Effect of high-insulin diet (P < 0.05).

Recently, monensin (Rumensin 80®, monensin sodium, Elanco Animal Health, Greenfield, IN) was approved for use in lactating dairy cattle to enhance milk production efficiency in the US. However, although not labelled for treatment of subclinical ketosis, monensin supplementation of transition dairy cows increases plasma glucose concentrations and reduces subclinical ketosis. Because monensin increases propionate production in the rumen and glucose concentrations in plasma, it is expected that monensin supplementation will improve plasma insulin concentrations and influence reproductive performance. When cows were treated with a controlled release capsule that delivers approximately 335 mg of monensin/d, risks for ketosis, displaced abomasum and multiple illnesses were reduced, but reproductive parameters were not altered (Table 3; Duffield *et al.*, 1999).

Table 3. Effect of monensin in a controlled release capsule on conception rates of dairy cows at different inseminations (AI) postpartum (adapted from Duffield *et al.*, 1999).

	Treatment	
	Monensin	*Control*
Cows, n	406	403
Conception rate, %		
First AI	35.2	34.5
Second AI	37.6	41.5
Third AI	40.7	38.6
> 3 AI	60.0	64.1

Feeding fat and fatty acids

Lipids are important molecules that serve as sources of energy and are critical components of the physical and functional structure of cells. Lipids present in cell membranes, such as fatty acids in phospholipids, play an important role in regulating the properties and activity of cell membranes. Changes in chain length, degree of unsaturation and position of the double bonds in the acyl chain of fatty acids can have remarkable impacts on their function and may affect reproduction in cattle (Mattos *et al.*, 2000; Staples *et al.*, 1998).

There is overwhelming evidence that fatty acids of dietary origin can influence reproductive events in cattle (Mattos *et al.*, 2000; Staples *et al.*, 1998), although the exact mechanisms are still unclear. Potential mechanisms may be associated with improved dietary energy concentration (Ferguson *et al.*, 1990), increased concentrations of progesterone (Staples *et al.*, 1998), suppressed luteolytic signals around maternal recognition of pregnancy (Mattos *et al.*, 2000), and improved embryo quality (Adamiak *et al.*, 2006; Cerri *et al.*, 2004). The use of fat in diets of dairy cattle usually increases the energy concentration of the ration and improves lactation and reproduction (Table 4; Ferguson *et al.*, 1990).

Some have suggested that feeding fat improves reproduction in spite of provision of energy (Staples *et al.*, 1998). These effects might be mediated by the fatty acid make up of the fat source, as different fatty acids can have distinct effects at the tissue and cellular level. However, a major impediment to the study of fatty acids and reproduction in cattle is the inability to predict the delivery of specific lipids, particularly polyunsaturated fatty acids (PUFA) to the small intestine for absorption and the specific needs of different tissues for fatty acids to modulate reproduction. Because microbial activity in the rumen, resulting in lipolysis and biohydrogenation of lipids containing unsaturated fatty acids, dramatically reduces the amount of these fatty acids leaving the rumen, future research with lipids and reproduction will have to utilize methods of delivery that reduce the susceptibility of fatty acids to rumen microbial activity, thereby increasing the supply of unsaturated fatty acids for absorption. Unfortunately, commercial methods available to protect lipids from microbial biohydrogenation are not very effective at preventing saturation of PUFA in the rumen (Figure 2; Juchem *et al.*, 2007).

Table 4. Effect of feeding 500 g of saturated free fatty acids (FA) on reproduction of dairy cows (adapted from Ferguson *et al.*, 1990).

| | *Treatment* | |
	No supplemental FA	*500 g/d saturated free FA*
Cows, n	138	115
Conception 1st AI, %	42.6[a]	59.1[b]
Conception all AI, %	40.7[a]	59.3[b]
Pregnant, %	86.2[c]	93.0[d]

[a,b] Superscripts in the same row differ (P < 0.05).
[c,d] Superscripts in the same row differ (P = 0.08).

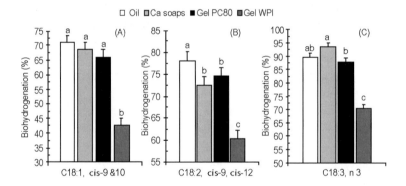

Figure 2. Biohydrogenation of unsaturated fatty acids from a blend of soyabean and linseed oils fed to lactating dairy cows as oil, Ca soaps, and two novel protein gels (Adapted from Juchem *et al.*, 2007).

In spite of the difficulties to deliver specific unsaturated fatty acids to ruminants, recent interest in the effects of lipids on reproduction of dairy cattle has generally indicated that fat supplementation improves fertility and effects differ with distinct fatty acid sources. More recently, there has been an increased interest in designing fat sources rich in omega-6 (linoleic acid, cis-9 cis-12 C18:2n6) and omega-3 (a-linolenic acid, C18:3n3; eicosapentaenoic - EPA, C20:5n3; docosahexaenoic - DHA, C22:6n3) PUFA for delivery to the lower gut for absorption with the ultimate goal of improving reproduction in dairy cows (Ambrose *et al.*, 2006; Cerri *et al.*, 2004; Fuentes *et al.*, 2007; Juchem *et al.*, 2007; Ambrose *et al.*, Fuentes *et al.*, 2007).

EFFECT OF FEEDING OMEGA-3 FATTY ACIDS ON REPRODUCTIVE PERFORMANCE OF DAIRY COWS

Omega-3 fatty acids have the ability to modulate the luteolytic signal and it is thought that they might enhance embryo survival in dairy cows (Mattos *et al.*, 2000). Ambrose *et al.* (2006) fed lactating dairy cows diets differing in supplemental fat sources from 28 days before to 32 days after the first postpartum insemination. Diets consisted of either rolled linseed, a source rich in linolenic acid or rolled sunflower seed, a source rich in linoleic acid. Fat sources provided approximately 750 g of oil/day. Although pregnancy to the first postpartum insemination did not differ between treatments, the proportion of cows calving (90.2 vs. 72.7%) was greater for those receiving omega-3 than omega-6 fatty acids, in part because of reduced pregnancy losses (9.8 vs. 27.3%).

Using a similar approach, Fuentes *et al.* (2007) altered the fatty acid composition of the diet of 356 lactating dairy cows by feeding either extruded linseed, a source of omega-3 fatty acids, or calcium soaps of palm fatty acids, a source rich in saturated and monounsaturated fatty acids. Although cows consuming the diet supplemented with omega-3 fatty acids experienced some suppression in release of prostaglandin after an experimental challenge, conception rates were not altered and time to pregnancy was similar between treatments (Figure 3).

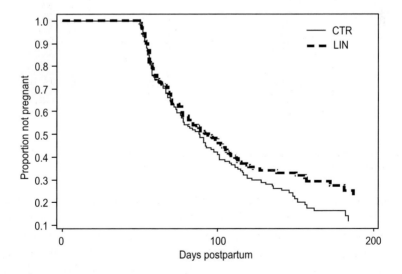

Figure 3. Survival curves for interval from calving to pregnancy in cows fed control (CTR) or linseed (LIN) diets. Median intervals from calving to pregnancy did not differ (P = 0.13) and were 88 days for CTR and 94 days for LIN (Fuentes *et al.*, 2007).

Other attempts to improve reproduction of dairy cows by feeding different fatty acid sources have been made by using calcium soaps of fatty acids. Juchem *et al.* (2007) conducted two experiments to evaluate the effects of feeding omega-3 PUFA as calcium salts on uterine synthesis of prostaglandin, pregnancy rates, and pregnancy losses. In experiment 1, 738 lactating multiparous cows were assigned in two replicates to the different treatment diets, whereas in experiment 2, 331 lactating multiparous cows were assigned to the dietary treatments. Treatments consisted of the totally mixed ration, except for the supplemental fat sources, calcium salt of fish and palm oils at 1.9 % of the diet dry matter, or tallow at 1.8 % of the diet dry matter to provide equal amounts of fatty acids. Rations were similar in total fat content in experiment 1 (5.6 vs. 5.3%) and experiment 2 (5.6 vs. 5.9%) for calcium soaps of fish and palm oils and tallow, respectively. Cows were time inseminated at 75 days postpartum in experiment 1, and oestrus-synchronized in experiment 2, and pregnancy was diagnosed at different intervals after insemination. Feeding fish oil fatty acids in a calcium soap form did not alter prostaglandin response to an oxytocin challenge in experiment 1 and pregnancy rates in experiments 1 and 2 (Table 5).

Table 5. Reproductive responses at first postpartum insemination in multiparous cows fed calcium salts of fish and palm oils (CaSFO) or tallow (Juchem *et al.*, 2007).

| | Treatment | | |
	CaSFO	Tallow	P
Experiment 1			
Cyclic, %	82.2	83.2	0.68
Pregnancy AI 1, %			
Day 28	35.9	40.7	0.19
Day 66	26.3	32.0	0.10
Pregnancy loss, %	23.5	20.4	0.55
Experiment 2			
Oestrous detection, %	52.2	58.6	0.24
Pregnancy AI 1, %			
Day 38	24.8	22.8	0.67
Day 66	22.4	21.6	0.87
Pregnancy loss, %	10.0	5.4	0.46

These results suggest that although feeding fat sources rich in omega-3 fatty acids can alter reproductive responses of dairy cows, they have not consistently improved establishment and maintenance of pregnancy in lactating dairy cows.

EFFECT OF FEEDING CA SALTS RICH IN OMEGA-6 AND TRANS FATTY ACIDS DURING TRANSITION ON LACTATION, HEALTH, AND REPRODUCTION OF DAIRY COWS

Fat sources rich in omega-6 fatty acids such as linoleic acid have the potential to increased synthesis of prostaglandins by dairy cows, which might be important to uterine involution and health. In addition, monoenoic trans fatty acids have the ability to suppress milk fat synthesis and upregulate hepatic gluconeogenic enzymes (Sellberg *et al.*, 2005). It was postulated that combining both groups of fatty acids would be beneficial to energy status of dairy cows, enhance uterine health, and consequently improve reproductive performance of dairy cows (Juchem *et al.*, 2007). Holstein cows (511) were assigned to one of two treatments consisting of calcium salts (2% of diet dry matter) of either palm oil or a combination of linoleic and trans-octadecenoic acids (LTFA) from 25 days prepartum to 80 days of lactation. Postpartum health was monitored daily and cows were time-inseminated at 69 days of lactation.

As expected, feeding LTFA reduced 3.5% fat-corrected milk (36.7 vs. 39.1 kg/d) as a consequence of decreased milk fat content (3.3 vs. 3.6%), which also decreased milk fat yield (1.24 vs. 1.37 kg/d). Body condition was not affected by fat source, and plasma concentrations of glucose, BHBA, and nonesterified fatty acids were similar across treatments. Concentration of liver triacylglycerol was similar between treatments. These data indicate that feeding LTFA did not alter energy status of dairy cows in spite of marked decreases in fat-corrected milk synthesis. However, feeding LTFA increased plasma concentrations of prostaglandin metabolites in the first days postpartum in primiparous, but not multiparous cows, and tended to decrease the incidence of puerperal metritis (15.1 vs. 8.8%). Pregnancy rate after first insemination tended to be greater at 27 days after AI, and was greater at 41 days after AI for cows fed LTFA compared with those fed palm oil (Table 6). These results indicate that unsaturated fatty acids fed in a rumen inert form have the potential to modulate reproductive events and improve pregnancy rates in lactating dairy cows in spite of similar effects on postpartum health.

EFFECT OF FAT SOURCES DIFFERING IN FATTY ACID PROFILE ON FERTILIZATION RATE AND EMBRYO QUALITY IN LACTATING DAIRY COWS

Because of the positive effects of LTFA on conception rates of lactating dairy cows, and indications that unsaturated fatty acids can improve embryo quality in superovulated dairy cattle (Thangavelu *et al.*, 2007), it was postulated that some of the positive effects of these fatty acids on fertility of dairy cows were

Table 6. Effect of feeding calcium salts rich of palm oil or calcium salts rich in linoleic and monoenoic trans fatty acids (LTFA) on health and reproduction of dairy cows (Juchem *et al.*, 2007).

| | *Treatments* | | |
	Palm oil	*LTFA*	*P*
Cows, n	246	255	- - -
Retained placenta, %	6.5	6.7	0.96
Uterine disease, %	22.3	24.4	0.68
Puerperal metritis, %	15.1	8.8	0.08
Cyclic cows, %	89.7	83.8	0.15
First ovulation, d	30.5	32.2	0.13
Pregnancy rate, %			
Day 27	28.6	37.9	0.07
Day 41	25.8	35.5	0.05
Pregnancy loss, %	9.8	6.3	0.50

mediated by changes in fertilization and embryo quality. Cerri *et al.* (2004) fed 154 lactating Holstein dairy cows one of the two treatment diets described in the studies of Juchem *et al.* (2007). After synchronizing the oestrous cycle and ovulation, cows were inseminated and uteri flushed 5 days after insemination. A total of 161 ovulations were detected in 154 cows, and 14 (18.7%) and 12 (15.2%) cows fed palm oil and LTFA, respectively, experienced double ovulation when inseminated. The number of structures recovered was 45 for palm oil and 41 for LTFA; the recovery rate (number of structures/number of corpora lutea) was similar for both treatments, averaging 53.4%. Fertilization rate tended to be higher for cows fed LTFA than those fed palm oil (87.2 vs. 73.3%). Similarly, the median number of accessory spermatozoa per structure collected was greater for cows fed LTFA than those fed palm oil (34.3 vs. 21.5), which might partially explain the greater fertilization rate. Cows fed Ca salts of LTFA throughout the transition period and early lactation had a greater proportion of embryos classified as high quality compared to cows fed Ca salts of palm oil (73.5 vs. 51.5%). Furthermore, the proportion of live cells (94.2 vs. 85.3%) tended to be greater for cows fed LTA than those fed palm oil. These results indicate that improvements in fertility of dairy cows at first postpartum insemination observed by Juchem *et al.* (2007) might be attributed to improvements in fertilization and embryo quality when cows are fed fat sources containing linoleic and monoenoic trans fatty acids during the transition period.

Improving postpartum health with supplemental rumen protected choline

Coordinated adaptation to lactation is critical to health and productivity of dairy cows. Lipid metabolism during the transition period plays a key role in this adaptive process. Excessive mobilization of adipose tissue to support milk and milk fat synthesis in early lactation results in increased incidence of subclinical and clinical ketosis (Duffield, 2000) and fatty liver (Drackley, 1999), both of which compromise reproductive performance of dairy cows. Nutritional manipulation during the periparturient period has proven to be the most effective means to minimize the incidence of lipid-related metabolic disorders in dairy cows and can potentially reduce prevalence of ketosis, thereby improving metabolism and subsequently reproduction.

Choline is normally synthesized using labile methyl groups donated by methionine in the process of transmethylation. In monogastric animals, choline deficiency has been shown to result in hepatic lipidosis. In lactating cows, the early postpartum period is characterized by high demands for energy and essential amino acids for synthesis of colostrum and milk. Furthermore, the early lactation period is characterized by increased fat mobilization and subsequent accumulation in the liver. Hepatic accumulation of fatty acids after re-esterification to triacylglycerol occurs because the rate of nonesterified fatty acid uptake by hepatocytes overcomes oxidation in the mitochondria or peroxisomes and export as very low density lipoprotein (Drackley, 1999). Because DMI is low in early lactation, which not only reduces protein intake, but also microbial synthesis of protein, it is plausible that cows in late gestation and early lactation might not consume sufficient quantities of methionine to synthesize phosphatidylcholine, thereby increasing the needs for dietary choline. Furthermore, because choline is important for synthesis of phospholipids, which are part of cell membranes and are also incorporated into hepatic lipoproteins, export of lipids from the liver as lipoproteins might be enhanced early postpartum when choline is supplemented in lactating diets.

Cooke *et al.* (2007) conducted two experiments to determine the effects of rumen protected choline on triacylglycerol accumulation and depletion from the liver of dairy cows. In experiment 1, 24 dairy cows between 45 and 60 days prepartum were subjected to a feed restriction protocol and fed or not 15 g/day of rumen protected choline. In experiment 2, 28 dairy cows between 45 and 60 days prepartum were subjected to a feed restriction protocol and fed or not 15 g/day of rumen protected choline. In experiment 1, cows fed rumen protected choline had hepatic tissue with reduced concentration of triacylglycerol during feed restriction and a period of negative energy balance. In experiment 2, cows fed rumen protected choline experienced a greater depletion of accumulated hepatic triacylglycerol after feed restriction was suspended and cows were allowed to consume feed ad libitum. These data suggest that feeding rumen-protected choline has the potential to improve hepatic lipid metabolism during period of inadequate energy intake.

Recently, Lima *et al.* (2007) conducted two extensive experiments to evaluate the effect of rumen protected choline fed during the transition period on incidence of health disorders, lactation and reproduction of dairy cows. In experiment 1, 362 Holstein cows were assigned to treatments at 253 days of gestation, and treatment diets were fed until 80 days of lactation. The diets were exactly the same, but cows receiving rumen protected choline were dosed daily with 15 g of choline/day. In experiment 2, 573 Holstein primigravid cows were assigned to treatments at 256 days of gestation, and treatment diets were fed only during the prepartum period. The diets were exactly the same, but cows receiving rumen protected choline were dosed daily with 15 g of choline/day.

In experiment 1, feeding rumen protected choline before and after calving reduced the incidence of clinical and subclinical ketosis and the proportion of cows with ketonuria (Table 7). Furthermore, cows receiving rumen protected choline throughout the transition period experienced less mastitis, although incidence of retained placenta, uterine diseases, and displacement of abomasum remained unaltered (Table 8). Because ketosis and mastitis were suppressed by feeding rumen protected choline, the overall morbidity of cows in experiment 1 was reduced. In experiment 2, in which primiparous cows were fed rumen-protected choline only prepartum, incidence of ketosis and other postparturient diseases were similar between treatments.

Reproductive performance of cows was generally not influenced by feeding choline. In experiment 1, feeding rumen protected choline did not affect the proportion of cyclic cows, conception rates at first insemination or pregnancy maintenance (Table 9). Similarly, in experiment 2, feeding rumen-protected choline did not influence fertility of dairy cows after the first postpartum insemination (Table 10). These data suggest that feeding rumen protected choline throughout the transition period improved postparturient health and minimized the risk for ketosis in dairy cows, but these benefits in health were not reflected in improved reproduction. Furthermore, when fed only prepartum to primigravid cows, rumen protected choline did not improve postpartum health or reproduction.

Conclusions

It is clear that events that take place during the transition period of dairy cows influence the risk of developing postpartum diseases and subsequent reproductive performance. Recent evidence suggests that changes in feeding behaviour and dry matter intake during late gestation are associated with risk of clinical and

Table 7. Effect of feeding rumen-protected choline (RPC) on ketosis in dairy cows – Experiment 1 (Lima *et al.*, 2007).

	Treatment (TRT)				P		
	Control		RPC				
	Primiparous	Multiparous	Primiparous	Multiparous	TRT	Parity	TRT*Parity
	% (no./no.)						
Ketonuria[1]	32.3 (21/65)	26.8 (30/112)	7.8 (5/64)	12.4 (14/113)	0.001	0.56	0.18
Clinical ketosis[2]	13.9 (9/65)	9.8 (11/112)	4.7 (3/64)	3.5 (4/113)	0.01	0.10	0.74
DIM at diagnosis (± SEM)	9.3 ± 1.9	7.4 ± 1.9	12.4 ± 3.0	6.8 ± 2.6	0.61	0.15	0.43
Relapse of ketosis[3]	4.6 (3/65)	5.1 (9/112)	0 (0/63)	3.5 (4/113)	0.05	0.14	0.50
Subclinical ketosis[4]							
1 d postpartum	23.5 (16/68)	45.2 (52/115)	20.3 (13/64)	33.0 (38/115)	0.07	0.001	0.52
14 d postpartum	12.3 (8/65)	40.0 (44/110)	15.9 (10/63)	22.1 (25/113)	0.35	0.001	0.05

[1] Ketonuria using Ketostix reagent strips (Bayer Diagnostics).
[2] Anorexia, depressed attitude, severe ketonuria using Ketostix, including some cases of nervous ketosis.
[3] Proportion of all cows with more than one case of clinical ketosis.
[4] Subclinical ketosis = plasma 3-OH-butyrate > 1,000 µMol/L.

Table 8. Effect of feeding rumen-protected choline (RPC) on health of dairy cows – Experiment 1 (Lima et al., 2007).

	Treatment (TRT)				P		
	Control		RPC				
	Primiparous	Multiparous	Primiparous	Multiparous	TRT	Parity	TRT*Parity
	% (no./no.)						
Retained placenta	9.2 (6/65)	12.3 (14/114)	9.4 (6/64)	10.5 (12/114)	0.72	0.51	0.78
Postpartum fever	33.9 (22/65)	29.5 (33/112)	37.6 (24/64)	28.3 (32/113)	0.77	0.19	0.64
Puerperal metritis	4.6 (3/65)	2.7 (3/112)	7.8 (5/64)	0.9 (1/113)	0.69	0.02	0.27
Metritis	18.5 (12/65)	7.1 (8/112)	15.6 (10/64)	3.5 (4/113)	0.33	0.001	0.57
Displacement of abomasum	1.5 (1/65)	6.3 (7/112)	3.1 (2/64)	1.8 (2/113)	0.77	0.23	0.12
Mastitis	20.0 (13/65)	24.1 (26/108)	17.2 (11/64)	13.4 (15/112)	0.06	0.79	0.40
Postpartum disease[1]	58.5 (38/65)	56.3 (63/112)	42.2 (27/64)	36.3 (41/113)	0.001	0.46	0.73
Death	4.4 (3/68)	8.7 (10/115)	0 (0/64)	7.0 (8/115)	0.27	0.05	
Left study[2]	8.8 (6/68)	10.4 (12/115)	4.7 (3/64)	9.6 (11/115)	0.48	0.16	0.99

[1] Includes retained placenta, metritis, clinical ketosis, displacement of abomasum, and mastitis.
[2] Cows leaving the study prior to 80 days postpartum because of death or culling.

Table 9. Effect of feeding rumen-protected choline (RPC) on reproduction of dairy cows – Experiment 1 (Lima et al., 2007).

	Treatment (TRT)				P		
	Control		RPC				
	Primiparous	Multiparous	Primiparous	Multiparous	TRT	Parity	TRT*Parity
	% (no./no.)						
Retained placenta	9.2 (6/65)	12.3 (14/114)	9.4 (6/64)	10.5 (12/114)	0.72	0.51	0.78
Cyclic	71.4 (45/63)	86.4 (89/103)	63.9 (39/61)	93.4 (99/106)	0.67	0.001	0.05
Conception rate 1st AI							
d 30	43.6 (27/62)	39.8 (41/103)	47.5 (29/61)	48.5 (50/103)	0.20	0.84	0.73
d 65	40.3 (25/62)	32.4 (33/102)	39.3 (24/61)	37.9 (39/103)	0.47	0.42	0.60
Pregnancy loss	7.4 (2/27)	17.5 (7/40)	17.2 (5/29)	22.0 (11/50)	0.30	0.25	0.55

subclinical uterine inflammation. Furthermore, impairment in innate and cellular immune functions seems to predispose cows to retained placenta and subsequent complications of uterine diseases that suppress fertility of cows. It is clear, therefore, that transition cow programs should be designed to minimize disturbance in feeding behaviour and optimize nutrient intake and immune function during late gestation and early lactation.

Table 10. Effect of feeding rumen-protected choline (RPC) prepartum on reproduction of primiparous dairy cows – Experiment 2 (Lima *et al.*, 2007).

	Treatment		*P*
	Control	*RPC*	
	% (no./no.)		
Pregnant 1st AI			
day 38	50.8 (132/260)	50.6 (134/265)	0.83
day 66	48.3 (125/259)	48.7 (129/265)	0.49
Pregnancy loss 1st AI	4.6 (6/131)	3.7 (5/134)	0.69

Because of the complications of inadequate nutrient intake and negative energy balance, cows can experience prolonged periods of anovulation, which reduces oestrous detection, conception rate and pregnancy maintenance. A practical marker for this is the change in body condition from calving to the end of the voluntary waiting period, and excessive losses of body condition at that time will delay resumption of postpartum ovulation and compromise fertility. Nutritional strategies to improve energy status and metabolism of dairy cows include feeding of fatty acids and supplementation with rumen protected choline, although fertility responses are not always consistent. It is clear that supplemental fat improves conception rates in dairy cows, but responses vary with type of fatty acid. Generally, unsaturated fatty acids seem to promote improved reproductive responses compared with more saturated fat sources, and mechanisms are associated with modulation of luteolytic responses and improved embryo quality. Therefore, supplementing the diet of postpartum cows with moderate amounts of unsaturated fatty acids is suggested to optimize fertility. Lastly, incorporating a source of rumen protected choline seems to improve measures of energy metabolism in dairy cows, and to minimize the risk of lipid-related disorders, but response is optimized when supplementation is implemented pre- and postpartum.

References

Adamiak, S.J., Powell, K., Rooke, J.A., Webb, R. and Sinclair, K.D. (2006) Body composition, dietary carbohydrates and fatty acids determine post-fertilisation development of bovine oocytes in vitro, Reproduction, 131, 247-258.

Ambrose, D.J., Kastelic, J.P., Corbett, R., Pitney, P.A., Petit, H.V., Small, J.A. and Zalkovic, P. (2006) Lower pregnancy losses in lactating dairy cows fed a diet enriched in alpha-linolenic acid, Journal of Dairy Science, 89, 3066-3074.

Butler, W.R. (2003) Energy balance relationships with follicular development, ovulation and fertility in postpartum dairy cows, Livestock Production Science, 83, 211-218.

Bruno, R.G., Sa Filho, M.F., Lima, F.S., Magalhaes, V.J.A., Santos, J.E.P. (2007) The effect of a single uterine infusion of ceftiofur in the immediate postpartum on lactation and reproduction in dairy cows. Journal of Dairy Science, 90 (Suppl. 1), 10 (Abstract).

Cerri, R.L.A., Bruno, R.G.S., Chebel, R.C., Galvão, K.N., Rutigliano, H., Juchem, S.O., Thatcher, W.W., Luchini, D., Santos, J.E.P (2004). Effect of fat sources differing in fatty acid profile on fertilization rate and embryo quality in lactating dairy cows. Journal of Dairy Science, 87 (Suppl. 1): 297 (Abstract).

Cooke, R.F., Silva Del Río, N., Caraviello, D.Z., Bertics, S.J., Ramos, M.H. and Grummer, R.R. (2007) Supplemental choline for prevention and alleviation of fatty liver in dairy cattle, Journal of Dairy Science, 90, 2413-2418.

Curtis, C.R., Erb, H.N., Sniffen, C.J., Smith, R.D., Powers, P.A., Smith, M.C., White, M.E., Hillman, R.B. and Pearson, E.J. (1983) Association of parturient hypocalcemia with eight periparturient disorders in Holstein cows. Journal of American Veterinary Medical Association, 183, 559-561.

Drackley, J.K. (1999) Biology of dairy cows during the transition period: the final frontier?, Journal of Dairy Science, 82, 2259-2273.

Duffield, T.F., Leslie, K.E., Sandals, D., Lissemore, K., McBride, B.W., Lumsden, J.H., Dick, P. and Bagg, R. (1999) Effect of a monensin-controlled release capsule on cow health and reproductive performance, Journal of Dairy Science, 82, 2377-2384.

Duffield, T. (2000) Subclinical ketosis in lactating dairy cattle. Veterinary Clinics of North America Food Animal Practice, 16, 231-253.

Ferguson, J.D., Sklan, D., Chalupa, W.V. and Kronfeld D.S. (1990) Effects of hard fats on in vitro and in vivo rumen fermentation, milk production and reproduction in dairy cows, Journal of Dairy Science, 73, 2864-2879.

Fuentes, M.C., Calsamiglia, S.S., Sánchez, C., González, A., Newbold, J., Santos, J.E.P., Rodríguez-Alcalá, L.M., Fontecha J. (2008) Effect of extruded linseed on productive and reproductive performance of lactating dairy cows. Livestock Production Science, In Press.

Galvão, K.N., Greco, L.F., Vilela, J.M., Santos, J.E.P. (2006). Effect of intrauterine infusion of ceftiofur on uterine health. Journal of Dairy Science, 89 (Suppl.

1), 9 (Abstract.).

Gilbert, R.O., Shin, S.T., Guard, C.L., Erb, H.N. and Frajblat, M. (2005) Prevalence of endometritis and its effects on reproductive performance of dairy cows, Theriogenology, 64, 1879-1888.

Gong, J.G., Lee, W.J., Garnsworthy, P.C. and Webb, R. (2002) Effect of dietary-induced increases in circulating insulin concentrations during the early postpartum period on reproductive function in dairy cows, Reproduction, 123, 419-427.

Goshen, T. and Shpigel, N.Y. (2006) Evaluation of intrauterine antibiotic treatment of clinical metritis and retained fetal membranes in dairy cows. Theriogenology, 66, 2210-2218.

Grant, R.J. and Albright J.L. (1995) Feeding behavior and management factors during the transition period in dairy cattle, Journal of Animal Science, 73, 2791-2803.

Hammon, D.S., Evjen, I.M., Dhiman, T.R., Goff, J.P. and Walters, J.L. (2006) Neutrophil function and energy status in Holstein cows with uterine health disorders. Veterinary Immunology and Immunopathology, 113, 21-29.

Hileman, S.M., Lubbers, L.S., Jansen, H.T. and Lehman, M.N. (1999) Changes in hypothalamic estrogen receptor-containing cell numbers in response to feed restriction in the female lamb, Neuroendocrinology, 69, 430-437.

Huzzey, J.M., Veira, D.M., Weary, D.M. and von Keyserlingk, M.A. (2007) Prepartum behavior and dry matter intake identify dairy cows at risk for metritis. Journal of Dairy Science, 90, 3220-3233

Juchem, S.O. (2007) Lipid digestion and metabolism in dairy cows: effects on production, reproduction and health. PhD thesis, University of California Davis.

Kasimanickam, R., Duffield, T.F., Foster, R.A., Gartley, C.J., Leslie, K.E., Walton, J.S. and Johnson, W.H. (2004) Endometrial cytology and ultrasonography for the detection of subclinical endometritis in postpartum dairy cows, Theriogenology, 62, 9-23.

Kendrick, K.W., Bailey, T.L., Garst, A.S., Pryor, A.W., Ahmadzdeh, A., Akers, R.M. (1999) Effects of energy balance on hormones, ovarian activity, and recovered oocytes in lactating Holstein cows using transvaginal follicular aspiration. Journal of Dairy Science, 82, 1731-40.

Kimura, K, Goff, J.P., Kehrli, M.E., Jr. and Reinhardt, T.A. (2002) Decreased neutrophil function as a cause of retained placenta in dairy cattle. Journal of Dairy Science, 85, 544-550.

Lima, F.S., Sa Filho, M.F., Garrett, J.E., Santos, J.E.P. (2007) Effects of feeding rumen-protected choline on health and reproduction of dairy cows. Journal of Dairy Science, 90 (Suppl. 1), 354 (Abstract).

Markusfeld, O. (1985) Relationship between overfeeding, metritis and ketosis in high yielding dairy cows. Veterinary Record, 116, 489-491.

NAHMS (1996) Dairy 1996 Part III: reference of 1996 dairy health and health management. Online. Available: http://nahms.aphis.usda.gov/dairy/dairy96/DR96Pt3.pdf

Mattos, R., Staples, C.R. and Thatcher, W.W. (2000) Effects of dietary fatty acids on reproduction in ruminants, Reproduction, 5, 38-45.

Radcliff, R.P., McCormack, B.L., Crooker, B.A. and Lucy, M.C. (2003) Plasma hormones and expression of growth hormone receptor and insulin-like growth factor-I mRNA in hepatic tissue of periparturient dairy cows, Journal of Dairy Science, 86, 3920-3926.

Rhoads, R.P., Kim, J.W., Leury, B.J., Baumgard, L.H., Segoale, N., Frank, S.J., Bauman D.E. and Boisclair Y.R. (2004) Insulin increases the abundance of the growth hormone receptor in liver and adipose tissue of periparturient dairy cows, The Journal of Nutrition, 134, 1020-1027.

Rutigliano, H. (2006) Effects of source of supplemental Se and method of presynchronization on health, immune responses, reproductive efficiency, uterine health, and lactation performance of high producing dairy cows. Master of Science thesis, University of California Davis.

Santos, J.E., Huber, J.T., Theurer, C.B., Nussio, C.B., Nussio, L.G., Tarazon, M. and Fish, D. (2000) Effects of grain processing and bovine somatotropin on metabolism and ovarian activity of dairy cows during early lactation, Journal of Dairy Science, 83, 1004-1015.

Santos, J.E., Thatcher, W.W., Chebel, R.C., Cerri, R.L. and Galvão, K.N. (2004) The effect of embryonic death rates in cattle on the efficacy of estrus synchronization programs, Animal Reproduction Science, 82-83:513-535.

Santos, J.E.P., Rutigliano, H.M., Sa Filho, M.F. (2008) Risk factors for resumption of postpartum cyclicity and embryonic survival in lactating dairy cows, Animal Reproduction Science, in press

Selberg, K.T., Staples, C.R., Luchini, N.D. and Badinga, L. (2005) Dietary trans octadecenoic acids upregulate the liver gene encoding peroxisome proliferator-activated receptor-alpha in transition dairy cows, Journal of Dairy Research, 72, 107-114.

Staples, C.R., Burke, J.M., Thatcher, W.W. (1998) Influence of supplemental fats on reproductive tissues and performance of lactating cows. Journal of Dairy Science, 81, 856-871.

Stevenson, J.S. (2001) Reproductive management of dairy cows in high milk-producing herds. Journal of Dairy Science, 84, E. suppl., E128-E143.

Thangavelu, G., M.G. Colazo, D.J. Ambrose, M. Oba, E.K. Okine, M.K. Dyck. 2007. Diets enriched in unsaturated fatty acids enhance early embryonic development in lactating Holstein cows. Theriogenology

Thangavelu, G., Colazo, M.G., Ambrose, D.J., Oba, M., Okine, E.K. and Dyck,

M.K. (2007) Diets enriched in unsaturated fatty acids enhance early embryonic development in lactating Holstein cows, Theriogenology, 68, 949-957.

Theurer, C.B., Huber, J.T., Delgado-Elorduy, A. and Wanderley, R. (1999) Invited review: summary of steam-flaking corn or sorghum grain for lactating dairy cows, Journal of Dairy Science, 82,1950-1959.

Urton, G., von Keyserlingk, M.A. and Weary D.M. (2005) Feeding behavior identifies dairy cows at risk for metritis. Journal of Dairy Science, 88, 2843-2849.

Villa-Godoy, A., Hughes, T.L., Emery, R.S., Chapin, L.T. and Fogwell R.L. (1988) Association between energy balance and luteal function in lactating dairy cows, Journal of Dairy Science, 71, 1063-1072.

Wade, G.N. and Jones, J.E. (2004) Neuroendocrinology of nutritional infertility. American Journal of Physiology – Regulatory, Integrative and Comparative Physiology, 287, R1277-1296.

Whiteford, L.C. and Sheldon, I.M. (2005) Association between clinical hypocalcaemia and postpartum endometritis. Veterinary Record, 157, 202-203.

2

NUTRITIONAL AND MANAGEMENT FACTORS AFFECTING REPRODUCTIVE EFFICIENCY IN U.S. DAIRY HERDS

MILO C. WILTBANK, HERNANDO LOPEZ, SIWAT SANGSRITAVONG, KENT A. WEIGEL, DANIEL Z. CARAVIELLO

University of Wisconsin, Department of Dairy Science and Endocrinology, 1675 Observatory Drive, Madison, WI15 3706, USA

Introduction

Reproductive efficiency is declining on U.S. dairy herds. There are numerous factors that affect reproductive efficiency on individual farms. These include heat detection rate, heat stress, semen quality, bull fertility, AI technique, nutrition, body condition score, clinical and subclinical mastitis, cow comfort, and many other factors related to whole farm management, individual farm managers and labourers, and individual cows (Lucy, 2001; Caraviello, 2005; Garnsworthy, 2006; Wiltbank, Lopez, Sartori, Sangsritavong, Gümen, 2006). This chapter will briefly summarize two recent research areas. The first section of the chapter is based on results of a recent study that evaluated numerous factors simultaneously to determine the management factors most related to reproductive performance. This study used a machine learning technique to simultaneously evaluate numerous factors that may be affecting reproductive efficiency on U.S. dairies (Caraviello, Weigel, Craven, Gianola, Cook, Nordlund, Fricke, Wiltbank, 2006a). The second section of this manuscript is based on recent research in our laboratory that has found an intriguing biological link between high feed consumption and reproductive efficiency caused by elevated metabolism of hormones (Wiltbank *et al.*, 2006). Although this elevated hormone metabolism does not explain all aspects of nutritional effects on reproduction in dairy cows, it is becoming clear that hormone metabolism is the key missing link between high milk production and certain changes in reproductive efficiency such as decreased expression of oestrus.

Some management factors affecting percentage of cows pregnant at 150 days

This section is based on the research of Daniel Caraviello that he did to receive his Ph.D. degree from University of Wisconsin-Madison (Caraviello, 2005). He used a machine learning technique (Freund and Mason, 1999) to analyze reproductive data from 153 large commercial dairies that participate in the Alta Advantage progeny-testing programme. After editing, the data set had 17,587 lactation records from 9,516 cows that calved from 2000 to 2004 on 153 large (average of 613±46 lactating cows), commercial dairies across the United States. We collected as many different variables as possible using production records from Dairy Herd Improvement (DHI), on-farm computer records of reproduction and other variables, temperature information from weather stations located within 25 miles of each farm, body condition score collected by a single trained evaluator, and finally a comprehensive survey completed with the help of Alta Advantage consultants. A total of 341 potential explanatory variables were included in the analysis including: general management issues, sire selection, reproductive management, inseminator training and techniques, heat abatement, facility design, nutrition, employee management, animal health etc. An alternating decision tree algorithm was used to determine the variables and relationships among variables that helped to explain the differences in reproductive performance among cows and among herds (for details see Caraviello *et al.*, 2006a).

There are many different measures of reproductive performance including: days open, conception rate at first service or other services, 21-day pregnancy rate, reproductive culling rate, days to first AI, and calving interval. For this study we chose to use percentage of cows that were pregnant at 150 days in milk (DIM). In our research this has been found to be a very robust variable for determining reproductive efficiency on farms. It is close to mid-gestation, and it encompasses heat detection efficiency and conception rate during multiple breeding periods. It also is robust to heterogeneity among farms in reproductive management methods (synchronization programmes, heat detection methods) and selected length of the voluntary waiting period. In addition, there are good economic reasons to select % pregnant at 150 DIM because after this time there are higher losses for each day open than found before this time (our unpublished results).

The decision tree that was eventually selected contained 25 key variables that best explained the percentage of cows pregnant at 150 DIM. To test the decision tree, a portion (10%) of the records were withheld during development of the model and then the model was used to test the accuracy of prediction using these records. The selected model was accurate in selecting pregnancy status at 150 DIM for 71.4% of cows. Overall, 60.7% of cows were pregnant at 150 days, but there were substantial differences between farms. The decision tree helped to predict accurately the variables that were associated with lack of pregnancy in the 39.3% of cows that were not pregnant at 150 DIM.

The complete report was published in Caraviello *et al.* (2006a) and only the most informative variables for predicting reproductive performance will be discussed here. Figure 1 contains the first 10 nodes that had the greatest influence on % pregnant at 150 DIM. The root node is greater than 0 because on average more than 50% of cows were pregnant at 150 DIM.

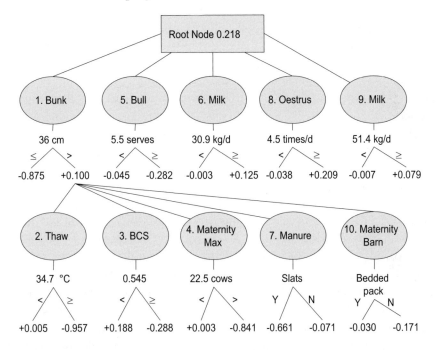

Figure 1. Diagram of the first 10 nodes of the decision tree relating farm variables to % pregnant at 150 days in milk. The nodes are: 1. Bunk space per cow in the breeding pen (cm/cow); 2. Thawing temperature used to thaw semen; 3. Percentage of "BCS Faults" in the herd (explained below); 4. Maximal number of cows in the maternity pen; 5. After how many services are cows moved into the bull breeding pen; 6. Milk production with cutoff point of 30.9 kg/d; 7. Method for handling manure; 8. Number of times per day that oestrus is detected; 9. Milk production with cutoff point of 51.4 kg/d; 10. Type of bedding used in maternity barn.

The first node (node 1) of the decision tree corresponded to amount of bunk space per cow in the breeding pen. Thus, cows that were overcrowded (<36 cm of bunk space/cow) had a much lower percentage of cows pregnant at 150 DIM than cows with more bunk space. The extremely low amount of bunk space (<36 cm/cow) is likely to be associated with overcrowded three-row barns. Nevertheless, there was a linear increase in predicted percentage of cows pregnant at 150 DIM as bunk space increased from 30 to 60 cm (from 35% to 70% pregnant at 150 DIM).

Other authors have suggested changes in eating behaviour, milk production and metabolic health when cows have inadequate bunk space (Calamari, Maianti and Stefanini, 2003). Thus, bunk space per cow seemed to be associated with reproductive efficiency by this machine learning methodology.

Nodes 2, 3, 4, 7 and 10 were built only on the node of cows with >36 cm of bunk space. Node 2 related to temperature that was used on the farm for thawing semen. Unfortunately, few cows could be evaluated because few producers reported this variable (only 965 cows). Thus, this was not a very useful node even though it appeared to have predictive value and could be critical for predicting reproductive performance. This demonstrates that nodes must be carefully evaluated because the machine learning technique is powerful in dealing with missing values but may overcompensate when a node has few values recorded.

Node 3 is body condition score (BCS) faults for the herd. In other words, the percentage of cows where BCS was too low at a given stage of lactation for a given herd. There is substantial evidence linking BCS to reproductive performance (for review see Garnsworthy 2006). Figure 2 shows BCS data from a single herd from this study. All of the data collected in this study were used to calculate a fourth-degree polynomial curve representing average BCS throughout the lactation, and this curve is superimposed on the BCS scatter plot from the individual herd (Figure 2). Mean BCS for dry cows was 3.22; this declined to 2.88 by 30 DIM and declined further to 2.70 by 50 DIM. Mean BCS subsequently increased to 2.75 by 80 DIM and stabilized at around 2.85 by 200 DIM. Based on these data, we selected a specific "BCS threshold" that is also shown in Figure 2. This threshold was 3.0 for dry cows and cows before 30 DIM, was 2.5 from 30 DIM to 180 DIM and then was 2.75 after 180 DIM. Cows that fell below this threshold were considered to have a "BCS Fault". We then calculated the percentage of cows with a "BCS Fault" in each herd. This methodology allowed us to evaluate an individual dairy herd for BCS status in a single visit. The herd shown in Figure 2 had 15% BCS faults overall. We used the BCS Fault information to compare BCS status of each herd with reproductive performance for that herd.

The herds in this study ranged from almost 0% to more than 60% BCS faults. The relationship between percentage of BCS faults and reproductive performance was evaluated at the herd level by comparing herd BCS status with percentage of cows pregnant at 150 DIM. Application of a logistic regression model at the herd level showed that the proportion of cows pregnant at 150 DIM decreased linearly as percentage of BCS faults increased (Figure 3). The probability of pregnancy at 150 DIM was 0.80 for herds with 15% BCS faults, compared with 0.53 for herds with ≥45% BCS faults.

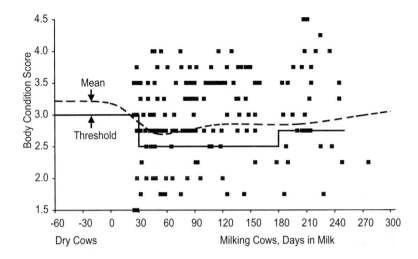

Figure 2. Scatter plot for an example herd with some BCS variation between different cows even when plotting data by stage of lactation. The lines indicate the calculated **Mean** (fourth degree polynomial) of BCS at different times postpartum for all herds in the study. The **Threshold** developed for this study is also shown. Each box represents the BCS for an individual cow.

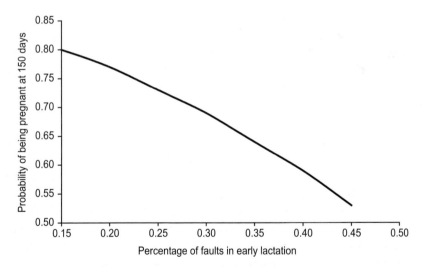

Figure 3. Probability of pregnancy by 150 d postpartum compared to percentage of BCS faults based on the herd level analysis. The plot is calculated from the logistic regression using lactation number = 1.5 and maximum daily temperature = 85 °F.

Thus, this research adds further evidence that BCS is an important factor in reproductive performance on dairy herds. Previous research has provided clear evidence that BCS of an individual dairy cow is associated with reproductive efficiency (Garnsworthy, 2006; Dechow, Rodgers, Klei, Lawlor and VanRaden, 2004). This study specifically indicated that differences in BCS Faults at a herd level may also be an important predictor of herd reproductive performance. It may be possible to use this "BCS Fault" system to help with differentiating herds with reduced reproductive performance primarily due to BCS compared to herds that have other underlying causes for reproductive inefficiencies.

Returning to the decision tree in Figure 1, other important variables were identified in this study that were predictors of reproductive performance. Node 4 represented a variable that was collected on the maximum number of cows in the maternity pen. When number of cows was more than 22.5 cows there was a negative effect on the predicted percentage of cows pregnant at 150 DIM. This value tended to have a linear decrease in value as number of cows in the maternity pen increased from 10 to 25.

Nodes 6, 9 and 15 (not shown) were all concerned with milk yield near first insemination. Cows that had lower milk yield (< 30.8 kg/d in Node 6 and < 51.3 kg/d in Node 9) tended to have lower percentage pregnant at 150 DIM, perhaps due to this value reflecting somewhat the disease state of some cows. The group with milk yield from 35.9 to 40.3 kg/d had the greatest percentage pregnant at 150 DIM (Node 15, not shown). In other analyses using the machine learning technique (Caraviello *et al.*, 2006a) we have found that lower milk yield (< 30 kg/d) is a strong predictor of dramatically increased percentage of cows that become pregnant to first AI (first service conception rate). Thus, although milk yield can cause some negative effects on reproductive performance, this negative effect can be observed when comparing conception rate data to milk production near the time of AI rather than overall reproductive performance. Most US herds are using timed AI programmes to assure that high producing cows have increased opportunity to become pregnant by 150 DIM (Caraviello *et al.*, 2006b).

Thus, there are many variables that are associated with reproductive efficiency in individual cows and on individual dairy farms. Clearly variables associated with overcrowding (bunk space, number of cows in maternity pens) were important predictors of reproductive performance. Body condition scores of the herd and milk yield of individual cows were also key predictors. It should be noted that the associations found in this study do not indicate a "cause and effect" relationship. There could be numerous reasons for these associations that are unrelated to the particular variables that we found associated with reproductive performance.

Additionally, we found in this study that pregnancy status at 150 DIM was a useful variable for measuring reproductive performance in research trials. However, this is unlikely to be a useful variable for monitoring current status of reproductive efficiency in an individual dairy. This variable has excessive delay or "lag" in indicating the current status of reproduction. On individual herds we generally use a variable that combines both heat detection rate (percentage of eligible cows that are bred every 21

d) with pregnancies per AI (sometimes called conception rate; percentage of cows that become pregnant to each AI) to produce a variable known as 21-day pregnancy rate (percentage of eligible cows that become pregnant every 21 d). We calculate this value for every 21-d period and closely monitor any decreases in this value. Thus, as soon as pregnancy diagnosis is complete we can calculate the percentage of eligible cows that became pregnant during the previous 21 d (Both % that received AI and % of those cows receiving AI that conceived). We find average values of about 14-15% for 21 day pregnancy rates on US dairies; however, we strive to design programmes that consistently produce 21 day pregnancy rates above 20%.

High feed consumption and reproductive efficiency are linked by high hormone metabolism

This section will not attempt to review all of the nutritional factors that can potentially alter reproductive efficiency in dairy cattle. This has been reviewed in numerous other publications and would require a complete volume for adequate review. We will focus on a critical link that has become increasingly relevant to our understanding of nutrition and reproduction. This link is different from the link discussed above concerning BCS and reproduction. Negative energy balance and the resulting low BCS cause a delay in time to first ovulation and thus increase the percentage of cows that are anovular (not ovulating). The increased percentage of anovular cows is not related clearly to milk production in most studies (see Lopez, Caraviello, Satter, Fricke and Wiltbank , 2005). However, there are other key reproductive efficiency measures that are related clearly to milk production. This review will focus on two key reproductive measures, efficiency of heat detection and double ovulation rate. These are chosen because of the clear relationship to milk production. We will use these measures to build a model for how reproductive efficiency can be altered dramatically by the high feed consumption associated with high milk production. These two measures are used to demonstrate a physiological model that can explain the relationship between high feed consumption and decreased reproductive efficiency. However, this model becomes more complicated when trying to explain a complex reproductive variable such as conception rate. Nevertheless, it seems likely that this model will also be important in explaining some aspects of this variable as well.

DURATION OF OESTRUS

It is clear that low rates of oestrous detection are reducing reproductive efficiency on commercial dairy farms. Indeed, Washburn *et al.* (2002) reported a decrease from 50.9% in 1985 to 41.5% in 1999 for oestrous detection rates in Holstein dairy herds in Southeastern U.S.A. However, studies have reported both a negative relationship between level of milk production (Harrison, Ford, Young, Conley, Freeman, 1990; Harrison, Young, Freeman, Ford, 1989) or no relationship (Fonseca, Britt, McDaniel, Wilk, Rakes, 1983; Van Eerdenburg, Karthaus, Taverne, Merics, Szenci, 2002) using visual observation twice daily to measure expression of oestrus. We have recently completed a study in which we evaluated duration of oestrus in a group of lactating dairy cows using the HeatWatch system (Lopez, Satter and Wiltbank, 2004). This system allowed continuous monitoring of all mounts 24 h per day and can be used to calculate duration of oestrus in individual dairy cows. Cows with milk production above the herd average (~ 40 kg/d) had shorter (P < 0.001) duration of oestrus (6.2 ± 0.5 h) than cows with lower milk production (10.9 ± 0.7 h).

The effect of milk production on oestrous expression was not due to a parity effect because separate analysis of primiparous and multiparous cows showed similar effects. Figure 4 shows the relationship between level of milk production and duration of oestrus. In order to consistently observe this strong negative relationship between level of milk production and duration of oestrus, it is critical that milk production data be collected close to the time of oestrus, only data from ovulations after the first postpartum ovulation be utilized (first ovulation has low expression of oestrus), all ovulations be consistently monitored throughout the observation period (to avoid false oestrus or missing data from ovulations), and that duration of oestrus be monitored on a continuous basis with an electronic heat monitoring system.

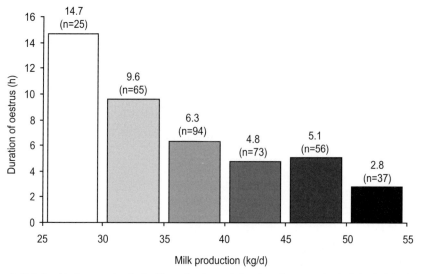

Figure 4. Relationship between level of milk production and duration of oestrus. Analysis included all single ovulations (n = 350) except first post-partum ovulations. Average milk production is for the 10 d before oestrus [From Lopez *et al.*, 2004].

As discussed below, we theorize that high milk production leads to decreased circulating oestradiol concentrations producing decreased duration of oestrus. Decreased oestradiol could also cause increased follicular size by delaying the time to oestradiol-induction of oestrus, GnRH/LH surge and ovulation in high-producing cows.

DOUBLE OVULATION RATE

Another reproductive trait that has been linked directly to milk production is double ovulation rate (see Lopez *et al.*, 2005; Wiltbank, Fricke, Sangritasvong, Sartori, Ginther, 2000). From a practical standpoint, double ovulation rate appears to be the underlying cause of increased twinning rate in lactating dairy cows, with 93% of twins being non-identical (del Rio, Kirkpatrick, Fricke, 2006). Numerous factors have been recognized as possible regulators of twinning rates, including age of dam, season, genetics, use of reproductive hormones or antibiotics, ovarian cysts, days open and peak milk production (reviewed in Wiltbank *et al.*, 2000). In a large study on risk factors for twinning, Kinsel, Marsh, Ruegg and Ethrington, 1998 concluded, "the single largest contributor (> 50%) to the recent increase in the rate of twinning is the increase in peak milk production". We performed a study in which we evaluated double ovulation rate in 240 dairy cows (Fricke and Wiltbank, 1999) that had ovulation synchronized with the Ovsynch protocol. Ovulation was determined by transrectal ultrasonography at the time of the second GnRH injection and 48 h later. The mean milk production, determined 3 d before ovulation, was 40.7 ± 0.8 kg/d and cows were segregated by whether they were below or above the mean value. Double ovulation rate in cows that were above average production was 20.2% compared with 6.9% in those below average ($P < 0.05$). This difference was similar regardless of lactation number. Recently, we reported results of a study (Lopez *et al.*, 2005) that evaluated naturally ovulating dairy cattle and found a similar relationship between milk production and double ovulation rate (Figure 5). Cows that produced less than 40 kg/d had a very low double ovulation rate, whereas, cows producing above 50 kg/d had more than a 50% double ovulation rate. It is surprising that there is such a dramatic inflection point in double ovulation rate as milk production increases above 40 kg/d, and it is still unclear what physiological changes occur as milk production increases above this critical value. This increase in double ovulation rate is likely to continue to increase twinning rate in dairy herds as milk production increases. It is also clear that this effect of milk production is most related to the level of production within the two weeks before the cow ovulates, and not to total milk production during the entire lactation. This effect was also similar when a more extensive regression model was used for analysis, and when multiparous and primiparous cows were analyzed separately (Lopez *et al.*, 2005). As with duration of oestrus, the first postpartum ovulation differed from other ovulations with a high double ovulation rate that was unrelated to milk production.

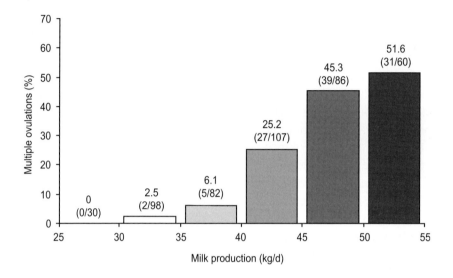

Figure 5. Relationship between incidence of multiple ovulation and milk production (From Lopez *et al.*, 2005). Analysis included all ovulations (n = 463) except first post-partum. Milk production for 14 d before ovulation.

CIRCULATING STEROIDS AND STEROID METABOLISM IN LACTATING DAIRY COWS

A number of studies have evaluated circulating hormone concentrations in lactating dairy cows. As discussed above, cows with higher milk production ovulate larger follicles, but have lower circulating oestradiol concentrations (Lopez *et al.*, 2004). In addition, higher producing dairy cows have a larger volume of luteal tissue, but reduced circulating progesterone (Lopez *et al.*, 2005). Table 1 shows a comparison of dairy heifers and lactating dairy cows that were monitored by daily ovarian ultrasonography and hormonal analyses (Sartori, Haughian, Shaver, Rosa and Wiltbank, 2004). It is clear that cows ovulated larger follicles but had reduced circulating oestradiol-17ß concentrations. This is somewhat surprising because it would be expected that cows with larger follicles would tend to have greater follicular oestradiol-17ß production. Again paradoxically, lactating cows had a much larger volume of luteal tissue but reduced circulating progesterone. This study also found much higher multiple ovulation rate in lactating cows.

Table 1. Comparisons (means ± SEM and percentages) between all (single- and multiple-ovulating) heifers (n = 27) and lactating cows (n = 14) with typical interovulatory intervals [From Sartori *et al.*, 2002]

	Heifers	*Lactating cows*	*P-value*
Interovulatory interval (d)	22.0 ± 0.4	22.9 ± 0.7	0.2774
Day of luteolysis	18.5 ± 0.4	18.9 ± 0.6	0.5261
Cycles with two waves; % (no./no.)	55.6 (15/27)	78.6 (11/14)	0.1468
Cycles with three waves; % (no./no.)	33.3 (9/27)	14.3 (2/14)	0.1918
Cycles with four waves; % (no./no.)	11.1 (3/27)	7.1 (1/14)	0.6847
Day of emergence of second follicular wave	8.9 ± 0.3	11.1 ± 0.6	0.0003
Interval (d) from emergence of last wave to ovulation	10.1 ± 0.5	10.9 ± 0.5	0.2927
Days from luteolysis to ovulation	4.6 ± 0.1	5.2 ± 0.2	0.0064
Incidence of co-dominant follicles during first wave; % (no./no.)	3.7 (1/27)	35.7 (5/14)	0.0127
Multiple ovulation rate; % (no./no.)	1.9 (1/54)	17.9 (5/28)	0.0162
Maximal size of largest ovulatory follicle (mm)	14.9 ± 0.2	16.8 ± 0.5	<0.0001
Oestradiol peak preceding ovulation (pg/mL)	11.3 ± 0.6	7.9 ± 0.8	<0.0001
Maximal luteal tissue volume (mm^3)	7303 ± 308	11120 ± 678	<0.0001
Progesterone peak (ng/mL)	7.3 ± 0.4	5.6 ± 0.5	0.0080

There appear to be two reasonable explanations for the disconnection between circulating steroid hormones and size of follicles and CL. The first possible explanation is that follicles and CL are less steroidogenically active in lactating dairy cows. This could be due to inadequate circulating stimulatory hormones, substrate for steroidogenesis, or intracellular steroidogenic pathways. There were more LH pulses in lactating than similar size non-lactating cows (Vasconcelo, Sangsritavong, Tsai and Wiltbank, 2003), suggesting that LH is not likely to be the cause of reduced steroidogenic output. In addition, the primary substrate for bovine ovarian steroidogenesis is high-density lipoprotein, and this is particularly elevated in lactating dairy cows (Grummer and Carroll, 1988). There is a reduction in circulating insulin-like growth factor-1 in lactating dairy cows and this could be related to reduced steroidogenic capacity (Lucy, 2001). Nevertheless, the hypothesis that ovarian structures in lactating dairy cows have reduced steroidogenic output has not yet been investigated adequately and therefore, cannot be disregarded or advocated at this time.

A more likely explanation is that lactating dairy cows have increased metabolism of steroid hormones as milk production increases. Circulating hormone concentrations are determined by rates of production and metabolism of the hormone. Increased feed consumption, such as during lactation, has been shown to alter circulating progesterone and excretion of progesterone metabolites during continuous delivery of progesterone (Parr, Davis, Miles and Squires, 1993; Rabiee, Macmillan and Schwarzenberger, 2001). Increased steroid metabolism due to high feed consumption could alter the reproductive physiology of any species, but may particularly alter reproduction in species with extreme increases in feed intake such as lactating dairy cows. We propose that some of the reproductive changes in lactating dairy cows are caused by dramatic increases in steroid metabolism due to elevations in feed consumption and liver blood flow.

In recent experiments, we tested the hypothesis that increased liver blood flow as a result of elevated feed intake in lactating dairy cows, would increase steroid metabolism (Sangsritavong, Combs, Sartori and Wiltbank, 2002). We found that prior to feeding, liver blood flow was greater in lactating (1561 ± 57 L/h) than similar size and age non-lactating (747 ± 47 L/h) cows. Liver blood flow and metabolism of progesterone and oestrogen increased immediately after any amount of feed consumption in both lactating and non-lactating cows. Metabolism of oestrogen and progesterone was much greater (2.3 X) in lactating than in non-lactating cows. In addition, changes in metabolism of oestrogen and progesterone in response to feeding were immediate and related to acute changes in liver blood flow. In lactating cows, a continuous high plane of nutrition appears to chronically elevate liver blood flow and metabolism of steroid hormones to approximately double the amount observed in non-lactating cows of similar size and age. These results indicate that even with a similar level of hormone production, there would be lower circulating hormone concentrations in lactating dairy cows.

Can elevated steroid metabolism explain the paradox of reduced circulating steroids in spite of larger follicular and luteal sizes? If we use the data in Table 1 to calculate an approximate index of circulating progesterone concentration divided by luteal volume, we find that heifers have approximately twice the value that is calculated in lactating cows (1.0 vs 0.5 ng/mL of progesterone per cm^3 of luteal volume). A similar calculation for circulating oestradiol and follicular volume also yields about a two-fold greater value in heifers than cows (6.5 vs 3.2 pg/mL circulating oestradiol per cm^3 of follicular volume). These values correspond closely to the approximately two-fold elevation in metabolism of oestrogen and progesterone that we have found in lactating versus non-lactating cows. A recent analysis of a larger group of individual lactating cows using this index showed a closer relationship of this index (circulating hormone/volume of tissue) to milk production (R^2 = 0.44 to 0.47; P < 0.01) than found when comparing either circulating hormones, follicular volume or luteal volume alone to milk production (Lopez *et al.*, 2005). Thus, although we cannot rule out the importance of changes in steroidogenic production by luteal and follicular tissue, it seems reasonable that the changes in circulating oestradiol and progesterone can be accounted for by increased rates of steroid metabolism in lactating cows.

We have synthesized this information into a simplified working model (Figure 6). Lactating cows have greater energy requirements than non-lactating cows (for example, a cow producing 50 kg/d of milk will require 53 Mcal/d (222 MJ/d) of net energy versus 12.5 Mcal/d (52 MJ/d) for a non-lactating cow; NRC, 2001). The high feed consumption required to meet these energy requirements leads to a dramatic increase in liver blood flow that leads to elevated metabolism of both oestrogen and progesterone. This would cause a reduction in circulating oestrogen and progesterone concentrations, even with high production of steroid hormones by the follicle or CL. This simple model potentially could explain some of the results described in the sections above.

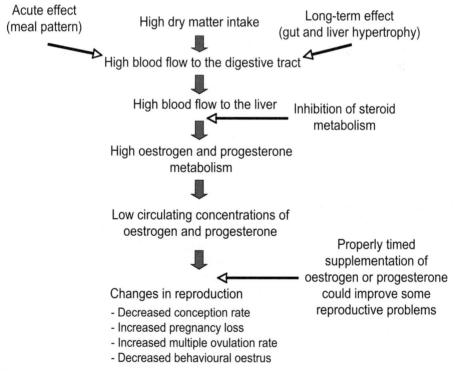

Figure 6. Schematic of the potential physiological pathway that may produce the changes in reproductive physiology observed in high-producing lactating dairy cows and possible ways to manipulate these pathways to improve reproduction.

Conclusions

It seems clear that numerous factors are affecting reproductive efficiency, both on a herd basis and on an individual cow basis. As discussed in the first section of this chapter, situations that result in overcrowding of dairy cows, either in the breeding pen or in the maternity pen seem to be important risk factors for reduced reproductive efficiency. As discussed in numerous previous studies, the nutritional status of the herd can have important effects on reproduction. The BCS status of the herd appears to be a way to monitor one aspect of the nutritional programme in the herd that can have a large effect on reproductive efficiency.

The effect of milk production on reproduction is clearly a complicated relationship. We have found that the increased steroid metabolism associated with high feed consumption can alter a number of reproductive values. For example, heat detection rate was reduced as dairy cows increased milk production. This has important practical implications. For example, in herds that use exclusively heat detection for identifying cows for AI, the lower producing cows have a greater likelihood of receiving AI than the higher producing cows. Thus, reproductive measures in herds using exclusively heat detection may not reflect the true problems of reproduction in some of the cows that would potentially have the highest values for pregnancy, the highest producing dairy cows in the herd.

Another practical implication of this research is that as herds increase milk production, they can expect to have increases in double ovulation rate that will result in increasing twinning rates. This relationship between milk production and double ovulation rate occurs whether natural oestrus or timed AI programmes are used to identify cows for AI. It seems clear that the main increase occurs after cows are producing about 40 kg/d. Thus, we must anticipate that we will have a dramatic increase in double ovulation rate in cows producing over 40 kg/d and this will result in an increase in twinning rate in cows that conceive during this time of high milk production. We must align our management procedures to deal with this increasing twinning rate if we are increasing milk production into this range in our dairies. First, we must set up a programme to diagnose twins. Second, we should set up procedures to manage cows that are likely to have twin births. Twinning cows will calve earlier (~7 d on average) and are likely to have more problems during the calving process. These twin calving cows were, on average, our highest producing cows during the previous lactation. Therefore, it is important to carefully design calving and early lactation procedures with these twinning cows in mind.

Finally, the relationship between milk production and conception rate (pregnancies per AI) is not as clear as found for the effects of milk production on expression of oestrus or double ovulation rate. In most studies in which cows are bred to standing oestrus there appear to be reductions in fertility due to high milk production, but this does not appear to be the case in studies in which cows are bred after ovulation synchronization programmes (see Wiltbank *et al.*, 2006). In addition, milk production is clearly not the only factor involved in reducing the fertility of high producing dairy cows (Lucy *et al.*, 2001; Garnsworthy, 2006). Reproductive management, nutrition and health programmes need to be designed to optimize fertility in dairy cows. These programmes need to be designed to assure that high producing cows have the maximal opportunity for being identified correctly for AI near the time of ovulation.

References

Calamari L, Maianti M.G. and Stefanini L. (2003) Effect of space availability at feed bunk and rest area on metabolic conditions and productive responses in dairy cows. *Italian Journal of Animal Science*, **2**(Suppl. 1), 281-283.

Caraviello D.Z., Weigel K.A., Craven M., Gianola D., Cook N.B., Nordlund K.V., Fricke P.M. and Wiltbank M.C. (2006a). Analysis of reproductive performance of lactating cows on large dairy farms using machine learning algorithms. *Journal of Dairy Science*, **89**, 4703-4722.

Caraviello D.Z., Weigel K.A., Fricke P.M., Wiltbank M.C., Florent M.J., Cook N.B., Nordlund K.V., Zwald N.R. and Rawson C.L. (2006b). Survey of management practices on reproductive performance of dairy cattle on large US commercial farms. *Journal of Dairy Science*, **89**, 4723-4735.

Caraviello D.Z. (2005). Development and evaluation of models for predicting reproductive performance in large commercial dairy herds. Thesis submitted as partial fulfillment of the requirements for the degree of Doctor of Philosophy. University of Wisconsin, Madison.

Dechow, C.D., Rogers G.W., Klei L., Lawlor T.J. and VanRaden P.M. (2004). Body condition scores and dairy form evaluations as indicators of days open in US Holsteins. *Journal of Dairy Science*, **87**, 3534-3541.

del Río N.S., Kirkpatrick B.W., Fricke P.M. (2006). Observed frequency of monozygotic twinning in Holstein dairy cattle. *Theriogenology*, **66**(5), 1292-1299.

Fonseca F.A., Britt J.H., McDaniel B.T., Wilk J.C., Rakes A.H. (1983). Reproductive traits of Holsteins and Jerseys. Effects of age, milk yield and clinical abnormalities on involution of cervix and uterus, ovulation, estrous cycles, detection of estrus, conception rate and days open. *Journal of Dairy Science*, **66**, 1128-1147.

Freund Y. and Mason L. (1999). The alternating decision tree learning algorithm. Pages 124-133 *in* Proceeding of the 16th International Conference on Machine Learning, Bled, Slovenia.

Fricke P.M. and Wiltbank M.C. (1999). Effect of milk production on the incidence of double ovulation in dairy cows. *Theriogenology*, **52**, 1133-1143.

Garnsworthy, P.C. (2006) Body condition score in dairy cows: targets for production and fertility. In *Recent Advances in Animal Nutrition - 2006*, pp. 61-86. Edited by P.C. Garnsworthy and J. Wiseman. Nottingham University Press, Nottingham, UK.

Grummer R.R. and Carroll D.J. (1988) A review of lipoprotein cholesterol metabolism: Importance to ovarian function. *Journal of Animal Science*, **66**, 3160-3172.

Harrison R.O., Ford S.P., Young J.W., Conley A.J. and Freeman A.E. (1990) Increased milk production versus reproductive and energy status of high producing dairy cows. *Journal of Dairy Science* **73**, 2749-2758.

Harrison R.O., Young J.W., Freeman A.E. and Ford S.P. (1989) Effects of lactational level on reactivation of ovarian function and interval from parturition to first visual oestrus and conception in high-producing Holstein cows. *Animal Production*, **49**, 23-28.

Kinsel M.L., Marsh W.E., Ruegg P.L., Etherington W.G. (1998). Risk factors for twinning in dairy cows. *Journal of Dairy Science*, **81**, 989-993.

Lopez H., Caraviello D.Z., Satter L.D., Fricke P.M., Wiltbank M.C. (2005). Relationship between level of milk production and multiple ovulations in lactating dairy cows. *Journal of Dairy Science*, **88**, 2783-2793.

Lopez H., Satter L.D., Wiltbank M.C. (2004). Relationship between level of milk production and estrous behavior of lactating dairy cows. *Animal Reproductive Science*, **81**, 209-223.

Lucy M.C. (2001) Reproductive loss in high-producing dairy cattle: where will it end? *Journal of Dairy Science*, **84**, 1277-1293.

Parr R.A., Davis I.F., Miles M.A. and Squires T.J. (1993). Feed-intake affects metabolic-clearance rate of progesterone in sheep. *Research in Veterinary Science*, **5,** 306-310.

Rabiee A.R., Macmillan K.L. and Schwarzenberger F. (2001). The effect of level of feed intake on progesterone clearance rate by measuring feacal progesterone metabolites in grazing dairy cows. *Animal Reproductive Science*, **67**, 205-214.

Sangsritavong S., Combs D.K., Sartori R. and Wiltbank M.C. (2002). High feed intake increases blood flow and metabolism of progesterone and estradiol-17ß in dairy cattle. *Journal of Dairy Science*, **85**, 2831-2842.

Sartori R., Haughian J.M., Shaver R.D., Rosa G.J. and Wiltbank M.C. (2004). Comparison of ovarian function and circulating steroids in estrous cycles of Holstein heifers and lactating cows. *Journal of Dairy Science*, **87**, 905-920.

Van Eerdenburg F.J.C.M., Karthaus D., Taverne M.A.M., Merics I. and Szenci

O. (2002) The relationship between estrous behavioral score and time of ovulation in dairy cattle. *Journal of Dairy Science* **58**,1150-1156.

Vasconcelos J.L.M., Sangsritavong S., Tsai S.J. and Wiltbank M.C. (2003) Acute reduction in serum progesterone concentrations after feed intake in dairy cows. *Theriogenology*, **60**, 795-807.

Washburn S.P., Silvia W.J., Brown C.H., McDaniel B.T. and McAllister A.J. 2002. Trends in reproductive performance in southeastern Holstein and Jersey DHI herds. *Journal of Dairy Science*, **85**, 244-251.

Wiltbank M.C., Fricke P.M., Sangritasvong S., Sartori R. and Ginther O.J. (2000). Mechanisms that prevent and produce double ovulations in dairy cattle. *Journal of Dairy Science*, **83**, 2998-3007.

Wiltbank M.C., Lopez H., Sartori R., Sangsritavong S. and Gümen A. (2006). Changes in reproductive physiology of lactating dairy cows due to elevated steroid metabolism. *Theriogenology*, **65**, 17-29.

3

A SCIENTIFIC APPROACH TO FEEDING DRY COWS

JAMES K. DRACKLEY[1], HEATHER M. DANN[2]
[1]*Department of Animal Sciences, University of Illinois at Urbana-Champaign, USA,* [2]*William H. Miner Agricultural Research Institute, Chazy, New York, USA*

Introduction

What constitutes optimal nutrition for dairy cows during the dry period has long been controversial. Although researched for several decades, the topic is unresolved and remains timely for several reasons. The continued increase in milk production per cow, and perhaps more importantly milk energy per cow, demands that each phase of the lactation cycle be optimized from a nutritional standpoint to maintain this productivity while keeping cows healthy. Perhaps as a result of continued selection for high productivity and high peak milk during early lactation, fertility of cows (particularly Holstein-Friesen) has continued to deteriorate in both confinement and grazing situations (Garnsworthy and Webb, 1999; Mee, 2004; Pryce, Royal, Garnsworthy and Mao, 2004). Most of the health problems encountered by dairy cows during lactation occur at or shortly after calving and may be influenced by prepartum nutrition. The feed industry has developed a large number of additives, products, and programs that perhaps is disproportionate to the length of the dry period. Although many of these products have merit in certain circumstances, they also in general are high-margin products that carry the potential for overuse when not indicated (Overton and Waldron, 2004). Overall, then, the dry period and transition to lactation play a critical role in profitability of individual cows and entire farming operations.

Given the importance of the dry period and the number of things that can go wrong during this time, it probably is to be expected that interest in nutritional management has been high. Advisors working with dairy farms develop strong opinions and biases that often are not substantiated by scientific data but perhaps are based on vast personal experience. A myriad of approaches have been advocated, including 'steaming up', limit-feeding, maximizing dry matter intake (DMI), feeding additional concentrates, feeding supplemental fats and oils, or feeding high-roughage low-energy diets. In most of these cases there is at least some logical scientific basis for why the approach might allow cows to make successful transitions from pregnancy to lactation. Although considerable research has been conducted, no clear scientific consensus has emerged on which strategy is preferred, or indeed whether there actually is an approach that produces the best results on average. A return to first principles seems in order.

Our objectives are to discuss some general difficulties with scientifically establishing optimal nutrition practices for the dry period and to review the scientific literature on dry period nutrition, with emphasis on energy nutrition. From this body of literature and recent research in our groups, we will develop the argument that controlling energy intake during the dry period (preventing either underfeeding or overfeeding) is the most scientifically defensible strategy.

Goals of dry period management

Although the optimal length of the dry period still is being revisited, the continuing need for a dry period for most cows on most farms has been re-affirmed by recent research (Collier, Annend and Fitzgerald, 2004; Rastani, Grummer, Bertics, Gümen, Wiltbank, Mashek and Schwab, 2005). One might question whether the scientific community and the nutrition industry have made the science and practice of nutrition during the dry period more complicated than it needs to be. After all, the dry cow is an animal with relatively simple and modest nutrient requirements. However, because dry period nutritional management may affect health and subsequent productivity, its importance extends far beyond the simple provision of nutrients to meet immediate requirements. In that context, then, a reasonable set of goals for nutritional management during the dry period might include: 1) meeting nutrient requirements for gestation and mammary development, 2) minimizing the risk for peripartal metabolic disorders and infectious diseases, 3) preparing the cow for high milk production and high subsequent fertility, and 4) optimizing input costs and maximizing profit.

Unfortunately, most producers, and many nutritionists and researchers, tend to look at these goals in isolation. This tendency is aggravated by the dynamic nature of dairy farming, in which seasons, feeds, weather, economic drivers, and labour change frequently, often before true results of a nutritional intervention can be assessed. What is desperately needed to bring sense to this confusing field is a more holistic or 'systems' approach that seeks to integrate effects of dry period nutrition on dairy profitability. In turn, profitability is a function of animal health and well-being, milk production and quality, feed conversion efficiency, reproductive success, and longevity, among others. A nutrition program optimized for only one parameter, such as high peak milk, may not be the most profitable overall approach for all dairy farms.

Challenges in research on dry period nutrition

A large body of original research and literature reviews has been produced dealing with dry cows through the transition to lactation. In non-pasture based systems, there is literature in which dry cows were fed forages and concentrates separately and more recent studies in which dry cows have been fed total mixed rations (TMR). Development and adoption of TMR for dry cows during the last 30 years or so has resulted in a major shift both in practice and in research. Use of TMR allows delivery of consistent nutrient profiles to cows. However, it is difficult for smaller herds to justify a separate TMR for just a few dry cows. Many studies published before the mid-1980s fed forages and concentrates separately. In some cases forages were fed for ad libitum intake without accurate determination of total feed intake. Consequently, extrapolating from older studies with component feeding to current situations where TMR are used is often difficult.

A more serious flaw with the majority of research studies both past and present is their limited cow numbers, which makes reliability and repeatability of results problematic. Coefficients of variation for many important outcome variables, such as DMI, are much greater during the transition period than during other times in lactation (Drackley, 1999), which increases numbers of cows needed to detect meaningful differences statistically. Cow numbers often are chosen to provide adequate replication for metabolic indicators (e.g., nonesterified fatty acids [NEFA] in blood, lipid in liver), but lack statistical power to truly detect meaningful (i.e., economically significant) differences in milk yield. Moreover, it is infeasible to conduct studies within university or research institute settings that include sufficient numbers of cows to determine influences of dry period nutrition on periparturient health disorders or subsequent reproductive efficiency. Thus, inferences are made from selected metabolic variables (or metabolic profiles) consistent with diseased cows, which are assumed to be highly predictive of, or correlated with, actual disease incidence on a population basis; the validity of this assumption has rarely been questioned.

Another major factor that may confound interpretation of nutritional manipulations is differences in the physical environments of cows from one research station to another. This may include differences in barn or stall design, bedding, grouping, floor surfaces, ventilation, environmental temperature and humidity, photoperiod, and disease challenge. Indeed, many of these factors could vary within a research station from month to month. In addition, whether housing and management conditions at research sites accurately reflect conditions that exist on commercial farms can be questioned.

The importance of the general area known as 'cow comfort' has emerged over the last two decades. The type of system (individual tie stalls vs. free stalls or cubicles; pasture-based vs. confinement) may affect transition success, or may interact with nutrition to determine transition success (Cook and Nordlund, 2004). Within types of systems, the quality of facilities and their management becomes a huge source of variation among studies or farms implementing various nutritional programs (Grant and Albright, 1995). A burgeoning number of studies has been conducted in recent years addressing aspects of cow behaviour and its interactions with feeding systems (Endres, DeVries, von Keyserlingk and Weary, 2005), feeding space (DeVries, von Keyserlingk and Weary, 2004), stall design and size (Tucker, Weary and Fraser, 2003, 2004); flooring surface (Tucker, Weary, de Passillé, Campbell and Rushen, 2006), bedding materials (Cook, Bennett and Nordlund, 2004; Fregonesi, Veira, von Keyserlingk and Weary, 2007), grouping size (Grant and Albright, 2001) and movements between groups (Cook and Nordlund, 2007). Together, these data allow for a strong argument to be made that non-nutritional aspects of dry period and transition management may be more important than diet amount or composition in determining transition success. If that is true, then it is probably also true that cows under excellent housing and management conditions can tolerate a much wider range of dietary conditions than cows under more difficult environmental conditions.

What is the optimal scientific approach to address dry period nutrition?

Given the inherent challenges of conducting sound research on dry cow nutrition from which conclusions can be drawn with confidence, what should be the scientific basis for determining optimal dry period nutrition? If research resources were not limited (which of course is highly unlikely to ever come to pass!), the logical scientific approach would be to conduct studies to titrate responses in these integrated outcome variables to different planes of nutrition, balances of nutrients, and diet composition. Studies would utilize adequate cows (hundreds per treatment) housed in industry-typical facilities and would provide statistically reliable results for productivity, disease incidence, fertility, and longevity. However, a further complication is that optimal nutrition may depend on or interact with dry period length, body condition, and age of the cows. As mentioned earlier, management factors such as overcrowding, poor comfort of stalls or cubicles, and frequent group changes probably will affect success on individual farms. A true factorial and systematic answer to these multifaceted questions is highly unlikely to ever be delivered from controlled university or institute-based facilities. The dairy industry may be better served by semi-controlled field trials conducted with large numbers of farms and cows to generate answers to these 'big-picture' questions. Such 'real-world' experiences often may be more meaningful to practicing nutritionists than controlled research studies with insufficient numbers of cows.

The preceding discussion is not intended to argue that controlled research is without value. On the contrary, dissection of the fundamental biology and principles of nutritional management is most appropriately conducted under highly controlled research environments. Many metabolic response variables that provide information about responses of cows to alternate dietary approaches are much less variable than dichotomous outcomes such as disease incidence or pregnancy outcome. Given the inability to research the question under the ideal proposed above, we are forced to make extrapolations from various metabolic and production responses in controlled research studies. The utility of these response variables is strengthened by our ability to profile responses across time, and to compare the different time trends that result from different nutritional treatments (i.e., use of treatment by time interactions in repeated measures designs).

Before turning to use of these variables to aid in evaluation of dry period nutritional approaches, a brief review of the fundamentals of periparturient biology in dairy cows seems prudent.

Fundamentals of cow biology during the transition period

As late-gestation cows approach parturition, nutrient demands by the near-term foetus and reproductive tissues reach a maximum, at a time when DMI may decrease. Consequently, cows may actually enter negative energy and protein balance during the last week prepartum (Grummer, 1995). However, the magnitude of this negative energy balance is usually very much less than that observed after calving (Bell, 1995). Regardless, at calving and into early lactation the processes of homeorhesis in support of lactation increase mobilization of NEFA from stored adipose tissue. Uptake of NEFA by the liver leads to increased triacylglycerol (TAG) deposition in liver and increased ketogenesis. With inappetance or stressors after calving that lead to extreme body lipid mobilization, the degree of TAG accumulation or ketone body synthesis may become pathologic (Drackley, Dann, Douglas, Janovick Guretzky, Litherland, Underwood and Loor, 2005). Increasing evidence implicates subclinical fatty liver and ketosis as risk factors for other disorders and disease (Breukink and Wensing, 1997; Duffield, 2000). Research consistently implicates DMI during the early postpartum period as the main variable defining the extent of negative energy balance, as the genetic and homeorhetic drive in early lactation to produce milk at nearly all costs is phenomenal (Drackley, 2006).

The capacity for hepatic gluconeogenesis increases markedly from late gestation to early lactation (Reynolds, Aikman, Lupoli, Humphries and Beever, 2003) as a result of increased enzymatic activity (Drackley, Overton and Douglas, 2001) but also due to some increase in hepatic mass (Reynolds, Durst, Lupoli, Humphries and Beever, 2004). The contribution of propionate to glucose synthesis is constrained by its supply and thus DMI. Alternate sources of glucogenic carbon such as lactate, alanine (and other amino acids) and glycerol assume greater relative importance during the transition to lactation. Body protein is mobilized to provide amino acids for milk protein synthesis and also to provide substrates for gluconeogenesis. The ability of greater supply of metabolizable protein (MP) to prevent or decrease this body protein mobilization seems limited (Phillips, Citron, Sage, Cummins, Cecava and McNamara, 2003).

The immune system is downregulated around parturition (Kehrli, Nonnecke and Roth, 1989a,b). Although the fundamental causes of this immunosuppression are not understood completely, there is evidence that adequate nutrition can lessen its decrease and help prevent infectious disease. Important factors are energy intake, protein supply, and adequate intakes of vitamins A and E, zinc, copper, and selenium, among others (Mallard, Dekkers, Ireland, Leslie, Sharif, Vankampen, Wagter and Wilkie, 1998; Goff, 1999). As the extent of negative energy balance increases and fatty liver develops, function of the immune system can decrease further (Breukink and Wensing, 1997).

The sudden onset of milk synthesis in the mammary gland results in a tremendous demand for calcium. As a result, blood calcium concentration can drop precipitously at calving, leading to milk fever or subclinical hypocalcemia. The latter is believed to be a contributing factor in disorders such as displaced abomasum and ketosis by decreasing smooth muscle function, which is critical for normal function of the digestive tract (Goff and Horst, 1997). Decreased smooth muscle tone also increases susceptibility to mastitis by impairing the closure of the teat ends after and in between milking (Goff and Horst, 1997). Hypocalcemia results in increased cortisol secretion, which may increase incidence of retained placenta (Goff, 1999). Until the ability of the digestive tract to absorb calcium can increase, calcium must be obtained by resorption from bone. Metabolic acidosis caused by a negative dietary cation-anion difference (DCAD) favours mobilization of calcium from bone, whereas high dietary potassium concentrations and positive DCAD suppress this process (Horst, Goff, Reinhardt and Buxton, 1997). What is less well defined is the role that declining DMI as parturition approaches may have on calcium supply and thus risk for hypocalcemia.

In summary, several factors that are quantifiable in intensive controlled research might be influenced by dry period nutritional strategies. These factors include: 1) DMI around and after parturition, 2) subsequent milk production and milk composition, or rate of change in these variables after calving, 3) degree of postpartal negative energy balance and body fat mobilization, 4) concentrations of energy-yielding compounds in liver (TAG and glycogen) and blood (NEFA, 3-hydroxybutyrate [BHBA], glucose), 5) calcium homeostasis, and 6) metabolic and ruminal adaptations to lactation. Because DMI during the immediate postpartum period and the resulting negative energy balance are central to these response criteria, factors that influence energy balance and the cow's response to this are the main focus in the following evaluation of the body of research on dry period nutrition. This focus is not meant to diminish the importance of other aspects.

Dry period nutrition and transition success

A fundamental principle of animal nutrition is that we generally strive to meet the animals' nutritional requirements, without either deficit or excess. Is there reason to suspect that dairy cows during the dry period should be any different? Or, looking at the question from a slightly different perspective, is there a benefit to providing more energy (or nutrients) than cows need absolutely?

NUTRIENT REQUIREMENTS

Estimates of metabolizable energy (ME) requirements for mature late-gestation cows are approximately 100 MJ/d (AFRC, 1993). In the National Research Council system (NRC, 2001), requirements are expressed in terms of net energy for lactation (NE_L), which is similar to net energy for maintenance (NE_M) at maintenance intakes. The NE_L for maintenance of late-gestation dairy cows is about 60 MJ/d, which with 0.60 efficiency of ME use equates to 100 MJ ME/d. With predicted DMI at various energy concentrations, the National Research Council has long stated that dry cows should receive a diet containing about 5.4 MJ NE_L/kg, or 9 MJ ME/kg DM (NRC, 1978).

Protein requirements are best expressed in terms of MP, which represents the sum of rumen microbial protein plus dietary rumen-undegradable protein plus endogenous protein reaching and digested in the small intestine (NRC, 2001). The NRC considers requirements for maintenance, pregnancy, and growth (if immature) that sum to approximately 800-850 g/d for dairy cattle weighing 625-700 kg. Addition of an estimated requirement for mammogenesis and initiation of lactation of 150-200 g/d (Bell, Burhans and Overton, 2000) would increase this amount to approximately 950-1050 g/d. It would seem that targeting a minimum of 1000 g/d in practice is a reasonable estimate, although many field nutritionists may strive to achieve 1100 g/d or more.

Protein nutrition in late gestation and its influences on postpartum health and lactational performance has been reviewed elsewhere (Bell *et al*, 2000; NRC, 2001; Friggens, Andersen, Larsen, Aaes and Dewhurst, 2004) and is not the focus of this discussion. Studies designed to evaluate the effects of protein nutrition during the dry period have yielded conflicting results (Chew, Murdock, Riley and Hillers,

1984; Huyler, Kincaid and Dostal, 1999; Moorby, Dewhurst and Marsden, 1996; Putnam and Varga, 1998; Putnam, Varga and Dann, 1999; Van Saun *et al.*, 1993; Van Saun and Sniffen, 1996). Bell *et al.* (2000) suggested that the uncertainty may be a result of the undefined relationship between dietary protein intake and MP supply in non-lactating, pregnant cows, and by the lack of understanding of the quantitative metabolism of amino acids in maternal and conceptus tissues. Overall there is little evidence that increasing MP supply beyond 1100 g/d will stimulate production. However, achieving adequate MP intake probably still is an important aspect of transition success and avoidance of disease (Friggens *et al.*, 2004; Drackley *et al.*, 2005).

DRY MATTER INTAKE

Factors affecting DMI of dairy cows have been extensively reviewed (Allen, 2000; Faverdin, 1999; Forbes, 2000; Grant and Albright, 1995; Ingvartsen and Andersen, 2000; NRC, 2001; Grummer, Mashek and Hayirli, 2004). Numerous models for predicting DMI have been developed (Hayirli, Grummer, Nordheim and Crump, 2003; NRC, 2001). Predicting DMI is complex because DMI is influenced by dietary, management, housing, environment, and animal factors (Grant and Albright, 1995; Ingvartsen and Andersen, 2000; NRC, 2001). Peak DMI usually occurs between 10 and 14 wk postpartum, well after peak milk production between 4 and 8 wk postpartum (NRC, 2001). The lowest DMI occurs at parturition, with the maximum increase at peak DMI being from 0.02 to 1.11 of that during wk 1 postpartum (Ingvartsen and Andersen, 2000). Research data indicate that DMI begins to decline gradually approximately 3 wk prior to parturition. The magnitude of the decrease is variable, but can be as much as 0.30 reduction on average (Grant and Albright, 1995; Grummer, 1995). In 699 Holstein heifers and cows fed 49 different diets during the last 3 wk of gestation, DMI decreased 0.32 during the last 3 wk of gestation; 0.89 of the decrease occurred during the last week of gestation (Hayirli, Grummer, Nordheim and Crump, 2002). More recent analyses indicate that the magnitude of decrease is greater with diets of greater energy concentration (Grummer *et al.*, 2004).

Forbes (2000) reviewed the physiological and metabolic aspects of feed intake control in ruminants and suggested that intake is regulated by a series of negative feedback signals from the digestive tract, liver, adipose tissue, and other organs. Ingvartsen and Andersen (2000) suggested that the drop in DMI in late gestation is caused not only by physical constraints, but also by changes in reproductive status, body condition, and metabolic changes associated with the onset of lactogenesis. Specifically, metabolic signals including nutrients, metabolites, reproductive hormones, stress hormones, leptin, insulin, gut peptides, cytokines, and neuropeptides play a role in intake regulation. More recently, Allen, Bradford and Harvatine (2005) developed the theory that increased fatty acid oxidation in the liver decreases feed intake in cattle, as in laboratory animals. The consequence of this mechanism would be that as plasma NEFA concentrations continue to increase, voluntary DMI might actually be decreased, which could worsen the spiral of negative energy balance complications.

Hayirli *et al.* (2002) modeled data from 699 cows and heifers used in 16 research trials conducted at eight universities and found that variation in prepartum DMI could be accounted for by day of gestation, animal factors [parity and body condition score (BCS)], and dietary factors [neutral detergent fibre (NDF), ether extract, ruminally degradable protein (RDP), and ruminally undegradable protein (RUP)]. Day of gestation, parity, BCS, NDF, ether extract, RDP, and RUP accounted for approximately 0.56, 0.10, 0.10, 0.15, 0.06, 0.01, and 0.01 of the variation, respectively.

Prepartum BCS is related to prepartum and postpartum DMI. Grummer (1995) reported correlation coefficients of -0.25 and -0.45 for prepartum BCS and DMI at 1 d prepartum and 21 d postpartum, respectively. Hayirli *et al.* (2002) found a modest negative correlation (r = -0.12) between prepartum BCS and prepartum DMI. The DMI of over-conditioned (> 4.0 BCS on a 1 to 5 scale) cows continuously and gradually decreased during the last 3 wk of gestation, whereas the DMI of under-conditioned (2 to 3 BCS) or properly-conditioned (3 to 4 BCS) cows was constant until the last week of gestation but then decreased sharply (Hayirli *et al.*, 2002).

Nutrient content of prepartum diets also influences prepartum DMI (NRC, 2001). Increasing energy content (Coppock, Noller, Wolfe, Callahan and Baker, 1972; Hernandez-Urdaneta, Coppock, McDowell, Gianola and Smith, 1976; Minor, Trower, Strang, Shaver and Grummer, 1998) or energy and protein content (VandeHaar, Yousif, Sharma, Herdt, Emery, Allen and Liesman, 1999) of prepartum diets increased DMI and energy intake. Hayirli *et al.* (2002) used data from 699 cows and heifers and found that reducing NDF from approximately 400 g/kg to 300 g/kg of dietary DM proportionally increased prepartum DMI by approximately 0.21. Increasing ether extract from 20 g/kg to 32 or 57 g/kg decreased prepartum DMI by approximately 0.11. Prepartum intake was not related to CP content of the diet. However, prepartum DMI increased quadratically as the level of RDP increased from 85 to 129 g/kg, whereas prepartum DMI decreased (by 0.06) linearly as the dietary content of RUP increased from 35 to 57 g/kg.

In a classic study, Bertics, Grummer, Cadorniga-Valino and Stoddard (1992) demonstrated that force-feeding cows in late gestation a forage diet through a ruminal cannula to maintain high prepartum DMI decreased postpartum liver TAG content, increased postpartum DMI, and increased milk yield. Grummer (1995) summarized 5 studies and found a positive correlation (r = 0.53) between DMI 1 d prepartum and DMI 21 d postpartum. Findings from the Bertics *et al.* (1992)

study and the Grummer (1995) summary resulted in many experts advocating that prepartum DMI be maximized so that postpartum DMI might be increased and also to improve postpartum performance and health. Many studies (Doepel, Lapierre and Kennelly, 2002; Mashek and Beede, 2000; Minor, Trower, Strang, Shaver and Grummer, 1998; Rabelo, Rezende, Bertics and Grummer, 2003; VandeHaar *et al.*, 1999) subsequently have tested the idea of maximizing prepartum DMI and energy intake but have found little if any benefit to postpartum metabolism and performance.

In contrast, other researchers (Agenäs, Burstedt and Holtenius, 2003; Douglas, Overton, Bateman, Dann and Drackley, 2006; Holcomb, Van Horn, Head, Hall and Wilcox, 2001; Holtenius, Agenäs, Delavaud and Chilliard, 2003; Tesfa, Tuori, Syrjälä-Qvist, Pösö, Saloniemi, Heinonen, Kivilahti, Saukko and Lindberg, 1999) found that restricting DMI or energy intake during the prepartum period was beneficial for postpartum metabolism and performance. The discrepancy in results led researchers (Drackley, 2003; Grummer *et al.*, 2004) to re-evaluate the idea of maximizing prepartum DMI and to evaluate the importance of the amount of decline in prepartum DMI. Drackley (2003, 2006) concluded that early postpartum DMI and hepatic lipid and TAG contents were more highly related to changes in DMI during the last 3 wk prepartum than to actual DMI during the last 3 wk prepartum. The proportional change in DMI during the last 3 wk was correlated to DMI at 3 wk postpartum (r = 0.43), lipid content in the liver at 1 d postpartum (r = -0.63), and TAG content in the liver at 1 d postpartum (r = -0.63; Drackley, 2003). Grummer *et al.* (2004) suggested that minimizing the decline in DMI is more important than maximizing DMI prepartum.

DIET COMPOSITION RECOMMENDATIONS FOR TWO-GROUP SYSTEMS

The confusion about optimal dry period nutrition exists despite the plethora of studies that have been conducted to determine dietary composition for periparturient cows. Only one set of nutrient requirements for dry, pregnant cows was listed in the 1989 edition of *Nutrient Requirements of Dairy Cattle* (NRC, 1989). By the mid 1990s, it was acknowledged by most nutritionists that these recommendations were outdated in that one set of recommendations was not appropriate for both far-off dry cows (early portion of the dry period) and close-up (last 3 wk prior to parturition) dry cows. Van Saun and Sniffen (1996) suggested increasing the dietary NE_L intake energy by 8 to 12 MJ above NRC (1989) recommendations for prepartum cows. The 2001 edition of *Nutrient Requirements of Dairy Cattle* (NRC, 2001) provided separate nutrient guidelines for far-off and close-up dry cows to account for the depression in DMI that occurs before parturition and the physiological and nutritional changes that occur in late pregnancy. Recommendations for composition of diets for multiparous cows during the far-off dry period were 5.2 MJ NE_L/kg DM (equivalent to 8.7 MJ ME/kg DM) and 120 g CP / kg (NRC, 2001). Recommendations for close-up diets for multiparous cows are 6.4 to 6.8 MJ NE_L/kg DM (equivalent to 10.7 - 11.3 MJ ME/kg DM) and 120 g CP/kg DM (NRC, 2001). Dietary recommendations for primiparous cows were 6.4 to 6.8 Mcal NE_L/kg DM (10.7 – 11.3 MJ ME/kg DM) and 135 to 150 g CP/kg (NRC, 2001). The NRC further specified that all diets should contain a minimum of 330 g NDF/kg, a minimum of 219 g ADF/kg, and a maximum of 420 g non-fibre carbohydrate (NFC) /kg (NRC, 2001). The origin of these recommendations seems to have been in the results of studies that showed improvements in prepartum DMI and reductions in plasma NEFA or liver TAG. Separate far-off and close-up groups were widely recommended as a way to improve management, target more expensive ingredients only to cows closest to calving, and minimize health disorders (Gerloff, 2000; Overton and Waldron, 2004).

ENERGY NUTRITION

Increasing the amount of non-structural carbohydrates in dry cow diets

Boutflour appears to have introduced the concept of "steaming up" the dry cow ration in 1928 (Boutflour, 1928). The concept of "steaming up" was to start feeding concentrates to the cow 6 wk before parturition and gradually increase the amount of concentrate fed. The amount of concentrate fed 1 wk prior to calving would be approximately 0.75 of the amount of concentrate the cow would get in her postpartum ration. Steaming up became common practice for farmers in Britain, but not in the United States, during the 1930s and 1940s (Greenhalgh and Gardner, 1958). Little research was available to support the claims of increased milk production when steamed-up dry cow diets were fed.

The concept of steaming up still receives some attention from time to time. Olsson, Emanuelson and Wiktorsson (1998) determined the effects of gradually increasing the proportion of concentrate before parturition to provide 110, 170, 200, or >200 MJ of metabolizable energy per cow by parturition. The low nutrition level (110 MJ) at parturition resulted in lower milk yield during the first month of lactation, and lower serum insulin and higher NEFA concentrations during the periparturient period.

During the late 1950s and 1960s, researchers studied the effect of feeding additional non-structural carbohydrates as concentrates to prepartum cows. Greenhalgh and Gardner (1958) found no increase in milk yield or udder edema when concentrates were increased gradually during the last 42 d of gestation. Because variable results were reported on the effect of dry period feeding on milk production, Schmidt and Schultz (1959) studied the effect of three rates of grain feeding on incidence of ketosis, severity of udder edema, and milk production. They found no differences in these outcome variables due to grain allocation. A study reported in 1962 (Swanson and Hinton, 1962) found that providing extra concentrates in the prepartum ration increased fat-corrected milk yield by 137 kg during the first 15 wk of lactation. However, Emery, Hafs, Armstrong and Snyder (1969) found that prepartum grain feeding starting at 21 d prepartum did not increase milk production in multiparous cows. Gardner (1969) evaluated the interaction of energy intake (115% and 160% of digestible energy required for maintenance) of diets fed prepartum and postpartum to cows on milk production and blood metabolites. Higher energy intakes prepartum did not affect milk production but increased blood ketone levels. However, higher energy intakes postpartum resulted in increased milk, protein, and lactose productions. The problem with many of these earlier studies was that cows were being fed a high plane of nutrition for too long during the dry period. Cows were often fed a high amount of grain starting 8 to 10 wk prior to parturition and often gained excess BCS, which increased the risk of metabolic problems.

One way to combat the decrease in nutrient intake associated with the decline in DMI before parturition is to increase the nutrient density of the diet. Numerous researchers have tested this approach. Adjusting the forage to concentrate ratio of the diet can alter energy content of the diet. Coppock *et al.* (1972) studied the effect of forage to concentrate ratio in a prepartum TMR on prepartum DMI and the occurrence of displaced abomasum (DA). This was one of the first studies using a TMR or complete feed for dry cows. Four TMR were fed starting 28 d prior to calving with forage to concentrate ratios of 75:25, 60:40, 45:55, and 30:70. The concentrations of protein (approximately 150 g CP/kg DM), Ca, and P were similar for all four diets. Mean DMI was not different among treatments, but DMI declined significantly as parturition approached for cows fed the 60:40, 45:55, and 30:70 diets. As the content of concentrate increased, so did the occurrence of DA. Coppock *et al.* (1972) suggested that lead-feeding dry cows with grain might be a contributing factor to the occurrence of DA.

Prepartum diets consisting of 1) alfalfa grass hay, 2) TMR of 0.41 maize silage, 0.47 alfalfa silage, and 0.12 high moisture maize grain, or 3) TMR of 0.25 maize silage, 0.28 alfalfa silage, and 0.47 high moisture maize grain were fed to cows starting 28 d before expected parturition (Johnson and Otterby, 1981). Dry matter intake was highest for cows receiving the diet containing 0.47 grain diet from 28 d to 13 d prior to parturition; there was no difference in DMI during the 2 wk prior to parturition. Milk production was not affected by treatment during the first 30 DIM. Johnson and Otterby (1981) concluded that TMR containing up to 0.47 cereal grain could be fed to cows for 1 month prior to parturition without causing DA.

Hernandez-Urdaneta *et al.* (1976) fed cows from 28 d prepartum to 4 d postpartum either a diet containing 0.95 forage: 0.05 concentrate or a diet of 0.80 forage: 0.20 concentrate. Cows fed the 0.80 forage diet had higher DMI and consumed more energy prepartum than the cows fed the 0.95 forage diet. They also found that cows could be changed abruptly from a high forage diet prepartum to a high concentrate (up to 0.60) diet postpartum without negative effects on DMI and milk production.

Data from 1,374 multiparous Holstein cows revealed that feeding diets with energy and protein concentrations higher than recommended by the NRC (1978) might reduce the incidence of metabolic and reproductive disorders (Curtis, Erb, Sniffen, Smith and Kronfeld, 1985). This paper led to more studies evaluating energy and protein concentrations in the diet.

Flipot, Roy and Dufour (1988) fed prepartum cows grass silage ad libitum and one of two rates of concentrate feeding, 2.5 or 7.5 g/kg body weight (BW). At parturition, cows were factorialized to one of three postpartum diets. Diets consisted of maize silage ad libitum, hay, and a concentrate containing 200 g CP/ kg fed at 2.5 g/kg BW, 7.5 g/kg BW, or ad libitum. Cows fed the higher amounts of concentrate during the prepartum and postpartum periods consumed more DM, energy, and protein. Prepartum treatments had no effect on milk production. Milk production was higher for cows fed higher amounts of concentrate postpartum. These results indicated that concentrate at 2.5 g/kg BW during the dry period was sufficient. During the postpartum period, cows fed concentrate ad libitum produced more milk.

Increasing the energy and protein concentrations from 5.4 MJ NE_L/kg and 122 g CP/kg to 6.7 MJ NE_L/kg and 160 g CP/kg in diets fed during the last 3 wk of gestation improved nutrient balance prepartum and slightly decreased the already low hepatic lipid content at parturition (VandeHaar *et al.*, 1999). There was no effect on postpartum DMI and milk production. Inclusion of steam-flaked maize grain source in high energy (6.7MJ NE_L/kg DM) close-up and lactation diets increased energy intake during the last 28 d prepartum and decreased NEFA and BHBA in plasma compared with cows fed diets containing less fermentable cracked maize grain (Dann, Varga and Putnam, 1999). However, no difference in NEFA or milk yield was detected postpartum, even though diets containing steam-flaked maize decreased ruminal acetate to propionate ratio postpartum and increased energy balance. Doepel *et al.* (2002) found that prepartum diets that contained 6.9 MJ NE_L/kg increased postpartum DMI and improved energy balance compared with prepartum diets that contained 5.4 MJ NE_L/kg, but did not increase milk yield during the first 42 d of lactation.

Mashek and Beede (2000) fed cows from 3 wk prepartum until parturition on diets with either no maize grain or 0.21 maize grain and found that cows in the third lactation or greater had higher milk and protein yields when fed the diet supplemented with maize grain. However, cows in the first or second lactation had lower milk yield when supplemented with maize grain. There was no difference in plasma NEFA or incidences of health disorders. In a subsequent study, Mashek and Beede (2001) found that primiparous and multiparous cows fed a high-energy (~6.7 MJ NE_L/kg) diet for greater than 26 d (36.6 ± 6.9 d) prepartum had improved energy status postpartum compared with cows fed the diet for less than 26 d (17.5 ± 4.1 d), as indicated by a tendency towards lower plasma NEFA and higher insulin concentrations and less BCS loss during the first 3 wk of lactation. Milk yield (first 60 d in milk) and incidences of ketosis and displaced abomasum were not affected by time spent on the diet. Contreras, Ryan and Overton (2004) fed multiparous cows a higher-energy close-up diet for either 21 or 60 d. Milk yield (first 150 d in milk), serum BHBA concentration (5 to 15 d in milk) and incidences of ketosis and displaced abomasum were not affected by time spent on the close-up diet.

Minor *et al.* (1998) showed that cows and heifers fed diets containing high NFC (> 400 g/kg of dietary DM) during the last 19 d of gestation and first 40 wk postpartum had a positive energy balance during the late gestation period, increased plasma glucose, increased liver glycogen, and tendencies for decreased plasma NEFA, plasma BHBA, and liver TAG compared with cows fed a standard NFC diet. Unfortunately, the experimental design did not allow the metabolic and performance results to be attributed to diets fed prepartum, postpartum, or during both periods.

Rabelo *et al.* (2003, 2005) compared a moderate-energy diet (6.6 MJ NE_L/kg, 400 g NDF kg, 380 g NFC/kg) and a high-energy diet (7.1 MJ NE_L/kg, 320 g NDF/kg, 440 g NFC/kg) during the last 28 d of gestation. Cows fed the high-energy diet tended to have greater DMI prepartum regardless of parity, but this failed to confer advantages in milk yield (Rabelo *et al.*, 2003). Cows fed the high-energy diet prepartum had greater concentrations of insulin and glucose both prepartum and postpartum (Rabelo *et al.*, 2005). Prepartal energy concentration had no effect on plasma NEFA or hepatic lipid accumulation, although cows and heifers fed the higher-energy prepartum diet had lower BHBA concentrations postpartum (Rabelo *et al.*, 2005).

Increasing the amount of fat as an energy source in dry cow diets

Skaar, Grummer, Dentine and Stauffacher (1989) increased energy concentration of prepartum and postpartum diets by using supplemental fat. Cows were fed diets without or with supplemental fat beginning 17 d prior to parturition and ending 15 wk postpartum. Dry matter intake and concentrations of glucose, NEFA, and BHBA in plasma were not affected by diet. Liver lipid and TAG contents tended to increase when fat was fed. In contrast, Grum *et al.* (1996) found that cows fed high fat diets during the dry period had little accumulation of TAG in liver and lower plasma NEFA at 1 d postpartum compared with cows fed diets with more grain. However, cows that were fed the high fat diet had lower DMI prepartum, which may explain the difference in liver composition compared with results of Skaar *et al.* (1989). Douglas, Overton, Bateman and Drackley (2004) found little benefit of adding fat to diets for dry cows on peripartal health and postpartum performance.

Importance of managing energy nutrition in dry cows

Prolonged over-consumption of energy during the dry period is clearly detrimental to cows. Fronk, Schultz and Hardie (1980) demonstrated that over-conditioned cows (BCS = 3.8 on a 5-point scale) were more likely to experience metabolic disorders than thinner cows (BCS = 3). Body condition significantly affects cow health, DMI, and milk production (Boisclair, Grieve, Stone, Allen and MacLeod, 1986; Garnsworthy and Jones, 1987; Garnsworthy and Topps, 1982; Reid, Treacher and Williams, 1986; Treacher, Reid and Roberts, 1986). Garnsworthy and Topps (1982) demonstrated that cows with a higher prepartum BCS (4 on a 5-point scale) lost more BW and BCS during early lactation; DMI was lower for the fat cows. Treacher *et al.* (1986) showed that fat cows (BCS = 4) at calving lost more BW and BCS, consumed less DMI, and produced less milk than thin cows (BCS = 2.5). Garnsworthy and Jones (1987) concluded that thin cows (BCS = 2) at parturition produce more milk from nutrient intake than do fat cows (BCS 3.5) and therefore were more biologically efficient.

Reid *et al.* (1986) compared cows that were either thin (BCS = 2.5) or fat (BCS = 4) at parturition and found no difference in adipose tissue mobilization from 4 wk prepartum to 26 wk postpartum. Lipogenic and lipolytic capacities of isolated adipocytes were not different between groups. However, fat cows had greater lipid content in liver and higher plasma NEFA concentrations than thin cows at 1 and 4 wk postpartum. Between 4 wk prepartum and 4 wk postpartum, fat cows lost more muscle fibre area than thin cows, indicating greater mobilization of muscle protein. Overconditioning also results in impairment of the immune system (Lacetera, Scalia, Bernabucci, Ronchi, Pirazzi and Nardone, 2005) and greater indices of oxidative stress (Bernabucci, Ronchi, Lacetera and Nardone, 2005).

As mentioned earlier, cows fed higher energy diets may have more pronounced decreases in DMI leading up to calving (Grummer *et al.*, 2004). The declining nutritional status before calving may be more of a negative signal metabolically than the absolute DMI (Drackley *et al.*, 2005). Consequently, limiting energy intake during the dry period has been explored as a practice to avoid overconditioning and to stabilize DMI.

Restricting dry matter or energy intakes

The effects of feeding cows either low or high amounts of energy before parturition on DMI, BW changes, and milk production have been studied (Kunz, Blum, Hart, Bickel and Landis, 1985). Cows fed ad libitum before parturition had a larger decrease in DMI prior to parturition than cows restricted to meet energy requirements. The restricted-fed cows had a faster increase in DMI and a smaller energy deficit in early lactation. Kunz *et al.* (1985) suggested that the endocrine and metabolic changes observed in early lactation improved glucose homeostasis, decreased fat mobilization, and decreased ketogenesis in cows fed restricted amounts during the dry period compared with cows fed ad libitum. Lodge, Fisher and Lessard (1975) fed cows a diet balanced to meet maintenance requirements or a diet to meet maintenance plus pregnancy requirements (1.8 × maintenance) starting 6 wk before expected parturition. Cows fed the maintenance diet lost more BW prepartum but less BW postpartum compared with cows fed the higher intake. There was no difference in milk production.

Restricting intake for 30 d before parturition to a level that supplied 0.66 of requirements for energy resulted in decreased NEFA and BHBA and increased milk yield postpartum (Lotan, Ziv, Levy, Marton and Adler, 1988). Cows fed a limited amount of feed that supplied 100% of their energy requirements for 10-14 wk prepartum resulted in lower concentrations of NEFA and BHBA in plasma, lower TG in liver, and higher glycogen in liver postpartum compared with cows allowed to consume higher-energy diets for ad libitum intake during the dry period (van den Top, Geelen, Wensing, Wentink, Van't Klooster and Beynen, 1996). In subsequent studies by the same research group, allowing excessive energy intake during a 10-wk dry period resulted in increased plasma NEFA, greater serum BHBA, and greater hepatic TG accumulation compared with cows that were restricted to approximately 80% of their energy requirement (Rukkwamsuk, Wensing and Geelen, 1998, 1999a,b). The overfed cows also had higher insulin concentrations during late gestation than the feed-restricted cows, with no differences in blood glucose (Rukkwamsuk *et al.*, 1998).

Holcomb *et al.* (2001) evaluated the effects of DMI (ad libitum or restricted to requirements) and forage content of the diet during the close-up period (last 19 d before calving) on postpartum performance of multiparous cows. Prepartum dietary treatments did not affect postpartum DMI, milk yield, BW, BCS, or plasma glucose. Feeding the higher forage diet (44% NDF) prepartum had less beneficial effect than restricting the amount of feed offered for decreasing plasma NEFA and increasing DMI postpartum (Holcomb *et al.*, 2001).

In a Swedish study, three groups of cows were used to compare plane of energy during the 10 wk before parturition (Agenäs, Burstedt and Holtenius, 2003; Holtenius, Agenäs, Delavaud and Chilliard, 2003). Cows were limit-fed 6, 9, or 14.5 kg DM to provide 0.71, 1.06, or 1.77 of their requirements for ME during the dry period. The cows fed the greatest amount of energy prepartum had greater BCS at calving but lost more condition in early lactation than cows in the other groups (Agenäs *et al.*, 2003). Prepartum dietary energy intake did not affect milk yield or concentrations of NEFA and BHBA postpartum (Holtenius *et al.*, 2003). Cows that consumed the most energy prepartum had higher plasma concentrations of insulin and glucose prepartum, but cows in the high energy group released more insulin and had lower glucose clearance rates in response to an intravenous glucose challenge prepartum compared with cows allowed to consume less energy (Holtenius *et al.*, 2003). These changes suggest the existence of insulin resistance in the overfed cows, similar to results of the Dutch studies (Rukkwamsuk *et al.*, 1998).

Roche, Kolver and Kay (2005) provided pasture allowances (DM) of 5.4, 8.2, 10.0, or 11.0 kg/d to grazing cows during the last 4 wk prepartum. Cows consumed 56, 84, 103, and 112 MJ ME/d. Cows that were underfed prepartum had greater mobilization of body reserves prepartum, were in lower BCS at calving, and had greater concentrations of NEFA, BHBA, and growth hormone but lower concentrations of glucose, insulin and leptin than cows that consumed adequate amounts of ME before calving. However, cows that were underfed prepartum had a lesser extent of negative energy balance after calving. Although initial milk yields were lower for the underfed cows, theses differences were confined to the first week postpartum

Our research group compared cows restricted in intake to 0.80 of the NRC energy requirements with those allowed ad libitum intake of a moderate energy diet (10.5 MJ ME/kg DM) during a 60-day dry period (Douglas *et al.*, 2006). Potential effects of supplemental energy source (fat verses non-fibre carbohydrates) also were evaluated at each energy intake. Diet composition had relatively few effects, but regardless of energy source, cows with restricted energy intake prepartum had greater postpartum DMI, lower concentrations of NEFA and BHBA in plasma, and less TG accumulation in the liver postpartum.

In contrast to these studies in which limiting DMI was positive or neutral, prepartum restriction of energy in a large herd study led to increased fat mobilization and evidence for adverse effects on lipoprotein metabolism (Kaneene, Miller, Herdt and Gardiner, 1997). Restricted cows had greater incidences of metritis and retained placenta. Differences between this study and the group of studies discussed previously may relate to the degree of nutrient restriction or differences in environmental and behavioural stressors in these group-fed cows.

Using high-bulk diets to limit energy intake

As a follow-up to the Douglas *et al.* (2006) study, Dann, Litherland, Underwood, Bionaz, D'Angelo, McFadden and Drackley (2006) determined the effects of energy intake during both far-off and close-up dry periods. During the far-off dry period (the first 5 wk of an 8-wk dry period), cows were fed 0.8, 1.0, or >1.5 of their energy requirements (NRC, 2001). The cows fed to meet their requirements received a high-straw diet to limit total energy intake at ad libitum DMI, while the restricted group was fed a limited amount of DM from a moderate energy diet. During the close-up period (the last 24 d before expected parturition) cows received a moderate-energy close-up diet either at restricted intake to provide 0.80 of energy requirements or for ad libitum intake. Similar to results of others (Rukkwamsuk *et al*., 1998; Holtenius *et al*., 2003), during the far-off period cows that over-consumed energy (>1.5 x energy requirements) had greater insulin concentrations in serum than did cows fed either 1.0 or 0.8 of their energy requirement, but glucose concentration was not different. During the close-up period, cows restricted to 0.8 of energy requirements had higher NEFA and BHBA in serum but lower glucose and insulin than cows fed for ad libitum intake. In addition, cows previously overfed during the far-off dry period had greater NEFA and BHBA concentrations in the close-up period than cows in the other groups, which is consistent with development of insulin resistance in the overfed cows. Regardless of close-up energy intake, cows that were allowed to over-consume energy during the far-off period had lower DMI, more negative energy balance, greater BHBA in serum, and greater TG accumulation in liver postpartum compared with cows fed controlled amounts of energy during the far-off period. Milk yield was >2 kg/d more for cows that consumed at their energy requirements during the far-off period compared with those consuming 1.5 or 0.8 x their requirements. Liver tissue obtained by biopsy at 1 d postpartum revealed that the cows that were allowed to consume in excess of their requirements during the far-off dry period had greater rates of fatty acid esterification and lower rates of oxidation, which would favour accumulation of TAG in liver (Litherland, Dann, Hansen and Drackley, 2003).

Minor *et al*. (1998) fed a high-NDF (49 g/kg of DM) diet (including 0.25 wheat straw) in the close-up period. As might be expected, DMI was lower prepartum compared with a lower-NDF diet (0.125 wheat straw and 0.30 NDF), but greater energy intakes by the lower-NDF diet did not increase DMI or milk yield and did not decrease hepatic lipid accumulation postpartum.

Beever (2006) recently reviewed results of feeding bulky high straw (ca. 0.50 of DM) diets during the entire dry period. These diets contained some maize silage or whole-crop cereal silage and supplied adequate ME and MP at ad libitum intakes but prevented overconsumption of energy during the dry period. Surveys of producers that adopted this practice indicated marked improvements in transition health problems. Recently our group compared such a high straw diet with either restricted or ad libitum intakes of a moderate energy diet (Janovick Guretzky, Litherland, Moyes and Drackley, 2006). Cows and heifers fed the high-straw diet during the dry period had more stable DMI during the dry period, had lesser increases in NEFA and BHBA in plasma, and less TAG accumulation in liver compared with overfed cows. Milk production was not statistically different among groups.

Dewhurst, Moorby, Dhanoa, Evans and Fisher (2000) fed three diets to dry cows during the last 6 wk before calving. Diets were ad libitum grass silage, a 60:40 (DM) mixture of grass silage and barley straw, or ad libitum grass silage plus 0.5 kg of prairie meal. Cows fed the grass silage – barley straw mixture had the lowest DMI prepartum, did not gain BCS during the dry period, and had the lowest BCS score after calving. The DMI by cows fed the grass silage – barley straw diet was more constant before calving and decreased less than cows fed the other two diets. Milk production and composition during the first 22 wk of lactation were not affected by dry period diet, although milk protein and lactose yields were lower during the first month postpartum for cows fed grass silage – barley straw. For that group, intake of ME averaged 81 MJ at 5 wk before calving but only 68 MJ during the last week prepartum. In contrast, in the other groups ME intakes averaged 132 MJ at wk 5 prepartum and 100 MJ during the final week before calving.

GENERAL CONCLUSIONS ON DIET COMPOSITION FOR DRY COWS

The impact of dry cow feeding on postpartum performance and health has been reviewed by others (Broster and Broster, 1984; Ingvartsen, Danfaer, Andersen and Foldager, 1996; Stockdale and Roche, 2002; Friggens *et al.*, 2004). Based on our review and synthesis of these previous reviews, some general conclusions can be made. No clear advantage or disadvantage can be defined concerning the optimum level of feeding (intake), nutrient density, types of forage, or proportions of non-structural carbohydrates that should be in prepartum diets to minimize the decline in prepartum DMI and optimize postpartum performance and health. However, the recommendations suggested by NRC (2001) seem reasonable as a conservative starting point. Cows with the highest prepartum DMI often had the greatest decline in DMI before parturition. Cows that were restricted-fed prepartum often had the greatest rate of increase in DMI immediately after parturition. The accumulated evidence indicates that these high bulk or low energy diets fed during the dry period do not increase subsequent milk production or energy balance other than during the first several days post-calving. Over-conditioned cows or cows that were over-fed during the entire dry period had greater BCS and BW change and more metabolic problems during the postpartum period. Cows with greater adipose lipid mobilization and greater serum or plasma NEFA during the periparturient period had greater fatty infiltration of the liver. Most studies in which the energy status of cows in late gestation was improved by higher nutrient density diets observed no effect on milk yield or composition. Most studies use too few animals to appropriately assess the effects of prepartum diet on the incidence of periparturient health disorders or reproductive success. Overall, little evidence supports feeding a close-up diet that is high in energy and protein concentrations for longer than approximately 3 wk prepartum. The additional cost of feeding a close-up diet for the entire dry period cannot be justified given the lack of milk production response or improvement in health. The potential for high straw or high bulk diets to limit energy intake and improve transition success is exciting.

A "biologically sensible" approach to dry period nutrition?

Obesity at calving is a well-known risk factor for health problems and suboptimal productive performance. Likewise, extreme under-nutrition may adversely affect postpartum outcomes. Based on the body of research conducted, it appears that feeding to approximately meet the requirements of cows for energy and protein (and of course other nutrients such as minerals and vitamins), without greatly exceeding energy requirements, is the approach most likely to achieve consistent success. This concept may be applied by several approaches and with varying dietary formulation, ranging from limit-feeding of moderate-energy diets to ad libitum feeding of high-roughage low-energy diets. Requirements for ME for dry cows and first-gestation heifers are quite modest (ca. 100 MJ) and can be met with surprisingly (perhaps) low-energy diets. Conversely, diets high in maize silage or whole-crop cereals and supplemented with additional concentrates will result in an excess of energy intake relative to requirements, as cows do not regulate intake to meet energy needs over the short-term. Energy over-consumption leads to marked decreases in DMI leading up to calving.

Our laboratory has obtained data from several lines of evidence to indicate that overfeeding results in changes analogous to obesity, with poor DMI, substantial body fat mobilization, increased fat deposition in the liver, and, if severe, impairment of liver function. Dann, Morin, Murphy, Bollero, and Drackley (2005) postulated that restricted feeding (to 0.80 of NE_L requirements) would make cows less susceptible to an induced ketosis after calving. To test this hypothesis, Dann *et al.* (2005) fed cows a moderate-energy diet for ad libitum intake or in restricted amounts to supply only 0.80 of energy requirements throughout the dry period. After calving, cows that were healthy according to a comprehensive health exam were assigned to either an ad libitum fed control group or to a group in which ketosis was induced by feed restriction (0.50 of the amount of TMR consumed during d 1-4 postpartum) beginning on d 5 postpartum. This feed restriction model of ketosis is simple, controlled and repeatable. As shown in Table 1, cows subjected to the postpartum feed restriction responded with strong increases in blood NEFA and BHBA, urine ketone excretion, and hepatic total lipid content as well as decreased serum glucose. However, the magnitude of these values was greater for cows that had been allowed to overconsume energy during the dry period. Thus, we suggest that cows that are subjected to less-than-ideal environmental conditions after calving, which cause decreased feed intake, are more likely to enter the downward spiral of ketosis and fatty liver if they have been allowed to overconsume energy throughout the dry period.

Table 1. Impact of dry period plane of nutrition on susceptibility to an induced ketosis during early lactation.

| | Dry period diet | | | |
| | *Ad libitum* | | *Restricted* | |
Dietary treatment > day 5:	*Ad libitum*	*Restricted*	*Ad libitum*	*Restricted*
Variables				
d 1-4 postpartum				
Serum glucose, mM	2.9	2.8	2.7	3.0
Serum NEFA, mM	1.25	1.09	1.11	0.99
Serum BHBA, mM	0.88	0.77	0.74	0.69
Liver total lipid, mg/g wet	61	69	62	60
d 14 or clinical ketosis				
Serum glucose, mM	3.0	1.9	3.0	2.4
Serum NEFA, mM	0.83	1.76	0.58	1.38
Serum BHBA, mM	0.72	2.05	0.59	1.40
Urine BHBA, mM	0.25	14.62	0.28	3.07
Liver total lipid, mg/g wet	54	155	55	116

Cows from both dry period groups were fed the same lactation diet for *ad libitum* intake starting at calving. At day 5, healthy cows were subjected to a feed restriction ketosis induction protocol (restricted) or continued to be fed *ad libitum*.
Data from Dann, Morin, Murphy, Bollero, and Drackley (2005) and unpublished.

Mechanistic reasons for these apparent improvements in resistance to disorders in response to controlling energy intake are becoming somewhat clearer. Some of these mechanisms were discussed by Beever (2006). Providing a consistent balanced diet of high bulk that will limit total energy intake with ad libitum DMI also seems to minimize the drop in DMI before calving. Data available to date indicate that these high-bulk diets, if formulated and fed to meet nutrient requirements of the cows, decrease body fat mobilization, blood ketones, and liver fat accumulation postpartum. Bulky feeds such as straw must be processed so that cows do not sort the TMR. A more thorough discussion of practical implementation aspects of these diets can be found elsewhere (Drackley, Janovick-Guretzky and Dann, 2007).

Our research group recently has explored changes in mRNA for thousands of genes in liver during the periparturient period using microarray and quantitative PCR techniques (Loor, Dann, Everts, Oliveira, Green, Janovick-Guretzky, Rodriguez-Zas, Lewin and Drackley, 2005; Loor, Dann, Janovick-Guretzky, Everts, Oliveira, Green, Litherland, Rodriguez-Zas, Lewin and Drackley, 2006). We have shown that diet can influence the relative expression of genes. In many cases these changes support changes observed in other variables. For example, the mRNA for several fatty acid oxidative genes was decreased by overfeeding during the dry period, whereas genes for esterification were increased (Loor *et al.*, 2006). There were also more unexpected findings, for example the expression of inflammation-associated gene products that were increased by excessive energy intake (Loor *et al.*, 2006). In addition, the gene products altered by an induced ketosis (Loor, Everts, Bionaz, Dann, Morin, Oliveira, Rodriguez-Zas, Drackley and Lewin, 2007) are providing exciting new avenues to pursue on the effects of dry period plane of nutrition.

Our conclusions here about the general advisability of feeding to meet requirements are in agreement with the concept of the 'biological sense" of 'priming the system' for subsequent metabolic adaptations and production as argued by Friggens *et al.* (2004), rather than attempting to suppress these adaptations by high energy feeding during the dry period. Controlling energy intake to near the cows' requirements also is consistent with observations in other animals and humans. For example, research evidence in pigs indicates that feed intake should be limited during gestation to avoid excessive loss of BCS after farrowing, with subsequent loss of fertility (e.g., Hoppe, Libal and Wahlstrom, 1990; Coffey, Diggs, Handlin, Knabe, Maxwell, Noland, Prince and Gromwell, 1994; Sinclair, Bland and Edwards, 2001). Medical recommendations for human pregnancy generally advocate modest gain in excess of foetal and maternal reproductive tissues, to avoid complications with delivery, decreased vitality of the newborn, and health problems in the mother (e.g., Hilson, Rasmussen and Kjolhede, 2006; Stotland, Cheng, Hopkins and Caughey, 2006; DeVader, Neeley, Myles and Leet, 2007).

Conclusions

Although the scientific literature is confusing and fraught with difficulties, we propose that the most likely way to achieve consistent and repeatable transition success is to aim to meet nutrient requirements for dry cows, without allowing cows to consume in excess of their requirements. In practice, a working range of 0.90 to 1.10 of required energy intake is tolerated well by cows, although the exact range cannot be determined from available literature. Use of high straw or other high bulk diets that allow ad libitum consumption while still controlling intakes of ME and MP to near requirements is a promising technique. There is continued need to evaluate these concepts under both research and field settings, particularly with regard to reproduction and longevity. On the basis of available scientific data as a whole, however, we conclude that requirements for energy (and other nutrients) should be met but not greatly exceeded during the dry period. Careful feeding management is necessary, of course, to ensure that formulated nutrient intakes are actually achieved in practice.

References

Agenäs, S., Burstedt, E. and Holtenius, K. (2003) Effects of feeding intensity during the dry period. 1. Feed intake, body weight, and milk production. *Journal of Dairy Science,* **86,** 870-882.

Agricultural and Food Research Council (AFRC). (1993) Energy and Protein Requirements of Ruminants. Agricultural and Food Research Council. CAB International, Wallingford, UK.

Allen, M. S. (2000) Effects of diet on short term regulation of feed intake by lactating dairy cattle. *Journal of Dairy Science* **83**, 1598–624

Allen, M.S., Bradford, B.J., and Harvatine, K.J. (2005). The cow as a model to study food intake regulation. *Annual Review of Nutrition* **25**, 523-247.

Bell, A.W. (1995) Regulation of organic nutrient metabolism during transition from late pregnancy to early lactation. *Journal of Animal Science,* **73,** 2804-2819.

Bell, A.W., Burhans, W.S. and Overton, T.R. (2000) Protein nutrition in late pregnancy, maternal protein reserves and lactation performance in dairy cows. *Proceedings of the Nutrition Society* **59**, 119-126.

Bernabucci, U., Ronchi, B., Lacetera, N. and Nardone, A. (2005) Influence of body condition score on relationships between metabolic status and oxidative stress in periparturient dairy cows. *Journal of Dairy Science,* **88**, 2017-2026.

Bertics, S.J., Grummer R.R., Cadorniga-Valino, C. and Stoddard, E.E. (1992) Effect of prepartum dry matter intake on liver triglyceride concentration and early lactation. *Journal of Dairy Science,* **75**, 1914-1922.

Beever, D.E. (2006) The impact of controlled nutrition during the dry period on dairy cow health, fertility and performance. *Animal Reproduction Science,* **96,** 212-226.

Boisclair, Y., Grieve, D.G., Stone, J.B., Allen, O.B. and MacLeod, G.K. (1986) Effect of prepartum energy, body condition, and sodium bicarbonate on production of cows in early lactation. *Journal of Dairy Science,* **69**, 2636-2647.

Boutflour, R.B. (1928) Limiting factors in the feeding and management of milch cows. In *Report of the Proceedings of the 8th World's Dairy Congress*, London, UK, pp 15-20. International Dairy Federation, Brussels, Belgium.

Breukink, H.J and Wensing, T. (1997) Pathophysiology of the liver in high yielding dairy cows and its consequences for health and production. *Israel Journal of Veterinary Medicine,* **52,** 66-72.

Broster, W.H. and Broster, V.J. (1984) Reviews of the progress of dairy science: long term effects of plane of nutrition on the performance of the dairy cow. *Journal of Dairy Research,* **51,** 149-196.

Chew, B. P., Murdock, R.R., Riley, E. and Hillers, J.K. (1984) Influence of prepartum dietary crude protein on growth hormone, insulin, reproduction and lactation. *Journal of Dairy Science,* **67,** 270-275.

Coffey MT, Diggs BG, Handlin DL, Knabe DA, Maxwell CV Jr, Noland PR, Prince TJ, Gromwell GL. (1994) Effects of dietary energy during gestation and lactation on reproductive performance of sows: a cooperative study. *Journal of Animal Science,* **72**, 4-9.

Collier, R.J., Annen, E.L. and Fitzgerald, A.C. (2004) Prospects for zero days dry. *Veterinary Clinics of North America – Food Animal Practice,* **20**, 687-701.

Contreras, L.L., Ryan, C.M. and Overton, T.R. (2004) Effects of dry cow grouping strategy and prepartum body condition score on performance and health of transition dairy cows. *Journal of Dairy Science,* **87**, 517-523.

Cook, N.B., Bennett, T.B. and Nordlund, K.V. (2004) Effect of free stall surface on daily activity patterns in dairy cows with relevance to lameness prevalence. *Journal of Dairy Science,* **87**, 2912-2922.

Cook, N.B. and Nordlund, K.V. (2004) Behavioral needs of the transition cow and considerations for special needs facility design. *Veterinary Clinics of North America – Food Animal Practice,* **20**, 495-520.

Cook, N.B. and Nordlund, K.V. (2007) The influence of the environment on dairy cow behavior, claw health and herd lameness dynamics. *Veterinary Journal,* Nov 5 (Epub ahead of print).

Coppock, C.E., Noller, C.H., Wolfe, S.A., Callahan, C.J. and Baker, J.S. (1972) Effect of forage-concentrate ratio in complete feed fed ad libitum on feed intake prepartum and the occurrence of abomasal displacement in dairy cows. *Journal of Dairy Science,* **55**, 783-789.

Curtis, C.R., Erb, H.N., Sniffen, C.J., Smith, R.D. and Kronfeld D.S. (1985) Path analysis of dry period nutrition, postpartum metabolic and reproductive disorders, and mastitis in Holstein cows. *Journal of Dairy Science,* **68**, 2347-2360.

Dann, H.M., Litherland, N.B., Underwood, J.P., Bionaz, M., D'Angelo, A., McFadden, J.W. and Drackley, J.K. (2006) Diets during far-off and close-up dry periods affect periparturient metabolism and lactation in multiparous cows. *Journal of Dairy Science,* **89**, 3563-3577.

Dann, H.M., Morin, D.E., Murphy, M.R., Bollero, G.A. and Drackley, J.K. (2005) Prepartum intake, postpartum induction of ketosis, and periparturient disorders affect the metabolic status of dairy cows. *Journal of Dairy Science,* **88**, 3249-3264.

Dann, H.M., Varga, G.A. and Putnam, D.E. (1999) Improving energy supply to late gestation and early postpartum dairy cows. *Journal of Dairy Science,* **82**, 1765-1778.

DeVader, S.R., Neeley, H.L., Myles, T.D. and Leet, T.L. (2007) Evaluation of gestational weight gain guidelines for women with normal prepregnancy body mass index. *Obstetrics and Gynecology,* **110**, 743-744.

DeVries, T.J., von Keyserlingk, M.A. and Weary, D.M. (2004) Effect of feeding space on the inter-cow distance, aggression, and feeding behavior of free-stall housed lactating dairy cows. *Journal of Dairy Science,* **87**, 1432-1438.

Dewhurst, R.J., Moorby, J.M., Dhanoa, M.S., Evans, R.T. and Fisher, W.J. (2000) Effects of altering energy and protein supply to dairy cows during the dry period. 1. Intake, body condition, and milk production. *Journal of Dairy Science,* **83**, 1782-1794.

Doepel, L., Lapierre, H. and Kennelly, J.J. (2002) Peripartum performance and metabolism of dairy cows in response to prepartum energy and protein intake. *Journal of Dairy Science,* **85**, 2315-2334.

Douglas, G.N, Overton, T.R., Bateman, H.G., II, Dann, H.M. and Drackley, J. K. (2006) Prepartal plane of nutrition, regardless of dietary energy source, affects periparturient metabolism and dry matter intake in Holstein cows. *Journal of Dairy Science,* **89,** 2141-2157.

Douglas, G.N., Overton, T.R., Bateman, H.G., Jr. and Drackley, J.K. (2004) Peripartal metabolism and production of Holstein cows fed diets supplemented with fat during the dry period. *Journal of Dairy Science,* **87**, 4210-4220.

Drackley, J.K. (1999) Biology of dairy cows during the transition period: the final frontier? *Journal of Dairy Science,* **82**, 2259-2273.

Drackley, J.K. (2003) Interrelationships of prepartum dry matter intake with postpartum intake and hepatic lipid accumulation. *Journal of Dairy Science,* **86**(Supplement 1), 104-105. (Abstract).

Drackley, J. K. (2006) Advances in transition cow biology. New frontiers in production diseases. In *Production Diseases in Farm Animals. Proceedings 12ᵗʰ International Conference,* pp. 24-34. Edited by N. Joshi and T. H. Herdt, Wageningen Academic Publishers, Wageningen, The Netherlands.

Drackley, J.K., Dann, H.M., Douglas, G.N., Janovick Guretzky, N.A., Litherland, N.B., Underwood, J.P. and Loor, J.J. (2005) Physiological and pathological adaptations in dairy cows that may increase susceptibility to periparturient diseases and disorders. *Italian Journal of Animal Science* **4**, 323-344.

Drackley, J.K., Janovick-Guretzky, N.A. and Dann, H.M. (2007) New concepts for feeding dry cows. In *Proceedings of the Tri-State Dairy Nutrition Conference,* Fort Wayne, IN, USA pp. 17-28. Edited by M. Eastridge, Ohio State University, Columbus.

Drackley, J.K., Overton, T.R. and Douglas, G.N. (2001) Adaptations of glucose and long-chain fatty acid metabolism in liver of dairy cows during the periparturient period. *Journal of Dairy Science,* **84**(Electronic Supplement), E100-E112.

Duffield, T. (2000) Subclinical ketosis in lactating dairy cattle. *Veterinary Clinics of North America – Food Animal Practice,* **16**, 231-253.

Emery, R S., Hafs, H.D., Armstrong, D. and Snyder, W.W. (1969) Prepartum grain feeding effects on milk production, mammary edema, and incidence of diseases. *Journal of Dairy Science,* **52**, 345-351.

Endres, M.I., DeVries, T.J., von Keyserlingk, M.A. and Weary, D.M. (2005) Short communication: Effect of feed barrier design on the behavior of loose-housed lactating dairy cows. *Journal of Dairy Science*, **88**, 2377-2380.

Flipot, P.M., Roy, G.L. and Dufour, J.J. (1988) Effect of peripartum energy concentration on production performance of Holstein cows. *Journal of Dairy Science,* **71**, 1840-1850.

Fregonesi, J.A., Veira, D.M., von Keyserlingk, M.A. and Weary, D.M. (2007) Effects of bedding quality on lying behavior of dairy cows. *Journal of Dairy Science,* **90**, 5468-5472.

Friggens, N.C., Andersen, J.B., Larsen, T., Aaes, O. and Dewhurst, R.J. (2004) Priming the dairy cow for lactation: a review of dry cow feeding strategies. *Animal Research,* **53**, 453-473.

Fronk, T.J., Schultz, L.H. and Hardie, A.R. (1980) Effect of dry period overconditioning on subsequent metabolic disorders and performance of dairy cows. *Journal of Dairy Science,* **63**, 1080-1090.

Garnsworthy, P.C. (2006) Body condition score in dairy cows: targets for production and fertility. In *Recent Advances in Animal Nutrition – 2006,* pp. 61-86. Edited by P.C. Garnsworthy and J. Wiseman. Nottingham University Press, Nottingham, UK.

Garnsworthy, P.C. and Jones, G.P. (1987) The influence of body condition at calving and dietary protein supply on voluntary food intake and performance in dairy cows. *Animal Production,* **44**, 347-353.

Garnsworthy, P.C. and Topps, J.H. (1982) The effect of body condition of dairy cows at calving on their food intake and performance when given complete diets. *Animal Production,* **35** 113-119.

Garnsworthy, P.C. and Webb, R. (1999) The influence of nutrition on fertility in dairy cows. In *Recent Advances in Animal Nutrition – 1999,* pp. 39-57. Edited by P.C. Garnsworthy and J. Wiseman). Nottingham University Press, Nottingham, UK.

Gerloff, B.J. (2000) Dry cow management for the prevention of ketosis and fatty liver in dairy cows. *Veterinary Clinics of North America – Food Animal Practice,* **16**, 283-292.

Goff, J.P. (1999) Mastitis and retained placenta - relationship to bovine immunology and nutrition. *Advances in Dairy Technology,* **11**, 185-192.

Goff, J.P. and Horst, R.L. (1997) Physiological changes at parturition and their relationship to metabolic disorders. *Journal of Dairy Science,* **80**, 1260-1268.

Grant, R.J. and Albright, J.L. (1995) Feeding behavior and management factors during the transition period in dairy cattle. *Journal of Animal Science,* **73**, 2791-2803.

Grant, R.J. and Albright, J.L. (2001) Effect of animal grouping on feeding behavior and intake of dairy cattle. *Journal of Dairy Science,* **84**(Electronic supplement), E156-E166.

Greenhalgh, J.F.D. and Gardner, K.E. (1958) Effect of heavy concentrate feeding before calving upon lactation and mammary gland edema. *Journal of Dairy Science,* **41**, 822-829.

Grum, D.E., Drackley, J.K., Younker, R.S., LaCount, D.W. and Veenhuizen, J.J. (1996) Nutrition during the dry period and hepatic lipid metabolism of periparturient dairy cows. *Journal of Dairy Science,* **79**, 1850-1864.

Grummer, R.R. (1995) Impact of changes in organic nutrient metabolism on feeding the transition dairy cow. *Journal of Animal Science,* **73**, 2820-2833.

Grummer, R.R., Mashek, D.G. and Hayirli, A. (2004) Dry matter intake and energy balance in the transition period. *Veterinary Clinics of North America – Food Animal Practice,* **20**, 447-470.

Hayirli, A., Grummer, R.R., Nordheim, E.V. and Crump, P.M. (2002) Animal and dietary factors affecting feed intake during the transition period in Holsteins. *Journal of Dairy Science,* **85,** 3430-3443.

Hayirli, A., Grummer, R.R., Nordheim, E.V. and Crump, P.M. (2003) Models for predicting dry matter intake of Holsteins during the prefresh transition period. *Journal of Dairy Science,* **86**, 1771-1779.

Hernandez-Urdaneta, A., Coppock, C.E., McDowell, R.E., Gianola, D. and N. E. Smith. (1976) Changes in forage-concentrate ratio of complete feeds for dairy cows. *Journal of Dairy Science,* **59**, 695-707.

Hilson, J.A., Rasmussen, K.M. and Kjolhede, C.L. (2006) Excessive weight gain during pregnancy is associated with earlier termination of breast-feeding among White women. *Journal of Nutrition,* **136**, 140-146.

Holcomb, C.S., Van Horn, H.H., Head, H.H., Hall, M.B. and Wilcox, C.J. (2001) Effects of prepartum dry matter intake and forage percentage on postpartum performance of lactating dairy cows. *Journal of Dairy Science,* **84**, 2051-2058.

Holtenius, K., Agenäs, S., Delavaud, C. and Chilliard, Y. (2003) Effects of feeding intensity during the dry period. 2. Metabolic and hormonal responses. *Journal of Dairy Science,* **86**, 883-891.

Hoppe, M.K., Libal, G.W. and Wahlstrom, R.C. (1990) Influence of gestation energy level on the production of Large White x Landrace sows. *Journal of Animal Science*, **68**, 2235-2242.

Horst, R.L., Goff, J.P., Reinhardt, T.A. and Buxton, D.R. (1997) Strategies for preventing milk fever in dairy cattle. *Journal of Dairy Science,* **80**, 1269-1280.

Huyler, M. T., Kincaid, R.L. and Dostal, D.F. (1999) Metabolic and yield responses of multiparous Holstein cows to prepartum rumen-undegradable protein. *Journal of Dairy Science,* **82**, 527-536.

Ingvartsen, K.L. and Andersen, J.B. (2000) Integration of metabolism and intake regulation: a review focusing on periparturient animals. *Journal of Dairy Science,* **83**, 1573-1597.

Ingvartsen, K.L., Danfaer, A., Andersen, P.H.and Foldager, J. (1996) Prepartum feeding of dairy cattle: a review of the effect on peripartum metabolism, feed intake, production, and health. *Stocarstvo,* **50**, 401-409.

Janovick Guretzky, N.A., Litherland, N.B., Moyes, K.M and Drackley, J.K. (2006) Prepartum energy intake affects health and lactational performance in primiparous and multiparous Holstein cows. *Journal of Dairy Science,* **89**(Suppl. 1), 267. (Abstract).

Johnson, D.G. and Otterby, D.E. (1981) Influence of dry period diet on early postpartum health, feed intake, milk production, and reproductive efficiency of Holstein cows. *Journal of Dairy Science,* **64**, 290-295.

Kaneene, J.B., Miller, R., Herdt, T.H. and Gardiner, J.C. (1997) The association of serum nonesterified fatty acids and cholesterol, management and feeding practices with peripartum disease in dairy cows. *Preventative Veterinary Medicine,* **31**, 59-72.

Kehrli, M.E. Jr., Nonnecke, B.J. and Roth, J.A. (1989a) Alterations in bovine lymphocyte function during the periparturient period. *American Journal of Veterinary Research,* **50**, 215-220.

Kehrli, M.E. Jr., Nonnecke, B.J. and Roth, J.A. (1989b) Alterations in bovine neutrophil function during the periparturient period. *American Journal of Veterinary Research,* **50**, 207-214.

Kunz, P.L., Blum, J.W., Hart, I.C., Bickel, H. and Landis, J. (1985) Effects of different energy intakes before and after calving on food intake, performance and blood hormones and metabolites in dairy cows. *Animal Production,* **40**, 219-231.

Lacetera, N., Scalia, D., Bernabucci, U., Ronchi, B., Pirazzi, D. and Nardone, A. (2005) Lymphocyte functions in overconditioned cows around parturition. *Journal of Dairy Science,* **88**, 2010-2016.

Litherland, N.B., Dann, H.M., Hansen, A.S. and Drackley, J.K. (2003) Prepartum nutrient intake alters metabolism by liver slices from peripartal dairy cows. *Journal of Dairy Science,* **86**(Supplement 1), 105-106 (Abstract).

Lodge, G.A., Fisher, L.J. and Lessard, J.R. (1975) Influence of prepartum feed intake on performance of cows fed ad libitum during lactation. *Journal of Dairy Science,* **58**, 696-702.

Loor, J.J., Dann, H.M., Everts, R.E., Oliveira, R., Green, C.A., Janovick-Guretzky, N.A., Rodriguez-Zas, S.L., Lewin, H.A. and Drackley, J.K. (2005) Temporal gene expression profiling of liver from periparturient dairy cows reveals complex adaptive mechanisms in hepatic function. *Physiological Genomics,* **23,** 217-226.

Loor, J.J., Dann, H.M., Janovick-Guretzky, N.A., Everts, R.E., Oliveira, R., Green,

C.A., Litherland, N.B., Rodriguez-Zas, S.L., Lewin, H.A. and Drackley, J.K. (2006) Plane of nutrition prepartum alters hepatic gene expression and function in dairy cows as assessed by longitudinal transcript and metabolic profiling. *Physiological Genomics,* **27,** 29-41.

Loor, J.J., Everts, R.E., Bionaz, M., Dann, H.M., Morin, D.E., Oliveira, R., Rodriguez-Zas, S.L., Drackley, J.K. and Lewin, H.A. (2007) Nutrition-induced ketosis alters metabolic and signaling gene networks in liver of periparturient dairy cows. *Physiological Genomics,* **32,** 105-116.

Lotan, E., Ziv, E., Levy, E., Marton, M. and Adler, J.H. (1988) Experimental manipulation of post partum energy partition in high yielding dairy cows. *Israel Journal of Veterinary Medicine,* **44,** 159-167.

Mallard, B.A., Dekkers, J.C., Ireland, M.J., Leslie, K.E., Sharif, S., Vankampen, C.L., Wagter, L. and Wilkie, B.N. (1998) Alteration in immune responsiveness during the peripartum period and its ramification on dairy cow and calf health. *Journal of Dairy Science,* **81,** 585-595.

Mashek, D.G. and Beede, D.K. (2000) Peripartum responses of dairy cow to partial substitution of corn silage with corn grain in diets fed during the late dry period. *Journal of Dairy Science,* **83,** 2310-2318.

Mashek, D.G. and Beede, D.K. (2001) Peripartum responses of dairy cows fed energy-dense diets for 3 or 6 weeks prepartum. *Journal of Dairy Science,* **84,** 115-125.

Mee, J.F. (2004) Temporal patterns in reproductive performance in Irish dairy herds and associated risk factors. *Irish Veterinary Journal,* **57,** 158-166.

Minor, D.J., Trower, S.L., Strang, B.D., Shaver, R.D. and Grummer, R.R. (1998) Effects of nonfiber carbohydrate and niacin on periparturient metabolic status and lactation of dairy cows. *Journal of Dairy Science,* **81,** 189-200.

Moorby, J. M., Dewhurst, R.J. and Marsden, S. (1996) Effect of increasing digestible undegraded protein supply to dairy cows in late gestation on the yield and composition of milk during the subsequent lactation. *Animal Science,* **63,** 201-213.

National Research Council (NRC) (1978) *Nutrient Requirements of Dairy Cattle,* 5th revised edition. National Academy Press, Washington, DC, USA.

National Research Council (NRC) (1989) *Nutrient Requirements of Dairy Cattle,* 6th revised edition. National Academy Press, Washington, DC, USA.

National Research Council (NRC) (2001) *Nutrient Requirements of Dairy Cattle,* 7th revised edition. National Academy Press, Washington, DC, USA.

Olsson, G., Emanuelson, M. and Wiktorsson, H. (1998) Effects of different nutritional levels prepartum on the subsequent performance of dairy cows. *Livestock Production Science,* **53,** 279-290.

Overton, T.R. and Waldron, M.R. (2004) Nutritional management of transition dairy cows: strategies to optimize metabolic health. *Journal of Dairy Science,* **87**(Electronic supplement), E105-E119.

Phillips, G.J., Citron, T.L., Sage, J.S., Cummins, K.A., Cecava, M.J. and McNamara, J.P. (2003) Adaptations in body muscle and fat in transition dairy cattle fed differing amounts of protein and methionine hydroxy analog. *Journal of Dairy Science*, **86**, 3634-3647.

Pryce, J., Royal, M.D., Garnsworthy, P.C. and Mao, I.L. (2004) Fertility in the high-producing dairy cow. *Livestock Production Science*, **86**, 125-135.

Putnam, D.E. and Varga, G.A. (1998) Protein density and its influence on metabolite concentration and nitrogen retention by Holstein cows in late gestation. *Journal of Dairy Science*, **81**, 1608-1618.

Putnam, D.E., Varga, G.A. and Dann, H.M. (1999) Metabolic and production responses to dietary protein and exogenous somatotropin in late gestation dairy cows. *Journal of Dairy Science*, **82**, 982-995.

Rabelo, E., Rezende, R.L., Bertics, S.J. and Grummer, R.R. (2003) Effects of transition diets varying in dietary energy density on lactation performance and ruminal parameters of dairy cows. *Journal of Dairy Science*, **86**, 916-925.

Rabelo, E., Rezende, R.L., Bertics, S.J. and Grummer, R.R. (2005) Effects of pre- and postfresh transition diets varying in dietary energy density on metabolic status of periparturient dairy cows. *Journal of Dairy Science*, **88**, 4375-4383.

Rastani, R.R., Grummer, R.R., Bertics, S.J., Gümen, A., Wiltbank, M.C., Mashek, D.G. and Schwab, M.C. (2005) Reducing dry period length to simplify feeding transition cows: milk production, energy balance, and metabolic profiles. *Journal of Dairy Science*, **88**, 1004-1014.

Reid, I.M., Roberts, C.J., Treacher, R.J. and Williams, L.A. (1986) Effect of body condition at calving on tissue mobilization, development of fatty liver and blood chemistry of dairy cows. *Animal Production*, **43**, 7-15.

Reynolds, C.K., Aikman, P.C., Lupoli, B., Humphries, D.J. and Beever, D.E. (2003) Splanchnic metabolism of dairy cows during the transition from late gestation through early lactation. *Journal of Dairy Science*, **86**, 1201-1217.

Reynolds, C.K., Durst, B., Lupoli, B., Humphries, D.J. and Beever, D.E. (2004) Visceral tissue mass and rumen volume in dairy cows during the transition from late gestation to early lactation. *Journal of Dairy Science*, **87**, 961-971.

Roche, J.R., Kolver, E.S. and Kay, J.K. (2005) Influence of precalving feed allowance on periparturient metabolic and hormonal responses and milk production in grazing dairy cows. *Journal of Dairy Science*, **88**, 677-689.

Rukkwamsuk, T., Wensing, T. and Geelen, M.J. (1998) Effect of overfeeding during the dry period on regulation of adipose tissue metabolism in dairy cows during the periparturient period. *Journal of Dairy Science*, **81**, 2904-2911.

Rukkwamsuk, T., Kruip, T.A.M. and Wensing, T. (1999a) Relationship between overfeeding and overconditioning in the dry period and the problems of high producing dairy cows during the postparturient period. *Veterinary Quarterly*, **21**, 71-77.

Rukkwamsuk, T., Wensing, T. and Geelen, M.J.H. (1999b) Effect of overfeeding during the dry period on the rate of esterification in adipose tissue of dairy cows during the periparturient period. *Journal of Dairy Science,* **82**, 1164-1169.

Schmidt, G.H. and Schultz, L.H. (1959) Effect of three levels of grain feeding during the dry period on the incidence of ketosis, severity of udder edema, and subsequent milk production of dairy cows. *Journal of Dairy Science,* **42**, 170-179.

Sinclair, A.G., Bland, V.C. and Edwards, S.A. (2001) The influence of gestation feeding strategy on body composition of gilts at farrowing and response to dietary protein in a modified lactation. *Journal of Animal Science,* **79**, 2397-405

Skaar, T.C., Grummer, R.R., Dentine, M.R. and Stauffacher, R.H. (1989) Seasonal effects of prepartum and postpartum fat and niacin feeding on lactation performance and lipid metabolism. *Journal of Dairy Science,* **72**, 2028-2038.

Stockdale, C.R. and Roche, J.R. (2002) A review of the energy and protein nutrition of dairy cows through their dry period and its impact on early lactation performance. *Australian Journal of Agricultural Research,* **53**, 737-753.

Stotland, N.E., Cheng, Y.W., Hopkins, L.M. and Caughey, A.B. (2006) Gestational weight gain and adverse neonatal outcome among term infants. *Obstetrics and Gynecology,* **108**, 635-643.

Swanson, E.W. and Hinton, S.A. (1962) Effects on adding concentrates to ad libitum roughage feeding in the dry period. *Journal of Dairy Science,* **45**, 48-54.

Tesfa, A.T., Tuori, M., Syrjälä-Qvist, L., Pösö, R., Saloniemi, H., Heinonen, K., Kivilahti, K., Saukko, T. and Lindberg, L.A. (1999) The influence of dry period feeding on liver fat and postpartum performance of dairy cows. *Animal Feed Science and Technology,* **76**, 275-295.

Treacher, R.J., Reid, I.M. and Roberts, C.J. (1986) Effect of body condition at calving on the health and performance of dairy cows. *Animal Production,* **43**, 1-6.

Tucker, C.B., Weary, D.M. and Fraser, D. (2003) Effects of three types of free-stall surfaces on preferences and stall usage by dairy cows. *Journal of Dairy Science,* **86**, 521-529.

Tucker, C.B., Weary, D.M. and Fraser, D. (2004) Free-stall dimensions: effects on preference and stall usage. *Journal of Dairy Science,* **87**, 1208-1216.

Tucker, C.B., Weary, D.M., de Passillé, A.M., Campbell, B. and Rushen, J. (2006) Flooring in front of the feed bunk affects feeding behavior and use of freestalls by dairy cows. *Journal of Dairy Science,* **89**, 2065-2071.

van den Top, A.M., Geelen, M.J.H., Wensing, T., Wentink, G.H., Van 't Klooster, A.Th. and Beynen, A.C. (1996) Higher postpartum hepatic triacylglycerol concentrations in dairy cows with free rather than restricted access to feed during the dry period are associated with lower activities of hepatic glycerolphosphate acyltransferase. *Journal of Nutrition,* **126**, 76-85.

Van Saun, R.J., Idleman, S.C. and Sniffen, C.J. (1993) Effect of undegradable protein amount fed prepartum on postpartum production in first lactation Holstein cows. *Journal of Dairy Science,* **76**, 236-244.

Van Saun, R. J. and Sniffen, C.J. (1996) Nutritional management of the pregnant dairy cow to optimize health, lactation and reproductive performance. *Animal Feed Science and Technology,* **59**, 13-26.

VandeHaar, M.J., Yousif, G., Sharma, B.K., Herdt, T.H., Emery, R.S., Allen, M.S. and Liesman, J.S. (1999) Effect of energy and protein density of prepartum diets on fat and protein metabolism of dairy cattle in the periparturient period. *Journal of Dairy Science,* **82**, 1282-1295.

4

LAMENESS IN DAIRY COWS: IMPACT OF PRACTICAL NUTRITIONAL AND ENVIRONMENTAL MANAGEMENT

J.N. HUXLEY

University of Nottingham School of Veterinary Medicine and Science, Sutton Bonington Campus, Loughborough LE12 5RD

Lameness is undoubtedly one of the most serious disease problems currently facing the UK (and world) dairy industries in terms of its impact on welfare and decreased productivity. This chapter will review the current UK situation and then describe the impacts of practical nutritional and environmental management on lameness.

Incidence

Over the last twenty years, the annual UK incidence of lameness recorded as cases per 100 cows per year has been reported to be between 22 and 24 (Esslemont and Kossaibati, 2002), 68.9 (Hedges *et al.,* 2001), 23.7 (Whitaker *et al.,* 2000), 24.0 (Esslemont and Kossaibati, 1996), 54.6 (Clarkson *et al.,* 1996) and 17.0 (Collick *et al.,* 1989). The wide variation in these figures probably reflects both variations in case description and how the data were collected - i.e. farmer records, veterinary treatment records or researcher observations. Lameness is notoriously under-recorded and the actually incidence is probably towards the upper end of the range reported here.

Prevalence

Locomotion scoring is currently the most widely accepted method for identifying lame animals and is correlated significantly with the level of hind limb sole and heel horn disease (Winckler and Willen, 2001). It involves a visual assessment of animals as they walk on a flat hard surface. Many different systems are described

(Manson and Leaver, 1988; Tranter and Morris, 1991; Sprecher *et al.,* 1997; Whay *et al.,* 1997; Winckler and Willen, 2001; Huxley and Whay, 2006), however, they all attempt to identify lame animals based on a combination of posture, and foot placement and cadence.

Based on the results of locomotion scoring the prevalence of lameness on UK dairy farms has recently been demonstrated as 30.0% (Huxley, 2005), 24.2% (Huxley *et al.,* 2004), 23.1% and 20.0% (Main *et al.,* 2003) and 25.0% (Clarkson *et al.,* 1996).

Currently, UK farmers underestimate considerably the number of lame animals in their herds; in one recent study the median prevalence estimated by farmer was 4.8% compared to an actual prevalence of 25.0% demonstrated by locomotion scoring (Huxley, 2005). This is in agreement with findings of other authors (Mill and Ward, 1994; Whay *et al.,* 2003).

Common foot lesion

There are many different causes of lameness in dairy cows. The vast majority are caused by foot lesions (~90%), with the remainder caused by lesions higher up the leg. Of the cases in the foot, one study reported that 92% were in the hind limb and that lesions affecting the hind foot occurred most commonly in the outer claw (68%) followed by the skin (20%) and then the inner claw (12%) (Murray *et al.,* 1996). Of the lesions that affected the fore foot, 46% were in the inner claw, 32% were in the outer claw and 22% were associated with the skin (Murray *et al.,* 1996). The same study also collected data on the causes of 9645 cases of lameness on 37 dairy farms between April 1989 and October 1991. The most common causes were sole ulcers (28%), white line disease (22%), local sole bruising (8%), digital dermatitis (8%), foul in the foot (5%), interdigital hyperplasia (5%) and foreign body penetrations (5%). At the time of this study, digital dermatitis was still a relatively new condition to the UK, having been reported first in 1988 (Blowey and Sharp, 1988). In the author's recent clinical experience, digital dermatitis has now joined sole ulcers and white line disease as one of the three most prevalent, and thus most important, causes of lameness in the UK.

Financial implications

Lameness is associated with a significant impact on farm profitability. It has been calculated that the average case of lameness currently costs the UK dairy industry £172 (Esslemont, 2005). Therefore, on a 100 cow unit with an incidence of 40 cases per 100 cows per year, lameness costs the business nearly £7000 per annum.

The impact of a case of lameness on future milk yield during that lactation has been calculated to be 390 kg total reduction in milk yield per 305-day lactation (Green *et al.,* 2002). Further analysis demonstrated that effects on production are influenced by the cause of the lameness. Lameness caused by a sole ulcer led to a mean reduction of 570 kg and a case of white line disease by 130 kg; digital dermatitis caused no reduction in yield (Amory *et al.,* 2006). Interestingly, animals that suffered a case of sole ulcer or white line disease had a reduction in milk yield for up to two months prior to the lesion being treated and animals that developed a sole ulcer initially produced more milk than unaffected cows (+1.5 kg / day) (Green *et al.,* 2002).

Welfare implications

The fact that animals alter their gait in response to the discomfort caused by lameness indicates that lameness is a painful condition. This has been confirmed by work which demonstrated that lame cows are more sensitive to pain (Whay *et al.,* 1997; Whay *et al.,* 1998).

Two recent surveys investigating the experience and attitudes of respondents to pain and the use of analgesics in cattle were distributed to 2391 named cattle veterinary surgeons (Whay and Huxley, 2005, Huxley and Whay, 2006) and 7500 named cattle farmers in the UK. As part of the survey, respondents were asked to estimate how painful they thought two causes of lameness (digital dermatitis and white line disease with a sub sole abscess) were on a ten point pain scale (1 – No pain at all; 10 – The worst pain imaginable). Results from questionnaires returned by 615 veterinary surgeons and 939 farmers were available for analysis. The pain scores assigned to both causes of lameness were similar between the two groups. The median pain scores estimated for digital dermatitis were 6 (veterinary surgeons) and 5 (farmers), whilst the median scores for white line disease with a sub sole abscess were 7 (veterinary surgeons) and 6 (farmers). Although these results are subjective estimates, they are the combined estimates of a large number of individuals with the most practical experience of bovine lameness. They indicate that two of the top three causes of lameness in the UK are considered painful conditions.

Many consider that lameness is currently the most significant welfare issue affecting dairy cattle in the UK because of the level of discomfort caused, the numbers of animals affected and the duration of clinical episodes (27 ± 19 days in one study (Tranter and Morris, 1991)).

Common causes of lameness in the UK

A detailed description of all the causes of lameness is outwith the scope of this paper; the reader is referred to standard texts or review papers (e.g. Blowey 1992b, a) for further details. This chapter will concentrate on the three most common causes of lameness in the UK, outlined above.

SOLE ULCERS (PODODERMATITIS CIRCUMSCRIPTA)

The horn on the sole of the foot is produced continuously by germinal cells in the soft tissue between the sole and the pedal bone. If these germinal cells are damaged (often by compression), horn formation is interrupted. A sole ulcer is a small circular lesion which most commonly occurs under the point where the flexor tendon attaches to the caudal edge of the pedal bone, which lies directly above the sole ulcer site. The effects of "subclinical laminitis" (see below), laxity within the suspensory structures of the foot around the time of calving, horn overgrowth and prolonged standing on concrete increases the pressure on the caudal edge of the pedal bone leading to pinching of the corium between bone and horn. In mild cases, blood is incorporated into sole horn as it is produced. In advanced cases, production of horn is completely arrested at the sole ulcer site.

The degree of lameness varies from slight to severe depending on the duration of the problem, the extent of the lesion and the presence (or absence) of secondary infection. Often both hind feet are affected, although one side is usually worse than the other. If animals are affected bilaterally, they often appear less lame because they are unable to favour an unaffected leg.

Treatment depends on reducing the pressure on the corium pinched between the pedal bone and solar horn. If overgrown, both claws are trimmed to restore normal weight bearing and the height of the affected claw is reduced to redistribute weight to the unaffected claw. In moderate to severe cases, the unaffected claw is blocked to shift weight bearing completely over to the unaffected side. Sole ulcers are associated with significant effects on production (see "Financial Implication") because even if they are successfully treated, it takes many weeks for the lesion to fully resolve.

WHITE LINE DISEASE (WLD)

The white line is the junction of the sole and the wall, and as such is an area of weakness. Dirt and stones may impact into the white line and eventually carry bacteria through the horn to the soft tissues of the corium beneath, causing infection and the production of pus. Often the white line and debris seal over the ensuing abscess that expands in the potential space between the corium and the horn. As the volume of pus increases it expands along the line of least resistance and the build up of pressure causes pain. In most cases this is under the sole; in extreme cases the whole sole can under run before the abscess breaks out and drains at the heel. Less commonly, the abscess expands and tracks up the wall before breaking out and draining at the coronary band.

WLD causes moderate to severe lameness, depending on the position and extent of the lesion and abscess that forms. The lateral claw of the hind foot is more commonly affected. Lesions are treated with a combination of corrective trimming to clear the lesion and drain any abscess which has formed, application of a foot block to the unaffected claw to reduce the pressure on the diseased side, and antibiotics by injection.

Cows are more likely to suffer WLD if their environment contains debris likely to impact in the white line. Small (2-10mm), sharp, hard gravel and stones (e.g. the aggregate used to cap roads), are the worst material, especially if it is lying on concrete or other solid surfaces. Additionally, anything that weakens the white line will predispose animals to disease. This can include the production of poor quality horn (see the next chapter – Galbraith, 2007) or physical damage to the white line if animals are forced to turn sharply on hard surfaces e.g. concrete. Sharp turns "tear" the white line open, making it easier for environmental debris to penetrate the resultant deficit.

DIGITAL DERMATITIS

Digital dermatitis was identified as a novel cause of lameness in cattle in Italy in 1972 (Cheli and Mortellaro, 1974) and was first reported in the UK in 1987 (Blowey and Sharp, 1988). The disease has spread nationwide since its introduction and is now endemic in most cattle-dense areas of the UK. The condition is thought to be caused by a spirochete (possibly *Treponema denticola*), although its exact aetiology has yet to be demonstrated conclusively.

In the initial stages, lameness is usually mild. However, if the condition is left untreated moderate to severe lameness ensues. The disease is characterised by small roughly circular (1 to 4 cm diameter) areas of moist browny-grey exudative areas of epidermal liquefaction. Lesions are usually in the interdigital area just behind the bulbs of the heel. Occasionally lesions can be found on the skin above one heel bulb only, in the interdigital space, at the coronary band at the front of the foot or around the accessory digits. If the diptheritic debris on the surface of the lesion is cleaned, an underlying bed of raw, intensely painful, dermal granulation tissue is exposed. Occasionally, if left untreated a "papilliform" or "hairy warts" form of the disease can develop in which long thick strands of keratin protrude from the underlying granulation bed.

Farms become infected either by purchasing infected cattle or the disease is introduced with dirty machinery or equipment. The causative agent(s) spreads between cows either via direct contact or in infected slurry. Individuals can be treated with topical application of antibiotics, although once disease is established in a herd most farms choose to control the disease with routine herd foot bathing using a combination of disinfectants, e.g. formalin, and antibiotics.

Aetiology of common claw lesions

Lameness in dairy cattle is a multifactorial condition both because of the different diseases that cause it and because of the huge differences that exist between farms. This section will concentrate on some of the ways that practical nutrition can influence lameness. Firstly, however, recent changes in our understanding of claw physiopathology will be discussed briefly.

"SUB-CLINICAL LAMINITIS"

A condition called "sub-clinical laminitis" ("SCL") has historically been proposed as one of the most significant underlying causes of claw lesions because it interferes with the integrity of claw horn tissues, predisposing animals to claw lesions, particularly sole ulceration and WLD. It is now recognised that "SCL" is a poor description of the underlying physiopathology and other terms have been proposed. As yet, however, none have become accepted widely. "SCL" was always supposed to be the result of the widely understood syndrome of subacute ruminal acidosis (SARA). It has recently become apparent that although SARA is undoubtedly important, the proposed mechanisms that lead to "SCL" have been difficult to reproduce experimentally and they do not explain fully the aetiology of disease. As a result, other mechanisms have been identified and proposed; e.g. it is now recognised that collogenases produced periparturiently affect the suspensory apparatus of the foot leading to sinkage of the pedal bone (Tarlton *et al.,* 2002). A complete review of the physiopathology of the bovine foot it outwith the scope of this paper and the reader is referred to the excellent recent review by Mulling and Greenough for further information (Mulling and Greenough 2006).

As stated previously, lameness is a multifactorial condition with many underlying predisposing causes. However, the most important impacts of practical nutrition and environmental management on lameness can be grouped into five areas that will be discussed in more detail:

SHEARING AND ABRASIVE FORCES APPLIED TO THE HOOF CAPSULE

Abrasion thins the sole, predisposing animals to sole ulceration and WLD, and shearing forces physically tear the white line apart, making it easier for environmental debris to penetrate the resultant deficit leading to WLD.

STANDING TIME ON CONCRETE AND OTHER HARD / ABRASIVE SURFACES

Standing time on concrete is thought increasingly to be one of the most important causes of sole ulceration and WLD because of the relentless pressure that is applied to the support structures of the foot (Mulling and Greenough, 2006). It is currently one of the principal intervention points being addressed in clinical veterinary practice to control lameness on farms.

WALKING SURFACES

The quality of the walking and standing surfaces has three principal impacts on lameness:

- Poor quality surfaces covered in debris, e.g. tracks used to access pasture, can predispose animals to WLD.
- Broken and damaged concrete can cause slips and trip, which increase pressure on the foot and can cause shearing forces as the animal attempts to maintain its balance. This can predispose the animal to sole ulceration and WLD. Additionally, the resultant pot holes retain stale slurry which becomes an excellent method of transmitting digital dermatitis.
- Smooth and glassy areas of concrete can cause animals to slip. This obviously increases the risk of significant injury if the animal falls, but also can cause shearing forces as the animal attempts to maintain its balance.

NUTRITIONAL MANAGEMENT

Practical aspects of nutritional management, particularly those involving SARA, still remain important causes of lameness.

CONTACT WITH SLURRY

Slurry softens the hoof capsule, which may predispose animals to WLD and sole ulceration. More importantly, slurry acts as a vector for the causative agent of digital dermatitis.

Shearing and abrasive forces

Shearing and abrasive forces usually result from either badly designed environments or negative social interactions. Poor environmental designs include building and alley layouts that force cows to turn sharply, particularly if animals are crowded, which may lead to racing and pushing e.g. narrow parlour exits with right angled turns.

Negative interactions occur as a result of social interactions within the herd. Cows within a group have a predominantly linear hierarchy, whereby animals are ranked in order from most dominant to most subordinate. Generally, older, larger and healthier animals are more dominant, although this is by no means always the case. Negative social interactions, e.g. butting and fighting, cause shearing and abrasive forces to the hoof capsule, particularly if they occur on concrete. Additionally, animals forced to retreat from more dominant group members are often forced to move rapidly and to turn sharply. Most negative social interactions occur when the social hierarchy is being established, e.g. when animals enter a group. During this time an animal will have to meet every other cow in the group and establish whether it is above or below them in the dominance order. Once a group is established, negative interactions will only occur between closely matched individuals competing for dominance and if animals are unable to remember their relative social rank when they encounter another individual within the herd. Additionally "bullying" of lower ranked animals can occur, particularly when competing for valued resources in the environment, e.g. water, access to feed space, prized cubicles etc.

POORLY DESIGNED BUILDING LAYOUTS

Feeding passageways should be as wide as practically possible, provide adequate space per cow (see below) and have entry and exit points at both ends to encourage good cow flow, i.e. they must not be blind ended. A passage width of at least 3 to 3.5m has been suggested as it allows two cows to pass each other whilst others are feeding (Bickert and Cermak 1997). Low ranking cows are much less likely to use blind ended passageways because of the fear of becoming trapped and "bullied" by more dominant herd mates who perceive their presence as competition for a limited resource. This can lead to substantial decreases in dry matter intake in low ranking animals and damage to the white line, predisposing them to lameness. Similarly, if out of parlour feeders are used, they should be sited in an open area of yard to encourage good cow flow and to avoid lower ranking animals becoming trapped.

FEED SPACE

Access to feed is one of the most valued resources in the environment. As a result animals will compete for access which often results in negative social interactions and bullying if feed space is inadequate. To minimise this and to maximise dry matter intakes, animals should be provided with at least 0.6m/cow of ad lib access trough space and preferably 0.8m/cow (Blowey 2005). The recent trend of fitting buildings with a double and a single row of cubicles for every run of trough space only provides 0.4m/cow, which is totally inadequate for the modern Friesian-Holstein cow. If low ranking cows and heifers are not able to feed, they do not go and lie down and try later, instead they mooch around waiting for access, thus dramatically increasing their standing time on concrete.

GROUP SIZE

As average herd size has increased, there has been a trend for group sizes to increase often, but not exclusively, as a result of a desire to simplify nutritional management. It is thought that cows can remember their social rank in groups of between 50 and 70 herd mates. Group sizes larger than this are likely to result in more negative social interactions because animals have to re-establish their rank each time they meet an individual they can not recall.

MOVEMENT BETWEEN GROUPS

Moving animals between groups is often driven by yield and nutritional management, e.g. high yielders and low yielders. Movements between groups cause unstable social hierarchies that increase negative social interaction. Moving animals between groups should be avoided, or at least minimised to one movement per lactation.

Standing time on concrete

Standing time on concrete is now thought to be one of the most important risk factors for the common causes of lameness, particularly sole ulceration and WLD.

COW COMFORT

Cubicle comfort is probably the single most important determinant of lying time and, therefore, the standing time on concrete. Cubicle comfort is currently a huge problem on many units because of under investment over the last decade and the relative increase in size of modern cows relative to the cubicles provided.

This will not be discussed further here as it has no direct link with nutritional management.

FEED FACE

- As discussed above, animals that are unable to access food, either because there is not enough space or they are too scared to enter confined areas occupied by dominant cows, will stand waiting for an opportunity to feed. This is true at all feeding areas (except in parlour feeders) if space is inadequate. The only way to limit this effect is to provide adequate feeding space (see above) with open access to minimise problems with cow flow.
- Cows spend many hours each day standing at the feed face and, along with the collecting yard, this represents the majority of standing time for most animals. Although it is difficult to reduce the time spent eating (and thus standing on concrete), the surface provided should be optimal (see "Walking Surfaces") and, ideally, feed should be presented on a surface 4-6" higher than the surface on which the cows are standing (John Hughes, Personal Communication) to reduce pressure on the front feet. Alternatively, the use of rubber floor matting, as an alternative to concrete, is now increasingly common in some parts of the world, particularly North America and parts of Scandinavia. There are now a number of units laying matting in the UK. Mats can be laid in areas where animals spend large amounts of time standing, e.g. feeding areas and collecting yards or throughout the entire environment. In theory, the provision of a soft standing surface as an alternative to concrete should lead to a reduction in lameness. Despite a number of trials, however, there is currently no experimental evidence to support this assertion.

COLLECTING YARD

As any herdsman will testify, cows enter the milking parlour in a similar order each milking. Animals that enter towards the end of milking are forced to stand on concrete in the collecting yard for many hours each day. This problem has been exacerbated recently as herd and particularly group sizes have increased. Group sizes are driven by management decisions often related in part to nutritional management. We have now reached the situation where some cows will stand for between two and three hours twice daily, inevitably leading to an increase in foot problems. Where practical and possible, group sizes should be reduced to decrease waiting times and limit negative interactions.

Walking surfaces

The quality of all walking and standing surfaces can have a significant impact on claw health as outlined above. They should be even, provide purchase, and be free of debris likely to cause WLD.

YARDS AND ALLEYWAYS AROUND FEEDING AREAS

The ideal surface for feeding areas and alleyways is even, free of debris and broken concrete, and grooved to provide purchase. These properties are especially important in feeding areas because cow traffic is dense and high, and they are areas where confrontations take place often. If necessary, all yards should be swept clean of gravel and other hard debris on a regular basis. This is particularly true in summer when animals carry debris from fields and deposit it on yards. Rubber floor matting (see above) may become more common in the future.

COW TRACKS

On some units, cow tracks used to access pasture can represent a significant risk for lameness. They are often of poor quality and are constructed with little thought for the animals that have to use them. Recent work has demonstrated that cows have a strong preference for soft (wood chip) tracks (Gregory and Taylor, 2002), although these are expensive to install and maintain. Recent suggestions include capping hard core tracks with soft (but surprisingly robust) substrates such as oolytic limestone. Soft stones such as oolytic limestone will bash to a smooth finish and are not hard (or sharp) enough to penetrate the white line. Where concrete roads and tracks are already in place, riveting a central band of second hand quarry belting is a relatively inexpensive method of significantly improving the quality of the track.

The use of tracks by heavy machinery causes significant problems because of the damage caused. Ideally, a separate (fenced off) cow track should be provided if heavy vehicle use is required also, although some of the newer surfaces, e.g. oolytic limestone, will stand some (but not excessive) vehicle use.

The loose sharp aggregate on roads and lanes is particularly dangerous. If animals have to use lanes to access pasture, they should be swept clean of loose chippings. If animals have to cross only from one side to the other, an old piece of carpet provides an ideal method of covering the road and can simply be rolled up after use.

Nutritional management

Despite recent changes in the proposed aetiology of "SCL", controlling SARA remains an important aspect of lameness control in cattle. The aetiology of SARA and its control are well understood and will not be covered here; rather the practical situation in which SARA can develop despite diets being formulated to avoid ruminal acidosis will be discussed.

Even if a diet is formulated to ensure adequate fibre intake, in practice this intake may never be met by some animals. This is especially true of heifers and subordinate animals fed on an in-parlour concentrate and an out-of-parlour forage / mixed ration system. In this situation, the animal will eat its entire parlour ration (because there is no competition), but may struggle to consume the forage component of the diet if the feeding area is inadequate or badly designed (see "Shearing and abrasive forces"). A similar situation arises when the concentrate component of the diet is introduced too rapidly after calving, before dry matter intake has peaked. In this situation, the animal will preferentially consume concentrates at the expense of adequate forage intake, and the forage to concentrate ratio will fall. Concentrates should be increased steadily after calving, especially in heifers, not peaking until at least four weeks into lactation. All too often in clinical practice, heifers are seen three to six months after calving with bilateral sole ulceration, from which they rarely recover.

Contact with slurry

Contact with contaminated slurry is one of the most significant risk factors for the acquisition of digital dermatitis. Although, of course, faecal production is related to nutrition, there is little that can be done practically to control or limit its production. However, as milk yields and dry matter intakes increase, the resultant increase in faecal volumes must be considered. Herd owners should be encouraged to increase the frequency with which housing is scraped to reduce the exposure of cows to large quantities of slurry.

Conclusions

Lameness in dairy cattle is multifactorial in origin and currently represents a significant challenge to the UK dairy industry. This chapter has reviewed some of the factors associated with claw and foot lesions in dairy cattle, particularly those associated with practical nutrition. For a more complete review of the causal factors, the reader referred to other papers on the subject (e.g. Vermunt 2004; Blowey 2005).

References

Amory J., Barker Z., Wright J., Blowey R.W. and Green L.E. (2006) The effect of hoof lesion type on the milk yield of dairy cows. In: *24th World Buiatrics Congress*, Nice, France.

Bickert W.G. and Cermak J. (1997) Housing considerations relevant to lameness in dairy cattle. In: *Lameness in Cattle*, pp. 300-307. Edited by P.R. Greenough. W.B. Saunders Company, Philadelphia.

Blowey R.W. (1992a) Diseases of the bovine digit. Part1: Description of common lesions. *In Practice*, **14**, 85-90.

Blowey R.W. (1992b) Diseases of the bovine digit. Part 2: Hoof care and factors influencing the incidence of lameness. *In Practice*, **14**, 118-124.

Blowey R.W. (2005) Factors associated with lameness in dairy cattle. *In Practice*, **27**, 154-162.

Blowey R.W. and Sharp M.W. (1988) Digital dermatitis in dairy cattle. *Veterinary Record*, **122**, 505-508.

Cheli R. and Mortellaro C. (1974) La dematite dgitale del bovino. In: *8th International Conference on Diseases of Cattle*, pp. 208-213, Milan.

Clarkson M.J., Downham D.Y., Faull W.B., Hughes J.W., Manson F.J., Merritt J.B., Murray R.D., Russell W.B., Sutherst J.E. and Ward W.R. (1996) Incidence and prevalence of lameness in dairy cattle. *Veterinary Record*, **138**, 563-567.

Collick D.W., Ward W.R. and Dobson H. (1989) Associations between types of lameness and fertility. *Veterinary Record*, **125**, 103-106.

Esslemont R. (2005) The cost of lameness in dairy herds. *UK Vet*, **10**, 41 - 49.

Esslemont R. and Kossaibati M. (2002) *The Costs of Poor Fertility and Disease in UK Dairy Herds. Trends in DAISY Herds Over 10 Seasons.* Intervet.

Esslemont R.J. and Kossaibati M.A. (1996) Incidence of production diseases and other health problems in a group of dairy herds in England. *Veterinary Record*, **139**, 486-490.

Galbraith, H. (2007) Lameness in dairy cows: influence of nutrition on claw composition and health. In *Recent Advances in Animal Nutrition – 2007*, pp ??? - ???. Edited by P.C. Garnsworthy and J. Wiseman. Nottingham University Press, Nottingham.

Green L.E., Hedges V.J., Schukken Y.H., Blowey R.W. and Packington A.J. (2002) The impact of clinical lameness on the milk yield of dairy cows. In: *XXII World Buiatrics Congress*, pp. 21-22, Hannover, Germany.

Gregory N.G. and Taylor O.D. (2002) Dairy cow preference for a soft track surface. *New Zealand Veterinary Journal*, **50**, 83-83.

Hedges J., Blowey R.W., Packington A.J., O'Callaghan C.J. and Green L.E. (2001) A longitudinal field trial of the effect of biotin on lameness in dairy cows.

Journal of Dairy Science, **84**, 1969-1975.

Huxley J., Burke J., Roderick S., Main D. and Whay H. (2004) Animal welfare assessment benchmarking as a tool for health and welfare planning in organic dairy herds. *Veterinary Record*, **155**, 237-239.

Huxley J.N. (2005) An investigation into the effects of herd health planning and health and welfare benchmarking on cattle health and welfare on organic dairy farms in South West England. Royal College of Veterinary Surgeons Diploma in Cattle Health and Production Thesis.

Huxley J.N. and Whay H.R. (2006) Cow based assessments Part 3: Locomotion scoring, claw overgrowth and injuries associated with farm furniture. *UK Vet*, **11**, 51-56.

Main D.C.J., Whay H.R., Green L.E. and Webster A.J.F. (2003) Effect of the RSPCA Freedom Food scheme on the welfare of dairy cattle. *Veterinary Record*, **153**, 227-231.

Manson F.J. and Leaver J.D. (1988) The influence of concentrate amount on locomotion and clinical lameness in dairy-cattle. *Animal Production*, **47**, 185-190.

Mill J.M. and Ward W.R. (1994) Lameness in dairy cows and farmers' knowledge, training and awareness. *Veterinary Record*, **134**, 162-164.

Mulling C.K.W. and Greenough P.R. (2006) Applied physiopathology of the foot. In: *24th World Buiatrics Congress*, pp. 103-117, Nice, France.

Murray R.D., Downham D.Y., Clarkson M.J., Faull W.B., Hughes J.W., Manson F.J., Merritt J.B., Russell W.B., Sutherst J.E. and Ward W.R. (1996) Epidemiology of lameness in dairy cattle: Description and analysis of foot lesions. *Veterinary Record*, **138**, 586-591.

Sprecher D.J., Hostetler D.E. and Kaneene J.B. (1997) A lameness scoring system that uses posture and gait to predict dairy cattle reproductive performance. *Theriogenology*, **47**, 1179 - 1187.

Tarlton J.F., Holah D.E., Evans K.M., Jones S., Pearson G.R. and Webster A.J.F. (2002) Biomechanical and histopathological changes in the support structures of bovine hooves around the time of first calving. *Veterinary Journal*, **163**, 196-204.

Tranter W.P. and Morris R.S. (1991) A Case-Study of Lameness in 3 Dairy Herds. *New Zealand Veterinary Journal*, **39**, 88-96.

Vermunt J. (2004) Herd lameness - A review, major causal factors, and guidelines for prevention and control. In: *13th International Symposium and 5th Conference on Lameness in Ruminants*, pp. 3-18, Maribor, Slovenia.

Whay H.R., Main D.C.J., Green L.E. and Webster A.J.F. (2003) Assessment of the welfare of dairy cattle using animal-based measurements: direct observations and investigation of farm records. *Veterinary Record*, **153**, 197-202.

Whay H.R., Waterman A.E. and Webster A.J.F. (1997) Associations between locomotion, claw lesions and nociceptive threshold in dairy heifers during the peri-partum period. *Veterinary Journal*, **154**, 155-161.

Whay H.R., Waterman A.E., Webster A.J.F. and O'Brien J.K. (1998) The influence of lesion type on the duration of hyperalgesia associated with hindlimb lameness in dairy cattle. *Veterinary Journal*, **156**, 23-29.

Whitaker D.A., Kelly J.M. and Smith S. (2000) Disposal and disease rates in 340 British dairy herds. *Veterinary Record*, **146**, 363-367.

Winckler C. and Willen S. (2001) The Reliability and repeatability of a lameness scoring system for use as an indicator of welfare in dairy cattle. *Acta Agriculturae Scandinavica, Section A - Animal Science*, **51**, 103 - 107.

5

LAMENESS IN DAIRY COWS: INFLUENCE OF NUTRITION ON CLAW COMPOSITION AND HEALTH

H GALBRAITH[1] AND J R SCAIFE[2]
School of Biological Sciences, University of Aberdeen, 23 St Machar Drive, Aberdeen, AB24 3RY, UK; [2]School of Equine and Animal Science, Writtle College, Lordship Road , Chelmsford , CM1 3RR, UK

Introduction

Lameness in dairy cattle is well recognised as a painful and internationally endemic production disease affecting up to 0.60 of animals in contemporary dairy herds (Vermunt, 2004). It has been associated with the selection of cows predominantly for milk yield and the intensification of nutritional supply, housing environments and management systems. Negative outcomes of such practices are suggested to include claw horn lesions which cause the majority of cases of non-infectious lameness, and infections due to digital dermatitis. Current thinking recognizes lameness produced by these and other lesions (Lamecow, 2007) as having a complex aetiology with risk factors related to 'intrinsic' animal characteristics of physiology and behaviour interacting with those derived from the 'extrinsic' external physical environment (Greenough, Weaver, Broom, Esslemont and Galindo, 1997)

An example of lesions which affect horn and internal tissues of a hind lateral claw of a dairy cow is shown in Figure 1. Major symptoms are bruising and haemorrhage which appear as compression injuries of soft tissues which are located between the pedal bone and horn of the sole and bulb. The causal mechanisms underlying production of such lesions are poorly understood but are currently considered to occur by complex processes related to (i) inflammation of the vascular dermal tissue as in acidosis-related laminitis (Nocek, 1997) and/or (ii) breakdown of dermal connective tissue particularly around calving in suggested response to physiological signalling by systemic hormones (Tarlton, Holah, Evans, Jones, Pearson and Webster, 2002). Such events are considered to increase load bearing on soft tissue and horn of the sole and decrease resistance to formation of damaged tissue (Tarlton *et al.*, 2002).

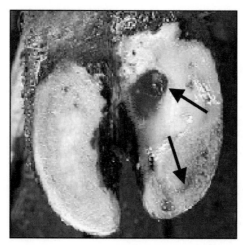

Figure 1. Image of hind claw of a dairy cow showing (arrows) solear ulcer and bruising. After: http://template. bio.warwick.ac.uk/E+E/lamecow/public_html/lesions.html

In considering how husbandry interacts with biology to compromise claw health, it is important to review the basic anatomy of the bovine digit and to consider how chemical and molecular composition contributes to physical function. There are clear implications for nutritional inputs which are required to support tissue homeostasis and integrity of the claw. These include amino acids, proteins, carbohydrates, lipids, minerals and vitamins which contribute to anatomical structure and metabolic catalysis. Additional considerations are the role of nutrients in influencing the mechanisms which regulate morphological development and physiological changes throughout the lifespan of the dairy cow and which may have secondary effects on claw structure and function. More detailed consideration will be given to these and other factors in the succeeding text.

Anatomy of the claw and biomechanical function

The basic anatomy of the bovine claw is shown in Figure 2. A major functional role is the transference of mechanical forces arising from the body weight of the animal, to the ground surface. Such transference occurs through the pedal bone which is suspended or supported within the horn capsule by the various components of the 'suspensory apparatus'. The positioning of the pedal bone is partly determined by the deep flexor tendon.

The suspensory component of this apparatus includes an intricate system of laminae in the dermis and epidermis of the claw wall which interdigitate to provide a strong yet flexible link between the pedal bone and the claw horn capsule

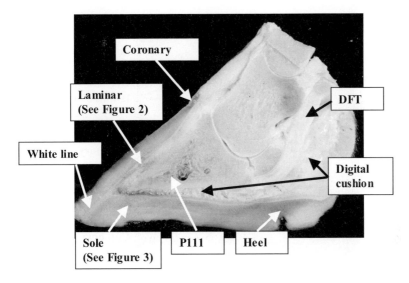

Figure 2. Sagittal section of bovine claw showing regions of the horn capsule and of horn production (coronary, laminar, sole and heel), the white line at the junction of sole and coronary (wall) horn, deep flexor tendon (DFT), pedal bone (P111) and digital cushion. After Galbraith *et al.* (2006b).

(Figure 3). The underlying soft tissue of the digital cushions of the hypodermis (Figure 2) also provides protection by acting as "shock absorbers" which lessen impact on underlying tissues. Major contacts between the ground surface and the body weight of the animal are coronary wall horn and, variably, depending on factors such as anatomical position, degree of erosion and trimming practice, horn of white line, sole and heel (Logue, Offer and Murray, 2005). Reductions in the efficacy of the suspensory system in preventing excessive impact of the pedal bone on dermal and epidermal soft tissue in sole and heel is considered a major cause of lesion formation. The solar and heel components of the horn capsule have an important role in protecting underlying soft tissue from the ground surface, and thin soles (5mm or less) have been associated with greater susceptibility to damage to underlying soft tissue (van Amstel, Shearer and Palin, 2004).

Loss of functionality in either the suspensory components of the claw wall or the digital cushions or both can lead to increased pressure of the distal phalanx on the corium and the development of sole ulcers. Browne, Hukins, Skakle, Knight, Hendry, Wilde and Galbraith (2007) have recently described differences in dimensions of different regions of the horn capsule between heifers of dairy and beef origins. Dairy heifers were shown to have lower dorsal wall angles, lower height of heel and thinner horn at solear sites and smaller dimension for soft tissue including the digital cushion at the heel (bulb) (Table 1 and Figure 4). These characteristics were considered to predispose to development of the claw horn

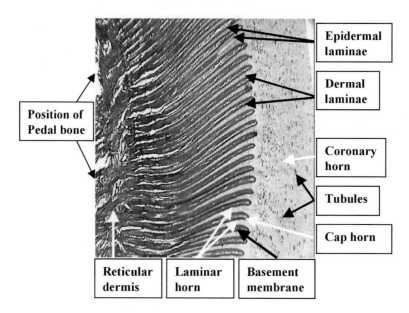

Figure 3. Horizontal section of mid-laminar region of a bovine claw showing the position of the pedal bone connecting to the reticular dermis and dermal laminae, epidermal laminae, cap horn and coronary wall horn with tubules. Stain: Verhoeff's van Giesen, X 40 magnification. (La Manna and Galbraith, unpublished)

Table 1. Mean values (with SEM) for external and internal claw measurements of dairy and beef heifers. After Browne *et al.* (2007).

Variable		Dairy	Beef	Statistical significance
Dorsal angle (°)		39 (2.0)	46 (0.82)	P < 0.001
Heel height (mm)		23.3 (4.65)	38.8 (7.14)	P < 0.01
Claw height (mm)		88.8 (1.5)	99.0 (3.16)	P < 0.05
Sole (apical):	horn tissue	5.3 (3.4)	13.5 (3.0)	P < 0.01
	soft tissue	2.3 (1.26)	3.0 (1.15)	n.s.
Sole -bulb :	horn tissue	6.25 (2.06)	13.8 (3.3)	P < 0.01
	soft tissue	6.5 (1.29)	8.0 (1.41)	n.s.
Bulb	horn tissue	7.5 (1.29)	9.5 (1.91)	n.s.
	soft tissue	6.5 (1.73)	13.0 (2.58)	P < 0.01

lesions typically observed in dairy cattle. Further information on the composition and role of the digital cushions is provided below.

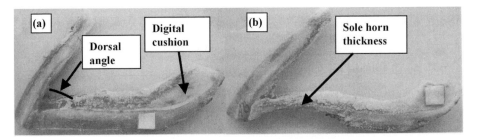

Figure 4. Digital images showing typical sections of claw from (a) beef and (b) dairy production types. After Browne *et al.* (2007).

In considering the properties of horn materials in relation to site-specific functional requirements, use has been made of the Durotech Shore D durometer, which measures impression hardness of materials by determining resistance to penetration by a sharply pointed probe. For example, pooled values for the sites of sole (apical, axial, abaxial) and wall (proximal and distal) for beef and dairy animals (Browne *et al.*, 2007) were 39.1, 37.4, 41.4, 67.5, 72.2 (SED = 2.84). These data demonstrate the similarities within wall and sole sites of measurement. They also show the greater hardness associated with the greater rigidity of wall in the suspensory system, while the lower values for sole are consistent with the requirement for greater flexibility. It is important therefore to be aware of site-specific characteristics when considering the cellular and extracellular biology of horn production in claw tissues.

Cell and molecular biology of horn production

In common with other tissues of the mammalian integument, horn is the end-product of continually renewing epidermis in the outermost layer of the claw. Much of the general information on claw horn biology has derived from knowledge of skin and hair follicle using investigative tools and approaches which have highlighted the conservation of structure and function across integumental tissues. As regards claw horn, its production occurs by proliferation and differentiation of specialised epithelial cells of the epidermis. These "keratinocyte " cells (e.g. Figure 3 for laminae and Figure 5 for solear epidermis and dermis) are positioned on a basement membrane in immediate contact with underlying dermis (Budras, Geyer, Maierl and Mülling, 1998; Galbraith, Rae, Omand, Hendry, Knight and Wilde 2006a).

The epidermis is avascular and keratinocytes receive nutrients, regulatory mitogens and morphogens across the basement membrane from the dermis.

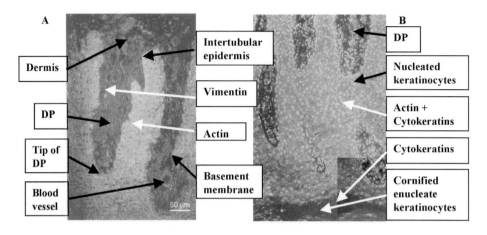

Figure 5. Sole crysosections showing epidermis, dermis, dermal papillae (DP) with (A) intertubular epidermis and site of tubule formation at tip of DP, dermal blood vessel and basement membrane. Immunohistochemical localisation shown for vimentin in dermal papillae, and actin predominantly in epidermis. Section B shows nucleitated (DAPI stained) keratinocytes with immunohistochemical signals co-localising for actin and cytokeratins. Cytokeratin signal only was maintained, with loss of actin signal, in cornified enucleiate keratinocytes in terminally differentiated horn. After Galbraith *et al.* (2006b).

The dermis in regions such as coronary, sole and heel extends into the epidermis in the formation of papillae (Figure 5). Intertubular horn is formed between papillae in addition to tubules of horn (Figure 3), which form from cells localised around the tips of papillae (Figure 5). The outermost cells form a well-differentiated approximately cylindrical cortex while the innermost medullated cells are poorly keratinized and may be shed in movement towards the outer surface. Tubular horn has similarities in structure to medullated hair produced by certain hair follicles, and signalling mechanisms responsible for its development are poorly understood (Galbraith, 2006). Tubular horn provides mechanical strength to the horn. In contrast, laminar horn in the laminar region is produced along the epidermal-dermal border of laminae in the absence of formation of the tubules which can be seen in coronary horn (Figure 3). The absence of tubules, along with the shorter transition to cornification in, for example 2-4 layers of cells compared with what may considerably exceed 20 in other anatomical regions, contributes to the formation of white line horn which has less mechanical strength than adjacent coronary and sole horn (Mülling, 2002). An additional source of horn formed by "cap" papillae at the terminus of laminae is "cap" horn which also contributes to the structure of the white line (Mülling, 2002). Proliferation of basal epidermal cells (Figure 5) occurs by cell division with one daughter cell normally remaining to divide further and the other committing to suprabasal migration to the outermost cornified layers (Tomlinson, Mülling and Fakler, 2004).

The increase in size of the epidermal-dermal unit during normal growth of the animal requires that mitosis is succeeded by further division of both daughter cells to increase the number of cells lining an elongated basement membrane and thus capacity for horn production. Such increases are seen in comparisons of claws of one week old calves with those of mature cows (Table 2). Concomitant with greater external physical dimensions are increases in internal measurements for height (extension into epidermis), cross-sectional width and length of the basement membrane of individual papillae.

Table 2. Comparison of external and internal dimensions of claws of three one-week-old calves and two mature dairy cows. Measurements were combined for medial and lateral claws of left front foot. Histological measurements for basement membrane and dermal papillae were made in triplicate at three solear sites by light microscopy using 1.0mm field of view. Data from Cross (1998).

Measurement (mm)	*Animal*		*Pooled standard*
	Calf	*Cow*	*deviation*
Claw:			
Dorsal length	45.3	73.8	6.37
Claw height	42.8	68.2	4.40
Heel height	25.2	37.2	6.24
Width	25.5	47.9	3.01
Toe angle (°)	50.2	39.0	6.90
Basement membrane (μm)	5208	7936	1302
Papillae:			
Height (μm)	210	405	69.94
Area (mm^2)	13810	37476	8034
Perimeter (μm)	469	892	158

Commitment to differentiation in mammalian epidermal cells involves sequential expression of a range of genes including those encoding for proteins which have been described on the basis of biochemical characteristics of molecular mass and iso-electric point (pI) as type I (acidic) and type II (basic) keratins. Properties of molecular mass and pI approximate to 40-65 kDa and 4.5-6.0 pH for type 1 and 50-70 kDa and 6.5-8.5 pH for type II keratins respectively (Bowden, 2005). The report by Moll, Franke, Schiller, Geiger and Krepler (1982) described eight type I keratins (K1-K8) and 11 type II keratins (K9-K19). Subsequent work (Heid, Werner and Franke, 1986) identified four members of type I and type II cytokeratin subfamilies (Ha1-4 and Hb1-4, "hair specific" hard keratins) from human, bovine and ovine hair follicles which differed from "cyto"keratins in the same species. Additional members have since been identified and changes in their nomenclature are under review (Bowden, 2006). There has been considerable recent focus, including that for the Human Genome Sequencing project, on proteins of human hair for which more than 100 keratin genes have been identified (Parry, Smith, Rogers and Schweizer, 2006). Information for the bovine genome is incomplete. Interestingly, Rogers, Edler, Winter, Langbein, Beckman and Schweitzer (2005) described the type II keratin domain on the human chromosome 12q13.13 as containing 27 keratin genes and 8 pseudogenes.

Certain keratins are associated with expression early in proliferation (e.g. cytokeratin 5 in basal cells) while others (e.g. cytokeratin 10) are synthesised in, and may be used as markers for, suprabasal cells. Such an approach has been applied by, for example, Hendry, Knight, Galbraith, and Wilde (2003) and Hepburn, Knight, Wilde, Hendry and Galbraith, (2008) in immunohistochemical studies using antibodies that cross-react across a range of animal species.

A common property of keratins is to form obligate heterodimers (type I dimerising with type II), which assemble further to form filamentous polymers of increasing size to give intermediate filaments (IFs) of ca. 10nm diameter. These IFs have been shown to form fibrous structures of defined three-dimensional shape. Recent work (Browne *et al.*, 2007) has shown, for bovine claw horn samples, X-ray diffraction patterns that indicated the presence of α-helical structures in fibrils which are typical of those occurring in other hard keratin-containing tissues of the integument (Figure 6). These workers also described the relationship between alignment of fibrils, their location in wall and solear horn and implications for their role in biomechanics of bearing of body-weight.

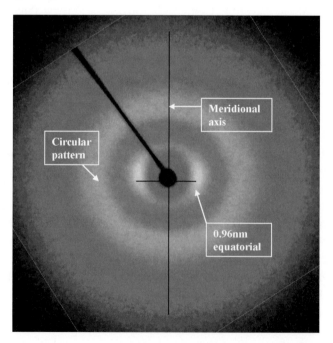

Figure 6. Typical X-ray diffraction pattern of a section of cornified coronary wall horn showing the presence of arcs on the equatorial (horizontal) axis at maxima of approximately 0.96nm (arrowed) typical of hard α-keratin. Note the diffuse disordered circular pattern (arrowed) and the absence of specific areas of intensity on the meridional (vertical) axis perpendicular to the equatorial axis. After Browne *et al.* (2007).

Intermediate filaments are known to interact with intermediate filament associated (non-filamentous matrix) proteins (IFAPs) or keratin associated proteins (KAPS) which form an important part of the cytoskeleton. Major components of IFAPS in keratinizing tissues (e.g. Gillespie, 1991: Parry *et al.*, 2006) belong to three molecular families comprising the high-sulphur proteins, the ultra-high sulphur proteins and the high-glycine-tyrosine proteins. Expression of IF proteins and IFAPs in the cytoskeleton of cells of animals is known to vary according to species, tissue, location of cells and nutritional and physiological status (Gillespie, 1991). A major chemical interaction between IFs and IFAPs involves the formation of disulphide bonds both within and between constituent molecules. This process is facilitated by the presence of high concentrations of cysteine molecules which for the "low" sulphur-containing proteins (keratin fraction) typically approximate (residues/100 residues) 4 to 7, and exceed 30 for certain ultra high sulphur matrix proteins in samples of hair and horn (Gillespie,1991). In addition to describing spontaneous disulphide bond formation under oxidative conditions, Hashimoto, Suga, Matsuba, Mizoguchi, Takamori, Seitz and Ogawa (2001) showed the process to be catalysed in rat skin epidermis by sulphydril (thiol) oxidase under terminal differentiation conditions. In basal cells undergoing mitosis, mechanisms involving phosphorylation and disassembly of IFs occur prior to eventual re-assembly after cell division. Additional components of the cytoplasm of eukaryote cells include microfilaments (7-9nm diameter) composed of polymeric F-actin filaments and microtubules (ca 24nm diameter) and polymers of globular tubulin (Steinert and Freedberg, 1991). Figure 5 shows cryosections of bovine claw solear tissue which illustrate the cellular nature of the epidermis and positive immunohistochemical signals indicative of expression of actin and cytokeratins in pre-cornified epidermis. It is interesting to note the apparent loss of expression of actin but not keratins following cornification.

Additional cell types in the epidermis are melanocytes which are neuroectodermal in origin and which produce the melanosomes which transfer to keratinocyes and produce the eumelanin and pheomelanin pigments in pigmented claw horn (Hepburn, Kinninmonth and Galbraith, 2007). Such synthesis depends on a supply of tyrosine and the presence of tyrosinase enzymes. These workers observed apparent delays due to pigmentation in attaining maximum values of impression hardness in pigmented coronary wall horn. Such an effect may be related to antagonism between the oxidative environment needed for cytoskeletal disulphide bond formation and the antioxidant properties of melanins.

Epidermal adhesion and communication, lipids and biotin

Although cytoskeletal structures have an important role in maintaining the physical integrity of individual cells, the functional integrity of integumental tissues depends also on effective adhesion between individual cells in tissues and between basal cells and the basement membrane (Odland,1991: Lodish, Baltimore, Berk, Zipursky, Matsudaira and Darnell (1995). Such adhesion involves desmosomal junctions which include plaque proteins and proteins such as cadherins and hemidesmosomes which connect cells to the basement membrane with anchorage by proteins such as integrins.   Intermediate filaments form internal anchorages at desmosomes and hemidesmosomes. Aherens junctions connect cells and form attachments with actin-microfilaments. Additionally, gap junctions comprised of connexion proteins have an important role in the avascular epidermis in the transport of nutrients and small signalling molecules between keratinocytes. They also have a role in signalling mechanisms which may exert effects by variation in concentration of molecules as in reaction-diffusion systems (Nagorcka & Mooney, 1982). Such mechanisms may explain how sequential gene expression and differentiation is controlled. Signalling molecules such as calcium or certain growth factors may be expected to regulate gene expression following such transport between cells. Proteins such as Connexin 43 have been identified immunohistochemically in sections of claw epidermis (Frohberg-Wang, Mülling, and Budras, 2004).

Additional proteins which are synthesised in late differentiating epidermal cells are those of the cell envelope which are located at the periphery and interact with IF and IFAP complexes to form structures which give rigidity to, and promote barrier function of, cells in final cornification. Candi, Tarcsa, Digiovanna, Compton, Elias, Marekov and Steinert (1998) described the importance of a lysine residue in the "head" domain of certain type II keratins which was essential for formation of isopeptide cross links to cell envelope proteins by calcium-dependent transglutaminase enzymes. Transglutaminases catalyse cross-linking of proteins such as loricin, involucrin and small proline-rich protein (Hitomi, 2005) in epidermal tissues such as skin although information on their presence in bovine claw tissue is limited. Immunohistochemical signals for Transglutaminase I have been described by Cowie and Galbraith (unpublished) predominantly in cells in locations beyond the interpapillary region and towards the cornified layer (Figure 7).

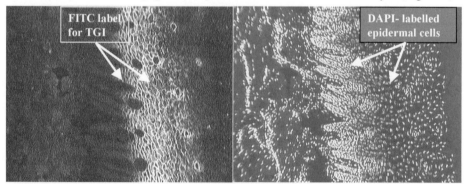

Figure 7. Vertical sections of coronary epidermis showing (a) positive signals for transglutaminase I (FITC-labelled antibody) on the internal periphery of epidermal cells and (b) same section with nuclei labelled with DAPI. Magnification X 200. (Cowie and Galbraith, unpublished)

Tomlinson *et al.* (2004) summarised the role of the intercellular cementing substance (ICS), which is composed of glycoproteins and complex lipids, and is centrally important in adhesion. This material is secreted into spaces between cells and provides a lipophilic water-resistant permeability barrier in cornified cells, such as that described in skin in a range of species (Wertz and Downing, 1991).

The lipid composition of epidermis from various species was first characterised by Gray and Yardley (1975a; 1975b). Subsequently, Lampe, Burlingame, Whitney, Williams, Brown, Roitman and Elias (1983a) and Lampe, Williams and Elias (1983b) described the presence of different lipid types in the germinative, differentiating and cornified layers of epidermis of human skin. They found that polar lipids decreased from 0.44 in the *stratum basale/spinosum* to 0.25 in the *stratum granulosum* and 0.05 in the *stratum corneum*. These results showed higher concentrations of phospholipids initially in the structure of the plasma membrane and organelle membrane bilayers in pre-cornified cells, and reductions during further differentiation and cornification of cells. Neutral lipids, composed mainly of sterols and triglycerides, increased from 0.51 in the germinative layer to 0.57 in the suprabasal differentiating layers and to 0.78 in the terminally differentiated cornified cells. Similarly, the sphingolipid fraction, containing ceramides, increased from 0.07 to 0.11 and to 0.26 with progressive differentiation. Total epidermal lipid was shown to constitute about 0.10-0.14 of the dry weight of skin epidermis (Gray and Yardley, 1975a). In the *stratum corneum*, approximately 0.08-0.1 of the dry weight is lipid.

Ueta, Kawamura, Kanazawa and Yamakawa (1971) first described the lipids of the bovine claw as comprising 0.31 cholesterol, 0.24 free fatty acid, 0.14 triacylglycerol, 0.10 cholesterol sulphate, 0.07 ceramide, 0.06 glucocerebroside and 0.03 diacylglycerol. The total lipid content of bovine claw horn was reported to vary from 0.015 for the wall to 0.03 for the heel and to contain very long chain fatty acids (>C24) which constituted up to 0.08 of the total fatty acid content (Scaife, Meyer and Grant, 2000). Offer and Logue (1998) reported that lipids from slivers of claw horn obtained from lame cows contained significantly more linoleic (C18:3n-6); linolenic (C18:3n-3) and arachidonic acid (C20:4n-6) than the claws of sound cows. Offer, Offer and Logue, (2000) subsequently showed that feeding cows a supplement of 300g/day fish oil for a period of three weeks resulted in significant increases in the long chain polyunsaturated fatty acid content of the total lipid in slivers of claw horn taken eight weeks after supplementation had ended.

The fatty acids of skin, in common with other epidermal tissues, have a number of unusual characteristics. Those in the sphingolipid fraction, which are predominantly ceramides and glucosylceramides, contain α- and ω-hydroxylated fatty acids that range in chain length from 24 to 32 carbon atoms (Hamanaka, Hara, Nishio, Otsuka, Suzuki and Uchida, 2002). These sphingolipids containing long chain fatty acids have been likened to 'molecular rivets' in providing adhesion between adjacent cornified epidermal cells (Wertz and Downing 1991). Such an unusual nature of composition of fatty acids indicates, for skin, the presence of considerable specialised synthesis followed by their incorporation into more complex lipids prior to deposition in the tissue. The very long chain nature of the fatty acids suggests extensive elongation of fatty acids *in situ* since none of these are components of the diet nor are they found in circulating lipoproteins. In this context, there is particular interest in the role of the B-vitamin biotin which has an essential role in fatty acid synthesis and elongation in acting as a cofactor in the enzyme acetyl-CoA carboxylase (Meyer, Koster, Mülling, Scaife, Birnie and Budras, 2003; Brownsey, Boone, Elliott, Kulpa and Lee, 2006). In a recent study (Meyer, 2004) examined the effects of biotin supplementation or depletion by avidin supplementation on the characteristics of claw horn from calves reared on a milk-based diet with limited access to forage for approximately 110days. Biotin depletion did not cause any major changes in the fatty acid composition of the claw horn in the depleted animals. However, the claw horn capsule was significantly heavier on a live-weight basis and the sole horn significantly thicker in the depleted animals. Expression of the cell proliferation marker Ki67 was increased significantly in the sole horn of the depleted animals, indicating that changes in the rate of proliferation of epidermal keratinocytes may be sensitive to biotin status.

Numerous studies have shown that a deficiency of biotin in farm animal diets is associated with abnormalities in keratinizing integumental tissues such as skin, hair, hoof and horn. In poultry, dermatitis, cracking and lesions of the feet and soft beak result from biotin deficiency (Whitehead, Bannister, Wight and Weiser, 1974). In pigs, progressive dermatitis and softening of the hoof horn are characteristic of biotin deficiency. The changes in hoof horn strength lead to 'concrete disease' typified by high rates of abrasion, lesions and secondary infections. This condition is responsive to biotin supplementation (Bryant, Kornegay, Knight, Webb and Notter (1985). In horses, poor quality hoof horn can be improved by dietary biotin supplementation, suggesting that marginal biotin deficiency can cause deterioration in hoof horn quality in this species. There is now a considerable body of evidence from epidemiological studies that daily supplementation of cow diets with 20mg biotin is effective in reducing lameness and foot lesions four to six months after starting supplementation (Green and Muelling, 2005). Although mechanisms by which biotin brings about this reduction in lameness are poorly understood, the data suggest inadequacy of supply from microbial synthesis in the digestive tract and from the diet. In addition to its role in lipid metabolism, biotin is also known to be involved in amino acid metabolism, cellular respiration and gluconeogenesis, and it has a number of non-carboxylase functions that may, in part, explain its effects in claw horn. These functions, which include regulation of gene expression, biotinylation of histones and effects on cellular proliferation have recently been reviewed by Zempleni (2005).

Basement membrane and dermis and claw health

The basement membrane is typically composed (Lodish *et al.*, 1995) of three layers that comprise of the *lamina lucida* which connects to the basal epidermal cells by hemidesmosomes involving integrins, and the underlying *lamina densa* by transvesely anchoring laminin proteins. The *lamina densa* layer connects via collagen VII to the *lamina fibroreticularis* which has continuity with collagens and elastin of the dermis. Crespo, Galbraith and Finn (1999) and subsequently Di Lucca and Galbraith (unpublished) have described immunohistochemically, the presence of Collagens I, IV and VII and fibronectin in sections of bovine claw dermis. The importance of an intact and undamaged basement membrane in the maintenance of normal keratization and claw horn health has been demonstrated by Hendry *et al.* (2003). These workers showed that solear ulceration was associated with (a) loss of basement membrane and abnormal expression of certain keratin proteins in the epidermis and (b) in the dermis, elevation in levels of matrix metalloproteinases and reductions in tissue inhibitor of metalloproteinase 2. In addition, treatment with anti-laminin antibody was shown to reduce protein synthesis in explant tissue cultures. Elevation of activity of matrix metalloproteinases is a typical response in damaged basement membrane and dermal tissues.

The major fibroblast cells of the dermis derive from the embryonic mesenchyme and differ from keratinocytes in epidermis which are ectodermal in origin. Among differences with keratinocytes is the presence in the cytoskeleton of type III IFs which contain vimentin (Figure 5).

Although fibroblasts in the dermal papillae of the mammalian hair follicle are known to belong to a stable population (Galbraith, 1998), their dynamics in claw dermis are not known. The fibroblasts have a range of roles which include production of paracrine and autocrine growth factors and extracellular proteins and other molecules of the extracellular matrix. These include proteoltytic metalloproteinase enzymes which are frequently elevated in expression in injured claw tissues and which require zinc for functional activity. Fibroblasts also synthesise connective tissue macromolecules, such as collagens and elastins, and adhesion molecules such as fibronectins, in addition to the ionically charged glycosaminoglycans and proteoglycans which have been studied in claw tissues (Tarlton *et al.*, 2002). The latter macromolecules have gel-like properties which are important in maintaining hydration and regulating retention and rate of release of other charged molecules such as those involving signalling.

It is also important to note that reticular, papillary and laminar dermis are vascularised (Hirschberg and Plendel (2001) and that blood supply is critical to health of both epidermis and dermis. Perturbation of the dermal vascular system is an important factor in the hypothesis relating inflammatory laminitis to formation of claw horn lesions. Symptoms are considered to include leakage of serum products into extra-vascular space to produce the characteristic yellowing of horn (Nocek, 1997). More severely, physical damage to blood vessels also produces symptoms of bruising, haemorrhage or ulceration (Figure 1) Another important property of the dermis is the presence of nerve fibres surrounding blood vessels (Buda and Budras (2004). These nerve fibres are considered to regulate vaso-constriction or vaso-dilation by the release of neurotransmitters and so may affect responses to inflammatory stimuli and regulate supply of signalling molecules and nutrients to both dermal and epidermal tissues. Enervation also has a role in the perception of pain arising from the presence of lesions.

It is well recognised that a major function of the dermis is to supply nutrients to support synthetic processes of horn production in the epidermis (Tomlinson *et al.,* 2004). In addition, exchange of chemical signals ("cross talk") between dermis and epidermal epithelia is known to regulate gene expression and epidermal synthesis in other tissues of the integument such as skin and hair follicle (Millar, 2002). The "double paracrine" mechanism demonstrated *in vitro* in skin by Maas-Szabowski, Shimotoyodome and Fusenig (1999) is one example. These workers showed that that interleukin-1 produced by keratinocytes stimulated the production of keratinocyte growth factor by dermal fibroblasts. The regulatory loop is completed by stimulation of proliferation of keratinocytes by keratinocyte growth factor derived from fibroblasts. Mulling, Wustenberg, Nebel, Hoffman, and Budras (2006) have recently described a similar mechanism occurring in bovine claw tissues.

The hypodermis, functional role and composition of lipids

The hypodermis in the claw is situated between the dermis and the pedal bone and its thickness varies (Budras and Habel, 2003: see Figures 2 and 4). Where absent, the dermis joins directly to the bone. The hypodermis is vascularised and is formed mainly of adipose tissue cells arranged in a fibro-collagenous matrix. It is particularly important in the claw, in locations under the perioplic and coronary segments (the coronary cushion), and in association with the bulb (the digital cushion). The latter (bulbar) tissues are composed of three parallel fat cylinders located axial, abaxial and middle with numerous transverse cushions connecting axial and abaxial (Lischer and Ossent, 2000). These act a shock absorbers which protect the sensitive underlying dermal and epidermal tissues from contusion damage produced by the pedal bone as weight is transferred to the ground through the claw horn capsule. Lischer and Ossent (2000) likened the structure of the bovine digital cushion to that of the triple cushion principle used in running shoes for humans. There is limited information on the size and lipid content of digital cushions in the cow or the extent to which they change in characteristics with breed, age, parity, reproductive status, presence or absence of lameness or diet. Lischer, Ossent, Raber and Geyer, (2002) examined the digital cushion in thirty six animals (Brown Swiss, Red Holsteins and Black and White Holsteins) that were sound or moderately lame with typical Rusterholz ulcers and concluded that the digital cushions appeared less evident in cows with ulcers than in sound animals. Histological examination of claws from 54 dairy cows (Brown Swiss, Simmental-Red Holstein and Black and White Holstein) (Raber, Lischer, Geyer and Ossent, 2004) suggests that the adipose tissue in the digital cushions of heifers is poorly developed and that the deposition of fat in the cushions increases over the first two to three parities but thereafter declines. Claws of front feet were shown to contain more fat than claws of hind feet. The lateral claws of the front feet contained more fat compared with the medial claws. This pattern was reversed in the hind feet and thus correlated inversely with distribution of load-bearing.

There is little detailed information on the fatty acid composition of digital cushions, although Raber, Scheeder, Ossent, Lischer and Geyer (2006) have recently reported preliminary data on the lipid content and fatty acid composition of digital cushions from Brown Swiss heifers and cows fed a maize silage, grass and hay diet. The mean lipid content of digital cushions was significantly lower in heifers (264 g/kg tissue) than in cows (367 g/kg tissue) and was markedly lower than typical values of 870 - 940g/kg tissue for the total fatty acid content of perinephric adipose tissue depots in the same animals. There were major differences in the lipid content of the six different fat pads isolated from each claw (74 - 431 g/kg tissue in heifers and 133 - 619 g/kg tissue in cows). Anatomically, two of the cushions which contained the lowest fat content were located in the region of the claw where sole ulcers are likely to develop. This observation suggested that there was inadequate cushioning to prevent impact damage to underlying soft tissue. The fatty acid content of the digital cushion was shown not to be typical of subcutaneous and perinephric adipose tissue in containing a higher proportion of monounsaturated fatty acids, predominantly C18:1n9, and lower proportions of saturated fatty acids. These data suggest tissue-specific synthesis of fatty acids or modification of absorbed fatty acids by desaturation to achieve the elevated monounsaturated fatty acid content. This may be important to ensure that digital cushions have the appropriate physical characteristics that enable them to deform under load.

To date there is no information on the way in which the fat content or fatty acid composition of digital cushions responds to nutritional influences and physiological state. Previous studies in non-ruminants have shown that dietary fatty acids can markedly influence the fatty acid composition of adipose tissue (Onibi, Scaife, Murray and Fowler, 2000); Scaife, Moyo, Galbraith, Michie and Campbell, 1994) and in ruminants the feeding of rumen protected lipids can achieve similar changes in the composition of adipose tissue depots (Scollan, Enser, Gulati, Richardson, and Wood, 2003). It is important to understand the factors that influence content and composition of fatty acids in digital cushions in order to better manage cow nutrition. If mobilisation of fat from adipose tissue depots in early lactation cows (Bauman and Currie, 1980) occurs also in digital cushions, this may have important consequences for development of lameness. The advent of functional foods and the greater interest in manipulation of milk fatty acid composition through targeted use of rumen protected fatty acids supplements (Jenkins and McGuire, 2006) may also have consequences for the functionality of digital cushions and occurrence of lameness.

Protein composition of claw tissue and implications for nutrition

Some aspects of protein nutrition and claw horn health have recently been considered by Livesey and Laven (2007). It is evident that protein is the major constituent of claw epidermis and dermis. In considering nutritional requirements for optimal production and maintenance of horn, it is therefore instructive to consider the composition of amino acids in horn tissue. Recent work (Galbraith *et al.*, 2006a) demonstrated higher concentrations of cysteine in dorsal wall than solear horn (Table 3). These results suggest the presence of a greater expression of proteins and peptides which contain greater concentrations of cysteine than in sole and heel. Such a greater expression of individual proteins and peptides has not been demonstrated.

Table 3. Relative composition of selected amino acids, (g amino acid/16 gN) in tissues and dietary protein sources. After Galbraith, (1995) and Galbraith *et al.* (2006a).

Amino acid	Wall horn	Sole horn	Muscle	Rumen microbial protein	Extracted soyabean meal	White fishmeal
Threonine	5.2	4.8	3.9	5.2	4.2	4.2
Leucine	8.1	8.9	5.8	7.4	8.2	6.7
Phenylalanine	2.3	1.4	3.1	5.5	5.5	3.9
Lysine	5.1	1.4	5.9	8.1	6.8	5.7
Methionine	0.70	1.04	1.8	2.5	1.4	3.0
Cyst(e)ine	6.51	4.05	1.1	1.0	1.4	0.9

Preliminary work using a proteomics approach (Galbraith, Flannigan, Swan and Cash, 2006b) has described patterns of expression of a range of protein species in extracts of cornified and soft tissues from coronary, laminar, sole and heel regions of cattle of beef and dairy origin. This approach involves the initial extraction of proteins into aqueous solutions. This process is made difficult by the inherent properties of chemical resistance conferred by helical keratin proteins which form polymers with linking by di-sulphide bond formation internally and externally to other proteins (Plowman, 2003). Following preparation of extracts, individual protein species are separated by 2-dimensional electrophoresis on the basis of molecular mass and isoelectric point, and processing by image analysis. Additional techniques, such as western blotting and peptide mass fingerprinting, are applied to the identification of individual proteins. Reference is made to libraries utilising information on known bovine gene sequences which, as indicated above, are incomplete for the bovine genome but which may show homology with other species particularly human. A typical pattern for extracts from dairy cow solear explant tissue is shown in Figure 8. Up to 400 individual spots are evident with a general profile of low and higher molecular mass species, which was similar to that described by Plowman (2003) for extracts of sheep wool. Results for a western blot probed with an antibody preparation with specificity against a range of cytokeratins showed dense expression of type I cytokeratins at pH 0 -5 and also a long "train" of those of type II extending beyond pH 6. This result was similar to that described for wool by Plowman, (2003).

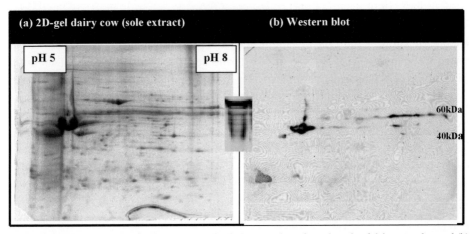

Figure 8. (a) Two-dimensional gel of extracts of soft tissue explants from the sole of dairy cow claw and (b) Western blot run using AE1/AE3 anti-cytokeratin antibody mixture and spots detected using Progenesis™ software. Insert shows a western blot from a 1-D gel (sole tissue extract) using AE1/AE3 anti-cytokeratin preparation. After Galbraith *et al.* (2006b).

Additional results derived from picking individual spots on gels from heel extracts followed by protein mass fingerprinting and reference to the *Bos taurus* database, provide a useful insight into expression of specific protein patterns for different sites (Figure 9).

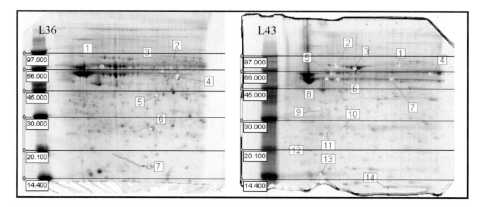

Figure 9. Gels (from heel extracts) used for spot picking and protein identification-based analysis of peptide fragments. Amersham marker used to show molecular mass. Circled spots indicate identified proteins using Progenesis™ software. Identification/similarity from Bos taurus database according to allocated spot number as follows: For L36 : 1. Keratin type II cytoskeletal 6A. 2. Keratin hair basic 5. 3. Selenium binding protein isoform 1. 4. Enolase 1. 5. 20a-hydroxysteroid dehydrogenase. 6. Heat shock protein B1. 7. Not identified. For L43: 1. Transferrin. 2. not identified. 3. Albumin. 4. Keratin complex 2 (gene 6a, isoform 4). 5. Cytoskeletal keratin 6C. 6. Cytoskeletal keratin 14. 7. Cytoskeletal keratin 14. 8. Cytoskeletal keratin 14. 9. not identified. 10. Heat shock protein B1. 11. Apolipoprotein. 12. not identified. 13. Adipocyte-type fatty acid binding protein. 14. Unidentified. After Galbraith *et al.* (2006b).

The results show the presence both cytokeratins (e.g. 6A and 6C, and 14) and trichocyte keratins (hair basic 5 identified) and proteins involved in metabolism of energy (enolase), steroids (20a-hydroxysteroid dehydrogenase), minerals (selenium binding protein isoform 1: transferrin (iron transport), adipose tissue (adipocyte-type fatty acid binding protein), cholesterol transport (apolipoprotein), metabolic stress and regulation (heat shock protein (HSPB1), the presence of which has been identified in extracts of wool (Plowman *et al.*, 2005)). The gel images also show the presence of protein species in the range of the lower molecular mass values expected of IFAPs, but these have not been identified. The presence of albumin is a reminder of the vascular nature of the dermal component of tissues studied and the possible provision of proteins from residual blood in tissue explants.

Given the importance of cysteine in the largely proteinaceous horn product there has been considerable interest in the supply of this amino to the claw epidermis. Sources are predominantly metabolisable protein from the digestive tract and methionine by post-absorptive metabolic transulphuration with the sulphur moiety supplied by methionine via homocysteine and the carbon skeleton from the non-essential amino acid serine (Reis, 1989). Analysis of horn tissue for a range of amino acids has allowed comparison with concentrations present in rumen microbial protein and common sources of ruminant feeds (Table 3). It is apparent that, of all of the amino acids, the proportion of cysteine from these sources is less (0.2-0.33) than that deposited in the horn samples studied. It is also of interest to note that methionine which, although a "sulphur-containing amino acid", is present to a considerably lower extent than cysteine and does not contribute directly to the formation of structurally-important disulphide bond formation. However, methionine is nutritionally essential and it has roles as the initial amino acid with starter codon (AUG) in peptide translation and synthesis, methylation, and synthesis of polyamines in addition to a role in structure of horn proteins, albeit at a lower concentration than cysteine (Reis, 1989). The low "working value" of 0.26 for the efficiency of utilisation of metabolisable protein for wool/hair production by ruminants reflects the relative imbalance between composition of supply of certain amino acids particularly cysteine, with that of keratinous end product (AFRC, 1993).

In this context, an important general consideration is the effect of competition between tissues and organs in the body for individual nutrients. This applies to all nutrients, whether derived from the diet or entering systemic circulation from endogenous sources. Mechanisms determining efficiency of uptake by individual cells include the presence of transport mechanisms. These in turn may be activated by hormones and growth factors in response to sensing of requirement and the need to maintain homeostatic concentrations in systemic circulation. Competition for claw tissues of the dairy cow may arise from demands of skin, digestive tract, skeleto-musculature and, according to physiological state, mammary gland and foetus and associated structures.

With regard to cysteine, the question also arises as to methods of optimizing supply to the claw tissue to ensure support of synthesis of keratin and IFAPs. Since the sulphydril group of molecular L-cysteine is susceptible to oxidation, there has been major interest in indirect provision by supplementing diets with L-methionine (in rumen-protected and intestinally digestible forms) or its analogues. Such an approach, utilising up to 5g/day, increased growth of hair fibre in goats (Souri, Galbraith, and Scaife, 1998; Galbraith, Mengal and Scaife, 1998) and rates of growth of wall horn in goats (Galbraith *et al.*, 1998) and dairy cows (15g/day) (Metcalf, Marsh, Johnston, May and Livesey, 1998) which were not sustained beyond the initial four or six weeks of study. More recently, Laven and Livesey (2004) and Livesey and Laven (2007) reported absence of effects of rumen protected methionine supplementation (15g/day) on development of haemorrhages or rates of growth and wear in claw horn of primiparous dairy cattle. Results from another study (Galbraith *et al.,* unpublished) showed that supplementation of dairy heifers throughout pregnancy with 5–6g/day rumen-protected L-methionine increased systemic blood concentrations (23.2 vs 19.2 μmol/litre) but had no effect on growth characteristics of, or concentrations of L-methionine or L-cysteine in, claw wall horn collected 2–3 days *post partum* (Galbraith *et al.*, 2006a). The above results contrast with those of Clark and Rakes (1982) who reported increases in rates of growth but reductions in the incorporation of cysteine into upper wall claw horn of dairy cattle supplemented with 30 g/day of methionine hydroxy analogue for

70–90 days. The efficiency of its conversion to methionine, which is required for the synthesis of cysteine, was not recorded. There are clear questions concerning the positive responses to methionine supplementation in wool and apparent absence in cattle horn. These may relate to the quantities required of methionine and more particularly cysteine to support animal fibre production of up to 5kg per year in small ruminants and the lesser production of an estimated 600g/year for dairy cattle claw horn (Hepburn *et al.,* 2008).

Recent studies (Hepburn *et al.,* 2008) investigated the characteristics of bovine claw tissues with respect to supply of methionine and cysteine using explants and *in vitro* tissue culture systems. In terms of uptake of methionine using its [35]S -labelled form, the data showed considerable capacity at mmol/litre concentrations, with uptake maximising at around 30 minutes. Subsequent investigation gave values for K_M (concentration at which uptake rate is 0.5 that of its maximal value) of 3.61 mmol/litre.

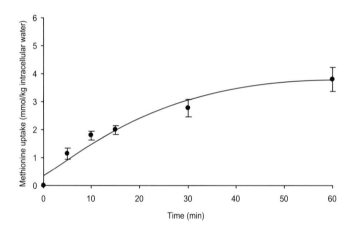

Figure 10. Time course for uptake of L-methionine by beef cattle solear tissue. Explants were incubated in DMEM/F12 L-methionine deficient medium supplemented with 1.0 mmol/litre methionine and 1.0 µCi/litre L-[35S]-methionine. Values shown are mean with SEM. After Hepburn *et al.* (2008).

Autoradiograhic measurements showed that the presence of radiographic label was concentrated in basal and suprabasal epidermis, when examined histologically, and gave normal patterns of protein banding typical of claw tissue extracts on electrophoretic separation. Autoradiographic signal on immunoblots also co-localised with those for cytokeratins known to be synthesised basally and suprabasally. This work also showed that estimates for synthesis of protein and DNA gave maximal rates in the range of 40-50 µmol/litre (Figures 11 and 12) which is ca. 0.1 that of maximum uptake capacity. These concentrations are within the normal physiological range of 20-50 µmol/litre (Shennan, Millar and Calvert, 1997; Hepburn *et al.,* 2008) and may provide a target at the upper concentrations, to be attained in systemic blood *in vivo.*

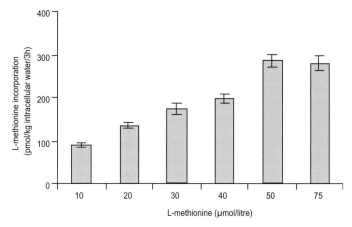

Figure 11. Effects of unlabelled L-methionine concentration on protein synthesis in dairy cattle solear tissue. Following 21h incubation, explants were incubated with 6.0 µCi/ml L-[35$_S$]-methionine and its incorporation was measured after 3 h. Values are shown as means with SEM. After Hepburn *et al*. (2008).

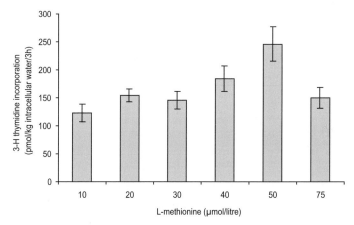

Figure 12. Effects of unlabelled L-methionine concentration on DNA synthesis in dairy cattle solear tissue. Following 21h incubation, explants were incubated with 2.5 µCi/ml [³H]methyl-thymidine and its incorporation was measured after 3 h. Values are shown as means with SEM. After Hepburn *et al*. (2008).

It was also shown that the presence of L-cysteine and L-cystine at varying concentrations in the culture medium had limited effect on uptake of ³⁵S-L-methionine or incorporation of ³⁵S-label into protein fractions. These data, in the context of other measures for effects on protein synthesis, indicate the effectiveness of conversion of methionine to cysteine in bovine claw horn tissues. The results are also consistent with those described by Reis (1989), who suggested that these amino acids had equivalent efficacy is supplying cysteine for wool production in sheep.

Additional studies that measured responses to provision of different concentrations of methionine to claw explant tissues from different anatomical regions utilised the proteomics approach. Conventional comparisons were made of "averaged" (i.e. protein spots present in at least 2 out of 3 or 3 out of 5 replicates) 2-dimensional gels of extracts of implants incubated for up to 48h in culture medium containing either 1.0 or 30.0 μmol/litre methionine. Typical profiles of extracts for coronary, laminar, sole and heel explants are shown in Figure 13. Analysis was made of numbers of spot counts which were unmatched (i.e. present on gels following incubation at 1.0 but not 30.0 μmol/litre methionine). The values obtained were 24, 36, 35 and 65 for coronary, laminar, sole and heel explants respectively. These results indicate differences both between source of explant and response to differences in supply of methionine. Further analysis to identify individual protein spots is ongoing.

Inflammation, lipids and implications for nutrition and claw health

Little is known about the nature of the inflammatory processes associated with the onset of laminitis or the development of other lesions. In terms of a prophylactic role for lipids, there is interest in increasing the quantities of n-3 polyunsaturated fatty acids (PUFAs) in tissues. These are known to decrease incorporation of arachidonic acid into cell membranes and, consequently, the quantities available for production of pro-inflammatory eicosanoids such as thromboxanes, prostaglandins, and leukotrienes.. These pro-inflammatory compounds stimulate production of other mediators including tumour necrosis factor, interleukin-1, and interleukin-6 as cytokines which have inflammatory effects in animal systems (Calder, 2006). Reductions in expression of adhesion molecules involved in inflammatory reactions between endothelial cells and leukocytes are also induced by the presence of n-3 polyunsaturates. Additional anti-inflammatory compounds induced by n-3 PUFAs include, from eicosapentaenoic acid (EPA) the resolvin mediators, and D-resolvins from docosahexaenoic acid (DHA). These relationships suggest the possibility of manipulating lipid profiles in claws by dietary means and of providing a means to reduce the severity of inflammatory processes associated with lameness. One approach could include supplementation of cow diets with protected fish oils to increase the content, in claw tissues, of the anti-inflammatory n-3 PUFAs, EPA and DHA. As indicated above, the results of Offer *et al.*, (1998) suggest that such an approach has potential to alter the spectrum of PUFA in bovine claw tissues.

Lameness due to infectious dermatitis

The major cause of lameness produced by microbial infections in dairy cattle is digital dermatitis Murray (2004). This condition is associated with indoor conditions, poor hygiene and exposure of skin above the heel of the claw to excreta.

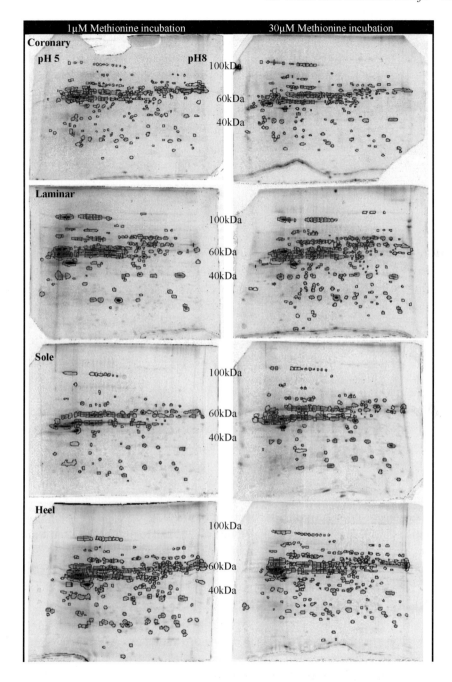

Figure 13. Averaged 2-D gels showing common spots for soft tissue explants from four anatomical regions incubated *in vitro* at 1.0 or 30µM (µmol/litre) methionine. Circled spots detected by Progenesis™ software. After Galbraith *et al.* (2006b).

Laven (2007) recently described relationships between heel height and toe length of claws and lesion score for first-calving Holstein heifers. Infection typically presents as lesions which penetrate through the epidermis and into dermis of the skin above the epidermal horn of the bulb. Lesions may be ulcerative and may display hyperplasia and hyperkeratosis of the epidermis with progression towards healing over time (Murray, 2004). There has been particular interest in a number of phylotypes of the genus *Treponema* which have been frequently isolated from lesions and which have similarities with those causing human dental infections. Virulence factors noted for treponemal isolates have included adhesion to dermal fibronectin and proteolytic properties of outer membrane and cytotoxic effects on epidermal cells (Edwards, Dymock and Jenkinson, 2003). The induction of the innate immune response by neutrophils has been suggested as a major contributor to the tissue damage observed in treponema-induced infections of the mouth. Chemical mediators of inflammation and cytokines have been shown to be released in addition to direct effects of the organisms on fibroblasts and production of a range of pro-inflammatory cytokines (Nixon, Steffen and Ebersole, 2000). It is not known to what degree such responses occur in bovine claw skin, nor whether such production is responsible for the proliferation and differentiation effects on epidermal keratinocytes. In addition, increasing activity of matrix metalloproteinases, which act to break down connective and other tissues, have been noted (Murray, 2004).

Nebel, Mülling, Nordhoff and Budras (2004) reported development of a system to investigate interactions of treponemal isolates with bovine skin explants *in vitro*. These workers showed (i) the adhesion of treponemes to isolated skin tissue keratinocytes and (ii) penetration, by the organisms, of epidermis of skin tissue explants via intercellular spaces of *stratum corneum* and *stratum spinosum*. The cornified epidermal barrier may be considered a major line of defence in protecting underlying tissues against attack by infectious treponema. Consequently, nutritional measures targeted at improving the supply of structural lipids in addition to those with anti-inflammatory activity may usefully be applied to optimise barrier function of cells, as suggested for the maintenance of claw horn epidermis.

Nutritional imbalances, physiological status and lameness

As stated above, the major cause of claw horn lameness is damage to tissues in dermis and epidermis of the claw. One suggested origin of such damage is that arising, in the vascular dermis, from disturbance in microcirculation and associated with inflammation of varying severity (Nocek, 1997). This symptom of "laminitis" has been associated in turn with ruminal acidosis produced by excessive provision, in the diet, of readily fermentable starch-based carbohydrates and production, in turn, of excessive quantities of ruminal lactic acid (Nocek, 1997). Inadequate provision of cellulosic fibre is also recognised as an important risk factor. Physiological responses include lowering of blood pH and systemic and local vasoactive effects causing inflammation on claw dermis, hypoxia and tissue damage. Recently, Gozho, Krause and Plaizier (2007) demonstrated that feeding fermentable grain-based diets induced sub-acute ruminal acidosis and increased quantities of pro-inflammatory lipopolysaccaride (LPS) in the rumen of lactating dairy cows. Ruminal lipopolysaccahride (LPS: endotoxin) was significantly increased but was not measurable in systemic blood. Serum amyloid A concentration was also increased, showing activation of an inflammatory response. Further evidence relating rumen fermentable carbohydrate nutrition to production of laminitis was provided by Thoefner, Pollitt, van Eps, Milinovich, Trott, Wattle and Andersen (2004) and by Thoefner, Wattle, Pollitt, French and Nielsen (2005). These workers gave an alimentary overdose of oligofructose to dairy-breed heifers and observed a number of responses, including acute laminitis and, on post mortem histological examination, stretching of laminae and changes in basement membrane structure. There are clear parallels with the equine model of diet-induced clinical and histological laminitis by oligofructose administration, as described by van Epps and Pollitt (2006).

Other nutritional inputs affecting claw health include the forage component of dairy diets. For example, Offer, Leach, Brocklehurst and Logue (2003) and Leach, Offer, Svoboda and Logue (2005) compared responses of heifers to diets varying in dry matter of the forage component at various stages during rearing, and for six months after subsequent calving. Low dry matter diets based on grass silage, gave rise to significantly worse lesions of white line and sole, and softer horn at abaxial sole and heel sites than diets with dry forage based on straw. These effects were associated with greater heel erosion and with standing longer in less-viscous slurry. "Direct dietary effects" on claw horn health due to digestive or post-absorptive effects, such as variation in end-products of rumen fermentation or production of rumen microbial protein, which may also have contributed to the results, remain to be explained.

Anatomical and physiological development, regulation and claw health

In terms of physiological regulation of development and maintenance of functionally healthy claws, important considerations are growth in utero and post partum, as the animals progress to mature body size and anatomical structure and composition. These processes are regulated by a range of signalling systems which orchestrate commitment to differentiation and proliferation and hypertrophy of cells and tissues. Little is known about the interactions between dermis and epidermis that give rise to specialised papillary and laminar structures in the claw. There may be parallels with development of structures in the hair follicle, which are thought to involve families of genes responsible for producing molecular signals that direct mitogenesis and morphogenesis in dermis and epidermis of the skin (Galbraith, 2006). These include a range of growth factors; there is particular interest in the WNT signalling pathway and the gene product sonic hedgehog.

Major events in the post-natal growth of the dairy cow include development of a functional reproduction system, and the changes, with suggested homeorhetic regulation of nutrient partition, (Bauman and Currie, 1981), in physiological state associated with pregnancy and subsequent lactation. Applied aspects with respect to nutrition and management of these physiological states and in relation to lameness are reviewed elsewhere in these proceedings (Huxley, 2007).

Some limited information is available on post-natal development of claw anatomy (Table 1), changes which may occur in claw horn quality during pregnancy, and effects on subsequent lactation. The latter have been studied by Kempson and Logue (1993) with respect to horn of the white line in heifers. These workers showed that good quality horn, which was characterised by good cellular structure, effective keratinisation and tight intercellular alignment, was associated with better claw horn health post partum.

This observation is important since the major incidence of claw horn lesions is known to occur in the first 10 weeks after calving (Tarlton *et al.*, 2002), concomitant with the changing physiological states of pregnancy, parturition and lactation (mammary development and milk production). Tarlton *et al.* (2002) compared post-mortem tissues of calving heifers with those of maiden heifer controls two weeks before, and four and 12 weeks after, calving. The results showed that calving heifers had a greater laxity of the laminar suspensory system than maiden heifers. The results suggested that such a weakening of laminar connective tissue predisposed the heifers to tissue damage indicative of solear ulcers and white line disease. Differences in properties of connective tissue at different sites of measurement were associated with altered chemical and macromolecular composition and variation in activities of matrix metalloprotease 2 and tissue inhibitor of metalloproteases. Widening and distortion of laminae atypical of inflammatory laminitis were also observed, on histological evaluation, with faster recovery evident for front compared with rear lateral claws. Tarlton *et al.* (2002) considered that systemic signalling for relaxin and oestradiol -17ß, which have been associated with connective tissue breakdown and remodelling in other tissues, may have a role in producing the observed effects. Current evidence therefore suggests that nutritionally-based laminitic effects and those of endogenous physiological signalling acting independently, may both give rise to lesions of the laminae and reduced protection against impact injuries of vascular dermis and soft tissue basement membrane and epidermis of the sole.

A possible role for systemic hormones such as insulin, cortisol, and prolactin which variously respond to nutritional supply has been investigated by Hendry, MacCallum, Knight and Wilde, (1999) using an *in vitro* claw tissue explant system. Insulin was shown to stimulate cell proliferation, and cortisol to inhibit protein synthesis, although prolactin had no effect on either. Other systemic hormones that respond to supply of absorbed nutrients or nutritional status and which have catabolic or anabolic actions on tissues include growth hormone, insulin-like growth factors and those associated with adipose tissue cells such as leptin. The effects of these on composition and functional properties of claw tissues is unknown.

Minerals and vitamins and claw health

A range of other essential nutrients that are expected to support the maintenance of good quality dermal and epidermal tissues and claw health have been reviewed by Tomlinson *et al.*, (2004). These include major minerals such as calcium, the blood concentrations of which are typically lowered in early lactation, and phosphorus, magnesium and trace minerals such as zinc, copper, manganese, cobalt and selenium. There is particular interest in selenium for enzymes such as glutathione peroxidase and (thyroxine) deiodinases which, for activity, depend on the presence of seleno-cysteine. Excessive quantities of seleno-cysteine in proteins may interfere with disulphide bonding in cytoskeletal structures. A range of vitamins is also essential for claw cell proliferation and metabolism. These include vitamins A and D and E, water-soluble B vitamins normally synthesised in the digestive tract, and vitamin C (endogenous synthesis) which is required for synthesis of collagens.

Where next?

This review has focused predominantly on the complexities of tissue, cell, extracellular and molecular aspects of lameness and nutrition in dairy cows in the context of data obtained from some applied studies. It has considered a range of nutrients required to meet requirements for production and maintenance of important anatomical structures and to provide substrate for production of horn. Certain nutrients were noted to support signal transduction and anabolic and catabolic enzyme systems. Examples were given where nutritional imbalances affect claw health, such as in ruminal acidosis, and the absence of responses to methionine suggest that this amino acid has not been limiting under the conditions of measurement. Biotin is known to have an essential role in health of integumental tissues and questions remain about the capacity of microrganisms in the digestive tract to contribute to fully meeting requirement of this and other vitamins. There is also scope for providing rumen-protected supplements containing precursors of anti-inflammatory fatty acids with a view to improving anti-inflammatory status in animals. The provision of adequate lipid to support maintenance of digital cushions of the claw, and protective barrier in the skin are also considered useful objectives but, as for other nutrients, competition with other tissues may interfere with desired partitioning. Interactions between nutrient supply and systemic physiological responses and health of claw horn are recognised as poorly understood as are endogenous mechanisms which may contribute to the growth of poor quality horn in pregnant heifers.

There are obvious gaps in our knowledge concerning the development and maintenance of dermal and epidermal structures needed to confer better resistance to the biomechanical challenges of contemporary husbandry and environments. Some animals avoid claw horn lesion formation better than others and the reasons for this, with respect to intrinsic integumental biology of the claw are essentially unknown. Genetic selection for such resistance, if the underlying biological factors were known, would be a useful approach to reducing the problem. Unfortunately, opportunities for improving knowledge of claw horn biology appear to be limited in the UK despite welfare issues concerning large numbers of animals affected with claw horn lameness. The limited funding for agricultural animal research was recently recognised by the UK Biotechnology and Biological Sciences Research Council with the CEDFAS (Combating Endemic Diseases of Farmed Animals for Sustainability) initiative. However, this initiative was targeted only at infectious endemic diseases and despite funding a project on bovine digital dermatis, did not apply to the major problem of non-infectious lameness. There would appear to be a requirement for further consideration, in an appropriate national forum, to correct this deficiency and to increase the priority in funding for such farm animal research.

References

AFRC (1993) Agricultural and Food Research Council. *Energy and Protein Requirements of Ruminants*. An Advisory Manual Prepared by the AFRC Technical Committee on Responses to Nutrients. CAB International, Wallingford.

Bauman, D.E. and Currie, W.B. (1980) Partitioning of nutrients during pregnancy and lactation: A review of mechanisms involving homeostasis and homeorhesis. *Journal of Dairy Science*, **63**, 1514-1529.

Bowden, P.E. (2005) The human type II keratin gene cluster on chromosome 12q13.13: Final count or hidden secrets? *Journal of Investigative*

Dermatology, **124 (3)**, XV-XVII.

Browne M. P., Hukins, D.W.L., Skakle J. M. S., Knight, C. H., Hendry, K. A. K., Wilde C. J and Galbraith, H (2007) X-ray diffraction and anatomical properties of claw tissues of beef and dairy cattle. *Journal of Agricultural Science*, **145**, 1-11.

Brownsey, R.W., Boone, A.N., Elliott, J.E., Kulpa, J.E. and Lee, W.M. (2006) Regulation of acetyl-CoA carboxylase. *Biochemical Society Transactions*, **34**, 223-227.

Bryant, K.L., Kornegay, E.T., Knight, J.W., Webb, K.E. and Notter, D.R. (1985) Supplemental biotin for swine. 3 Influence of supplementation to corn-based and wheat-based diets on the incidence and severity of toe lesions, hair and skin characteristics and structural soundness of sows in confinement during four parities. *Journal of Animal Science*, **60**, 154-162.

Buda, S and Budras, K-D. (2004) Nature of the innervation of dermal blood vessels in the claw suggests a central and local co-regulation of microcirculation. In *13th International Symposium of Lameness in Ruminants*, p 7 Edited by B. Zemljic. Maribor, Slovenia.

Budras, K.D., Geyer, H., Maierl, J. and Mülling, C.K.W. (1998) Anatomy and structure of hoof horn (Workshop report). In *10th International Symposium on Lameness in Ruminants,* pp 176-199. Edited by C. J. Lischer and P. Ossent. University of Zurich, Zurich.

Budras, K.D. and Habel,R.E. (2003). *Bovine Anatomy, An Illustrated Text*. Schlütersche GmbH & Co. Hanover, Germany.

Calder, P.C. (2006) n-3 polyunsaturated fatty acids, inflammation, and inflammatory diseases. *American Journal of Clinical Nutrition*, **83**, 1505S-1519S.

Candi, E., Tarcsa, E., Digiovanna, J.J., Compton, J.G., Elias, P.M., Marekov, L.N. and Steinert, P.M. (1998) A highly conserved lysine residue on the head domain of type II keratins is essential for the attachment of keratin intermediate filaments to the cornified cell envelope through isopeptide crosslinking by transglutaminases. *Proceedings of the National Academy of Sciences of the United States of America*, **95 (5),** 2067-2072.

Clark, A. K. and Rakes, A. H. (1982) Effect of methionine hydroxy analog supplementation on dairy cattle hoof growth and composition. *Journal of Dairy Science,* **65**, 1493–1502.

Crespo, R., Galbraith, H. and Finn, D. (1999). Expression of extracellular matrix proteins in solear tissues of Holstein-Friesian dairy cattle. In *Proceedings of the Symposium on Metabolic Stress in Dairy Cows*, pp 209 – 214. BSAS Occasional Publication no. 24. British Society of Animal Science, Edinburgh.

Cross, D.E. (1998) A survey of claw measurements and histological studies in relation to lameness in young dairy animals and comparison of these animal with older cows. M.Sc Thesis. University of Aberdeen.

Edwards, A.M., Dymock, D., Woodward, M.J, and Jenkinson, H.F. (2003) Genetic relatedness and phenotypic characteristics of Treponema associated with human periodontal tissues and ruminant foot disease. *Microbiology-SGM*, **149 (5)**, 1083-1093.

Frohberg-Wang, D., Mülling, C.K.W. and Budras, K.D. (2004) Cellular communication channels in bovine claw epidermis and their functional role for horn formation. In *13ᵗʰ International Symposium on Lameness in Ruminants*. pp. 234–236. Edited by B. Zemljic. Maribor, Slovenia.

Galbraith, H. (1995) The effects of diet on nutrient partition in Scottish Cashmere and Angora goats. In *The Nutrition and Grazing Ecology of Speciality Fibre Animals*, pp 23-50. Edited by J.P. Laker, and A.J.F. Russel. European Fine Fibre Network Publication No. 3. Macaulay land Use Research Institute, Aberdeen.

Galbraith, H. (1998) Nutritional and hormonal regulation of hair follicle growth and development. *Proceedings of the Nutrition Society,* **57,** 1-12.

Galbraith H. (2006) A current perspective on the biology of fibre production. In *Progress in South American Camelids Research, Volume 2*, pp 195-207. Edited by M.Gerken and C. Renieri, Wageningen Academic Publishers, The Netherlands.

Galbraith, H., Mengal, M. and Scaife, J.R. (1998) Effect of dietary methionine and biotin supplementation on growth and protein and amino acid composition of caprine hoof horn. In *10th International Symposium on Lameness in Ruminants,* pp. 227–229. Edited by Ch. J. Lischer and P. Ossent. Lucerne, Switzerland

Galbraith, H., Rae, H., Omand, T., Hendry, K.A.K., Knight, C.H. and Wilde, C J. (2006a) Effect of supplementing pregnant heifers with methionine or melatonin on the anatomy and other characteristics of their lateral hind claws. *The Veterinary Record* **156**, *21-24.*

Galbraith, H., Flannigan, S., Swan,L. and Cash, P. (2006b) Proteomic evaluation of tissues at functionally important regions in the bovine claw. *Cattle Practice,* **14**, 127-137.

Gillespie, J.M. (1991) The structural proteins of hair. Isolation, characterisation and regulation of biosynthesis. In *Physiology, Biochemistry and Molecular Biology of Skin*, pp. 625-659. Edited by L.A. Goldsmith, Oxford University Press, New York.

Gray, G. M., and Yardley, H. J. (1975a) Different populations of pig epidermis cells: isolation and lipid composition. *Journal of Lipid Research,* **16**, 441-47.

Gray, G. M., and Yardley, H. J. (1975b) Lipid composition of cells isolated from pig, human and rat epidermis. *Journal of Lipid Research,* **16,** 434-440.

Gozho, G.N., Krause, D.O. and Plaizier, J.C. (2007) Ruminal lipopolysaccharide concentration and inflammatory response during grain-induced subacute ruminal acidosis in dairy cows. *Journal of Dairy Science*, **90 (2)**, 856-866.

Green, L. and Muelling, C.K.W. (2005) Biotin and lameness – a review. *Cattle Practice*, **13**, 145-153.

Greenough, P. R., Weaver, D.A., Broom, D.M., Esslemont, R.J. and Galindo, F. A. (1997) Basic concepts of bovine lameness. In *Lameness in Cattle, Third Edition,* pp 71-86. Edited by P.R. Greenough. and A. D. Weaver. W.B. Saunders, Philadelphia.

Hamanaka S., Hara M., Nishio, H., Otsuka, F., Suzuki, S. and Uchida, Y. (2002) Human epidermal glucosylceramides are major precursors of stratum corneum ceramides. *Journal of Investigative Dermatology*, **119** 416-23.

Hashimoto, Y., Suga, Y., Matsuba, S., Mizoguchi, M., Takamori, K., Seitz, J. and Ogawa, H. (2001) Inquiry into the role of skin sulfhydryl oxidase in epidermal disulfide bond formation: Implications of the localization and regulation of skin SOx as revealed by TPA, retinoic acid, and UVB radiation. *Journal of Investigative Dermatology*, **117**, 752–754;

Heid, H.W., Werner, E., Franke, W.W. (1986) The complement of native α-keratin polypeptides of hair forming cells: A subset of eight polypeptides that differ from epithelial cytokeratins. *Differentiation,* **32** 101–119.

Hendry, K.A.K., Knight, C.H., Galbraith, H. and Wilde C.J. (2003) Basement membrane integrity and keratinisation in healthy and ulcerated bovine hoof tissue. *Journal of Dairy Research*, **70**, 19-27.

Hendry, K.A.K., MacCallum, A.J., Knight, G.H. and Wilde,C.J. (1999) Effect of endocrine and paracrine factors on protein synthesis and cell proliferation in bovine hoof tissue culture. *Journal of Dairy Research,* **66,** 23–33.

Hepburn, N.L., Kinninmonth, L. and Galbraith, H. (2007) Pigmentation, impression hardness and the presence of melanosomes in bovine claw tissue. *Journal of Agricultural Science,* **145**, 283-290.

Hepburn, N. L., Knight, C. H., Wilde, C. J., Hendry K. A.K. and Galbraith, H. (2008) Methionine uptake, incorporation and effects on proliferative activity and protein synthesis in bovine claw tissue explants in vitro. *Journal of Agricultural Science*, **146**, 103-115.

Hirschberg, R.M. and Plendel, J. (2004) Pododermal angiogenesis- new aspects of development and function of the bovine claw. In *13ᵗʰ International Symposium of Lameness in Ruminants*, pp 67-69. Edited by B. Zemljic, Maribor, Slovenia.

Hitomi, K. (2005) Transglutaminases in skin epidermis. *European Journal of Dermatology,* **15 (5)**, 313-319.

Huxley, J. (2007) Lameness in dairy cows: impact of practical nutritional and environmental management. In *Recent Advances in Animal Nutrition –*

2007, pp 75 - 98. Edited by P.C. Garnsworthy and J. Wiseman. Nottingham University Press, Nottingham.

Jenkins, T.C. and McGuire, M.A. (2006) Major advances in nutrition: impact on milk composition. *Journal of Dairy Science,* **89**, 1302-1310.

Kempson, S.A.,and Logue, D.N. (1993) Ultrastructural observations of hoof horn from dairy cows - changes in the white line during the 1st lactation. *Veterinary Record ,* **132 (21)**, 524-527.

Lamecow (2007) http://template.bio.warwick.ac.uk/E+E/lamecow/public_html/lesions.html. Accessed August 2007.

Lampe, M. A., Burlingame, A. L., Whitney, J., Williams, M. L., Brown, B. E., Roitman, E. and Elias, P. M. (1983a) Human stratum corneum lipids: characterisation and regional variations. *Journal of Lipid Research,* **24**, 120-30.

Lampe, M.A., Williams, M. L., and Elias, P. M. (1983b) Human epidermal lipids: characterisation and modulations during differentiation. *Journal of Lipid Research,* **24**, 131-40.

Laven, R.A. (2007) The relationship between hoof conformation and digital dermatitis in dairy cattle. *Cattle Practice,* **15**, 93-95.

Laven, R.A. and Livesey, C.T. (2004) The effect of housing and methionine intake on hoof horn hemorrhages in primiparous lactating holstein cows. *Journal of Dairy Science,* **87 (4**), 1015-1023.

Leach, K.A., Offer, J.E., Svoboda, I. and Logue, D.N. (2005) Effects of type of forage fed to dairy heifers: Associations between claw characteristics, clinical lameness, environment and behaviour. *Veterinary Journal,* **169 (3)**, 427-436.

Lischer, C. J. and Ossent, P. (2000) Sole ulcers in dairy cattle – what's new about an old disease. In *Proceedings of the XI International Symposium on Disorders of the Ruminant Digit*, pp 46-55. Edited by C.M. Mortellaro, L. De Veechis and A. Brizzi. Brescia, Italy

Lischer, C. J., Ossent, P., Raber, M. and Geyer, H. (2002) Suspensory structures and supporting tissues of the third phalanx of cows and their relevance to the development of typical sole ulcers (Rusterholtz ulcers). *Veterinary Record,* **151**, 694-698.

Livesey, C.T. and Laven, R.A. (2007) Effects of housing and intake of methionine on the growth and wear of hoof horn and the conformation of the hooves of first-lactation Holstein heifers. *Veterinary Record,* **160 (14),** 470-476.

Lodish, H., Baltimore, D., Berk, A., Zipursky, S.L., Matsudaira, P. and Darnell, J. (1995) *Molecular Cell Biology*, Third Edition. W. H. Freeman, New York.

Logue, D. N., Offer, J.E. and Murray, R.D. (2006) Improving claw trimming in cattle: Onwards from the Dutch Technique. *The Veterinary Journal,* **172 (2):** 204-206.

Maas-Szabowski, N., Shimotoyodome, A. and Fusenig, N.E. (1999) Keratinocyte growth regulation in fibroblast cocultures via a double paracrine mechanism. *Journal of Cell Science*, **112**, 1843-1853.

Metcalf, J.A., Marsh,C., Johnston, A.M., May, S.A. and Livesey, C.T. (1998) Effect of dietary methionine supplementation on hoof horn growth in primiparous cows. *Proceedings of the British Society of Animal Science*, p.200. Penicuik.

Meyer, K (2004) Dairy cow lameness: biotin, lipids and the structural integrity of hoof horn. PhD thesis, University of Aberdeen.

Meyer, K., Köster, A., Mülling, C., Scaife, J.R., Birnie, M. and Budras, K-D. (2003) Influence of biotin supplementation on the fatty acid pattern in bovine claw horn and its role for the function and integrity of the bovine hoof. In *Proceedings of the XXII World Buiatrics Congress*, pp. 78. Hannover, Germany.

Millar, S.E. (2002) Molecular mechanisms regulating hair follicle development. *Journal of Investigative Dermatology*, **118**, 216-225.

Moll, R., Franke, W.W., Schiller, D.L., Geiger, B.and Krepler, R. (1982) The catalogue of human cytokeratins: Patterns of expression in normal epithelia, tumours, and cultured cells. *Cell,* **31**, 11–24,

Mülling, C. (2000) Three-dimensional appearance of bovine epidermal keratinocytes in different stages of differentiation revealed by cell maceration and scanning electron microscopic investigation. *Folia Morphologica,* **59**, 239-46.

Mülling, C. K. W. (2002) Theories on the pathogenesis of white line disease. In *12th International Symposium on Lameness in Ruminants*, pp 90-98. Edited by J.K.Shearer. University of Florida, Orlando.

Mülling, C.K.W., Wustenberg, R.Y., Nebel, U., Hoffmann, D. and Budras, K.D. (2006) Innovative in vitro and ex vivo models in multidisciplinary European lameness research. *Cattle Practice*, **14,** 115-121.

Murray, R.D. (2004) Aetio-pathogenesis of anaerobic infections associated with bovine lameness and some human diseases. In *13th International Symposium of Lameness in Ruminants*, pp 138-141. Edited by B. Zemljic, Maribor, Slovenia.

Nagorcka B.N. and Mooney, J.R. (1982) The role of a reaction diffusion system in the formation of hair fibers. *Journal of Theoretical Biology,* **98 (4)**, 575-607.

Nebel,U., Mülling, C.K.W., Nordhoff, M. and Budras, K.D. (2004) In vitro infection of bovine epidermal cells and bovine skin explants with treponemes. In *13th International Symposium of Lameness in Ruminants*, pp 141-143. Edited by B. Zemljic, Maribor, Slovenia.

Nixon, C.S., Steffen, M.J., Ebersole, J.L. (2000) Cytokine responses to Treponema pectinovorum and Treponema denticola in human gingival fibroblasts.

Infection and Immunity, **68 (9)**, 5284-5292.

Nocek, J.E. (1997) Bovine acidosis: implications on laminitis. *Journal of Dairy Science*, **80**, 1055-1028.

Odland, G.F. (1991). Structure of the skin. In *Physiology, Biochemistry and Molecular Biology of the Skin,* pp 3-62. edited by L.A.Goldsmith. Oxford University Press, Oxford.

Offer, J.E. and Logue, D.N. (1998) The effect of lameness in the dairy cow on the fatty acid profile of claw horn lipids. In *Proceedings of the 10th International Symposium on Ruminant Lameness.* pp 220-221. Edited by C.J. Lischer and P. Ossent. University of Zurich, Zurich.

Offer, J.E., Offer, N.W. and Logue, D.N. (2000) Effects of dietary fish oil supplementation on the hoof lipid fatty acid profiles of dairy cattle. In *Proceedings of the XI International Symposium on Disorders of the Ruminant Digit*, pp 322-324. Edited by C.M. Mortellaro, L. De Veechis and A. Brizzi. Parma Italy.

Offer, J.E., Leach, K.A., Brocklehurst, S. and Logue, D.N. (2003) Effect of forage type on claw horn lesion development in dairy heifers. *Veterinary Journal*, **165 (3)**, 221-227.

Onibi, G. E., Scaife, J. R., Murray, I. and Fowler, V. R. (2000) Supplementary a-tocopherol acetate in full-fat rapeseed-based diets for pigs: influence on tissue a-tocopherol content, fatty acid profiles and lipid oxidation. *Journal of the Science of Food and Agriculture*, **80**, 1625-1632.

Parry, D.A.D., Smith, T.A., Rogers, M.A. and Schweizer, J. (2006) Human hair keratin-associated proteins: Sequence regularities and structural implications. *Journal of Structural Biology,* **155 (2),** 361-369.

Plowman, J. E. (2003) Review. Proteomic database of wool components. *Journal of Chromatography B*, **787**, 63-76.

Raber, M., Lischer, C, J., Geyer, H and Ossent, P. (2004) The bovine digital cushion - a descriptive anatomical study. *The Veterinary Journal*, **176**, 258-264.

Raber, M., Scheeder, M.R.L., Ossent, P., Lischer, C, J. and Geyer, H. (2006) The content and composition of lipids in the digital cushion of the bovine claw with respect to age and location-a preliminary report. *The Veterinary Journal*, **172**, 173-177.

Reis, P.J. (1989) The influence of absorbed nutrients on wool growth. In *The Biology of Wool and Hair*, pp. 185-204. Edited by G.E. Rogers, P.J. Reis, K.A. Ward and R.C. Marshall. Chapman and Hall, Cambridge.

Rogers, M.A., Edler, L., Winter, H., Langbein, L., Beckmann, I. and Schweizer, J. (2005) Characterization of new members of the human type II keratin gene family and a general evaluation of the keratin gene domain on chromosome 12q13.13. *Journal of Investigative Dermatology*, **124 (3)**: 536-544.

Scaife, J., Meyer, K. and Grant, E. (2000) Comparison of the lipids of the bovine and equine hoof horn. In *Proceedings of the XI International Symposium on Disorders of the Runinant Digit*, pp 125-127. Edited by C.M. Mortellaro, L. De Veechis and A. Brizzi. Parma, Italy.

Scaife, J. R., Moyo, J., Galbraith, H., Michie, W. and Campbell, V. (1994) Effect of different dietary supplemental fats and oils on the growth performance and tissue fatty acid composition of female broilers. *British Poultry Science*, **35**, 107-118.

Scollan N.D., Enser M, Gulati S.K., Richardson I. and Wood J.D. (2003) Effects of including a ruminally protected lipid supplement in the diet on the fatty acid composition of beef muscle. *British Journal of Nutrition*, **90**, 709 -716.

Shennan, D.B., Millar, I.D. and Calvert, D.T. (1997) Mammary-tissue amino acid transport systems . *Proceedings of the Nutrition Society*, **56 (1A)**, 177-191.

Souri, M. Galbraith, H. and Scaife, J.R. (1998) Comparisons of the effect of protected methionine supplementation on growth, digestive characteristics and fibre yield in Cashmere-yielding and Angora goats. *Animal Science*, **66**, 217–223.

Steinert, P.M. and Freedberg, I.M. (1991) Molecular and cellular biology of keratins. In *Physiology, Biochemistry and Molecular Biology of Skin*, pp. 113-167. Edited by L.A. Goldsmith. Oxford University Press, Oxford.

Tarlton, J.F., Holah, D.E., Evans,K.M., Jones, S., Pearson, G. R. and Webster, A.J.F. (2002) Biomechanical and histopathological changes in the support structures of bovine hooves around the time of first calving. *The Veterinary Journal*, **163**, 196-204.

Thoefner, M.B., Pollitt, C.C., van Eps, A.W., Milinovich, G.J., Trott, D.J., Wattle, O, Andersen. P.H. (2004) Acute bovine laminitis: A new induction model using alimentary oligofructose overload *Journal of Dairy Science*, **87 (9)**, 2932-2940.

Thoefner, M.B., Wattle, O., Pollitt, C.C., French, K.R. and Nielsen, S.S. (2005) Histopathology of oligofructose-induced acute laminitis in heifers. *Journal of Dairy Science*, **88 (8)**, 2774-2782.

Tomlinson, D. J., Mülling, C.H. & Fakler, T.M. (2004) Formation of keratins in the bovine claw: Roles of hormones, minerals and vitamins in functional claw integrity. *Journal of Dairy Science* 87, 797-809.

Ueta, N., Kawamura, S., Kanazawa, I. and Yamakawa, T. (1971) On the nature of so-called ungulic acid. *Journal of Biochemistry.* **70**, 881-883.

Van Amstel, S. R., Shearer, J.K and Palin, F.L. (2004) Moisture content, thickness and lesions of sole horn associated with thin soles in dairy cattle. *Journal of Dairy Science,* **87**, 757-763.

van Eps, A.W.and Pollitt, C.C. (2004) Equine laminitis induced with oligofructose. *Equine Veterinary Journal,* **38 (3),** 203-208.

Vermunt, J.J. (2004) Herd lameness - a review, major causal factors and guidelines for prevention and control. In *13ᵗʰ International Symposium on Lameness in ruminants,* pp 3-18. Edited by B. Zemljic, Maribor, Slovenia.

Wertz, P.W. and Downing, D.T. (1991) Epidermal lipids. In *Physiology, Biochemistry and Molecular Biology of the Skin, 2ⁿᵈ Edition,* pp205-236. Edited by L.A. Goldsmith. Oxford University Press, Oxford.

Whitehead, C.C., Bannister, D.W., Wight, P.A.L. and Weiser, H. (1974) In *Proceedings of XV World Poultry Congress,* pp 70-72. New Orleans.

Zemplini, J. (2005) Uptake, location and noncarboxylase roles of biotin. *Annual Reviews of Nutrition,* **25, 175-196.**

6

TSEs AND BLUETONGUE – WHERE ARE WE NOW?

PAUL ROGER
Veterinary Consultancy Services, Reeth, N Yorks DL11 6SZ

Introduction

This paper concentrates on issues concerning two specific disease threats to our livestock industry. In the present climate it is inevitable that the lion's share goes to bluetongue, but the Transmissible Spongiform Encephalopathies (TSEs) should not be ignored. The importance of understanding the aetiology and pathogenesis of disease is highlighted by these two examples. They emphasise the need to promote good science and to learn more about disease so that we have the ability to support our necessary wholesome and local production of food, to ensure protection of consumers, and to support the welfare of livestock.

These two very different diseases present threats to our livestock industry in different ways. Control methods are difficult and imprecise, but the overall approach needs to be consensual with all the relevant "stakeholders" contributing to an agreed strategy based on a sound scientific approach and recognising the finite means available for disease control.

TSEs

The TSEs that occur naturally include diseases that affect Man (Table 1). The unknown nature of the infective transmission of these diseases creates concern, as the primary control is through genetic selection for decreased susceptibility. Genetically resistant stock do not express clinical disease but they may do if they live long enough – the resistance is to development of clinical disease rather than to disease itself. Vaccination is not a possible option for prevention because there is no measurable immune response and there are no preventive or therapeutic treatments available to treat affected animals.

Table 1. Naturally occurring scrapie-like diseases

Name of disease	Species affected
Scrapie	Sheep, Goat, Mouflon
Chronic wasting disease	Mule deer, White-tailed deer, El
Transmissable mink encephalopathy	Farmed mink
Bovine spongiform encephalopathy	Cattle, Nyala, gemsbok, oryx, eland, kudu, ankole, bison
Spongiform encephalopathy in primates	Lemur
Feline spongiform encephalopathy	Domestic cat, Puma, cheetah, ocelot, lion, panther
Kuru	Man
Creuzfeldt-Jakob disease	Man
Variant CJD	Man
Gerstmann –Staussler syndrome	Man
Fatal familial insomnia	Man

(After Jeffrey and González, 2007)

SCRAPIE

Scrapie in small ruminants is typical of the TSEs. Symptoms vary but develop in the final stages of disease and include trembling, pruritus and increasing incoordination. Diagnosis can only be carried out post-mortem. The current control strategy has been to select for the more resistant genotypes and against the two most susceptible genotypes. The aim is to produce lamb meat containing at least one of the more resistant genes, thus trying to reduce the tiny chance of TSE transmission into the human food chain.

The situation has been complicated by the emergence of atypical scrapie – a newly identified form of the TSE – identified by post-mortem surveillance of the central nervous system in sheep. With this form, there is no reported clinical sign and all genotypes appear susceptible.

The EU and the Standing Committee on Food Chain and Animal Health (SCoFCAH) have advised increased surveillance, but this has had the effect of suspending the drive towards prohibiting the use of the previously recognised high-risk genotypes.

It remains important for the industry that we continue to adequately fund research into TSEs and to support the scientific expertise that we have developed in the investigation of this disease complex within the UK and with other colleagues in Europe and beyond.

Bluetongue

Bluetongue is an arthropod-borne viral disease of ruminants. There is no zoonotic implication. There are 24 different identified serotypes causing differing symptoms, but all depend on the presence of competent vectors for spread of disease.

OCCURRENCE

Wild ruminant species are considered a potential reservoir for the Bluetongue virus (BTV). The disease is seen in white-tailed deer (*Odocoileus virginianus*) and pronghorn (*Antilocapra americana*) in the United States. However, only BTV-1, BTV-2, BTV-10, BTV-11, BTV-13 and BTV17 have been recorded in the United States. The first case of BTV-1 reported in 2006 was from a white-tailed deer.

White-tailed deer and pronghorn in the United States are affected much more severely than cattle and often even more severely than sheep. In deer and pronghorn, the mortality rate can be extremely high. Bluetongue signs in white-tailed deer are identical to those from infection with epizootic hemorrhagic disease (EHD) viruses. Both bluetongue and EHD virus infections cause a fulminating hemorrhagic disease and sudden death in white-tailed deer.

There has only been a limited amount of surveillance of BTV-8 in wildlife in the continuing BTV outbreak in Europe. The only positive serological samples were recorded in the Federal State of Northrhine-Westfalia, in the area where livestock were most severely affected. A total of 18 individuals tested positive, including red deer, roe deer and mouflon (*Ovis musimon*). These preliminary results indicated that the seroprevalence with regards to BTV-8 in wild ruminants was low in Germany in 2007. However a potential role of these animals in the epidemiology of the disease cannot be excluded.

In 2006, 70 deer (species not recorded) were tested in Belgium. 68 were negative by PCR and antibody ELISA. Two were positive by antibody ELISA alone, but the origin of these positive results was uncertain.

The recent experience in Europe suggests that "spillover" into deer occurs only when there are high infection levels in farmed ruminants.

In 2006, BTV 8 arrived in Northern Europe, a jump of some 700km from where BTV had previously been known and where competent vector populations of midges were thought not to exist (and even further as the source of this sub-saharan serotype 8 has been suggested as Nigeria). In 2006, the disease spread in Northern Europe and has worryingly recrudesced in 2007 with large numbers of infections being reported daily. The symptoms, which are classically reported as being worst in sheep with cattle often as symptomless carriers, are seemingly more severe in this naïve population and cattle often show severe symptoms. Recently the clinical disease has also been seen in goats and a fatal case has also been reported in a camelid in Germany.

There is anecdotal evidence of different breed susceptibility, but no analysis of the current outbreak has yet been published.

SYMPTOMS AND CAUSES

The wide range of clinical signs makes it difficult to recognise an index case, as similar symptoms can be seen with a number of other diseases, including photosensitivity, and Foot and Mouth Disease. Indeed researchers from The Institute for Animal Health, Pirbright highlight the difficulty in detecting bluetongue virus by clinical signs alone. It has been suggested in the initial core group meetings that if the infection is found first in a native animal rather than in an imported one, that that would be sufficient evidence that there was circulating virus in the domestic midge population. The limiting factor of recognition in the field will necessarily involve investigation of cases that do not yield virus. It remains essential that all farmers, veterinary practitioners and livestock keepers of all hues remain alert to the threat of the incursion of disease.

Control is fraught as insecticides are not particularly effective at controlling *Culicoides* spp and *C. dewulfi*, which has been identified as a vector, is found inside buildings as well as outside. There is a need to understand more about the biology of the midge vector and to develop control strategies to limit the opportunities to enable these midge populations to become infected.

These factors make the disease a frightening prospect for our livestock industry but, due to the time-lag between the arrival of the disease in Northern Europe and the arrival in the UK, we are in a much stronger position to control or eradicate the disease than our European neighbours.

The viral load in this country is currently low, and the reported cases found equally through report and surveillance indicate a contained area of infection. This advantage could all be wasted if freer movements are allowed during the "Vector Free Period" (VFP) when the midge species involved in transfer and spread of the virus are inactive. This is thought to be when the environmental temperature drops below 10°C. It is uncertain whether infected adults can effectively overwinter or whether there is vertical transmission of virus in the vector population, although this is thought to be unlikely.

SPREAD

Bluetongue (BTV) was first diagnosed in Suffolk on 22 September 2007. This followed an intense outbreak on the near continent originating at the end of July.

This continental outbreak followed an outbreak in 2006. As at 23 December 2007, there have been 66 premises confirmed positive for BTV divided equally between report (clinical cases) and those identified by serology.

BTV was diagnosed in July 2006 in animals in southern Holland. Subsequently it appears that the disease was present in Belgium and parts of Germany prior to this date. Morbidity and mortality were low but, unusually cattle were affected and displayed clinical signs.

In 2007, when the disease re-emerged at the end of July, it first appeared in flocks and herds known to have been infected in 2006.The disease this time was far more severe with a high morbidity and far higher mortality, reaching 20% in some flocks and resulting in the destruction on welfare grounds of many cattle which became recumbent and remained so due to severe coronitis.

BTV then spread rapidly westwards to affect all Holland and into Denmark; in Germany it spread eastwards and southwards. In France (largely clear in 2006), it spread southwards from the Belgian border eventually reaching Switzerland. Morbidity and mortality mirrored that in Holland.

In the UK, BTV has now affected farms in Norfolk, Suffolk, Essex, Kent and East Sussex, essentially the eastern and south-eastern counties of England. The UK was declared a BTV infected country late in September 2007 and the appropriate controls were put in place. The disease has largely been confined to its original location, except for an as yet unexplained case in Peterborough. The outbreak is following the same pattern as that which affected Europe in 2006, with initially low morbidity and low mortality. Of the 66 confirmed UK cases, only eight are in sheep. Notice should be taken of the Dutch experience, in which recrudescence occurred in flocks/herds infected the previous year.

Movement of animals that were antibody positive but antigen negative may have played a role in both spreading disease and increasing the viral load in Northern Europe in 2007. Judging by the differing interpretation by various Member States of the testing requirements laid down in the EU Bluetongue Directive, it may be that 2008 will see a further initial spread of disease triggered through these movements.

CONTROL MEASURES

The initial incursion of disease triggers the three-phase approach to the disease:

- **Phase One** - Rigorous controls in the very early stages of an incursion with the aim of containing disease and eradicating it if possible.
- **Phase Two** – Relaxation of controls once the impact of rigorous controls becomes disproportionate to the likelihood or benefits of eradication (i.e. evidence no longer supports the Phase One approach).

- **Phase Three** – Learning to live with disease with free movement and an acceptance of endemic infection.

Vaccination with a specific vaccine against the strain may be a useful weapon, but this is still in development and the frightening prospect that the Industry may need to live with the disease is looming. Three manufacturers indicate that an effective killed vaccine should be available from May 2008 onwards.

Defra have quickly tendered for 22.5 million doses. Cost is not yet available and vaccination programs vary from manufacturer to manufacturer. Defra have accepted the need to ensure that the 66 infected premises are vaccinated immediately after vaccine becomes available. They insist that vaccination must be on a voluntary basis. This raises serious doubts as to whether such a policy will quickly rid the UK of BTV.

In other EU member states, BTV incursions into southern Europe have occurred over the last few years with other serotypes, notably BTV1, 2 and 4. The use of inactivated vaccines has been reported (Savini et al., 2007). They demonstrated that where blanket vaccination was imposed, the disease was effectively controlled whilst the neighbouring country, which failed to vaccinate, encountered a serious outbreak. More recently, Spain has confirmed an outbreak of BTV1 in the Basque country. In response to this outbreak in Guipuzcoa province, the Spanish authorities intend to vaccinate all animals in the adjoining provinces of La Rioja, Navarra, Castilla and Catulunya

If we are to eradicate BTV 8 from the UK a voluntary vaccination is unlikely to be effective. Many diseases of both sheep and cattle can be controlled by vaccination, e.g. infectious abortion, respiratory disease etc., but every year many cases continue to be diagnosed and are recorded by veterinary surgeons and the VLA laboratories.

Control sheep scab when initially treatment was made voluntary just before deregulation failed spectacularly, and sheep scab is still common place in UK flocks. Only by compulsory blanket vaccination will there be any hope of eradicating BTV 8 swiftly from the UK.

Defra is loath to institute a compulsory scheme, quoting precedent. However, precedent for successful compulsory treatments was set in 1978 with the Warble Fly (England and Wales) Order 1978 (SI 1197). Under this order every owner had to compulsorily treat all their cattle with an approved insecticide in the spring. Owners were also encouraged, but not forced, to treat animals again in the autumn. The owner was responsible for the cost of the treatment and administration. Compliance was checked by Veterinary Officers from MAFF. In addition, some regional offices required the supplying veterinary practice to furnish a list of clients purchasing product. This was a remarkably successful operation and warble fly soon became a rarity.

If Defra consider that the early eradication of BTV from the UK is desirable, a vaccination scheme based on one similar to that for warble fly in the late 1970s would seem to fulfil the criteria. In the BTV Protection Zone (PZ) vaccine would be purchased from the owner's veterinary surgeon, who could inform the local Defra office of uptake. Checks could be arranged through the Cattle Passport Scheme, and sheep flocks are registered. Such checking of compliance would not be an expensive exercise.

All animals entering the PZ would also be required to be fully vaccinated before entry, thus reducing the reservoir of susceptible animals available for viral maintenance and replication.

Movement of animals other than to slaughter in the current PZ is at a minimum in late May to mid July. If it were compulsory, such a scheme would be far more likely to attract EU funding, thus reducing the overall implementation costs to both Defra and the Industry. Precedent has been established, thus enabling all susceptible animals in the current PZ to be compulsorily vaccinated. Such vaccination will greatly reduce the chance of recrudescence in the 66 infected premises and will protect those susceptible animals in the PZ from further incursions from the continent.

We have a narrow window of opportunity to control and eradicate this disease in the UK and in the Northern EU whilst viral load in the UK is relatively low, provided that we have sufficient vaccine to cover our livestock population and are prepared for a campaign which will have to last for 2 -3 years.

Compensation is payable in accordance with the *Animal Health Act 1981* (or the *Disease of Animal (NI) Order 1981*) for animals destroyed for the purpose of disease control, including animals destroyed for diagnosis. Compensation should not be payable in the following circumstances:

• Imported infected animals slaughtered on a discretionary basis (under Import Regulations) as a disease risk; seriously affected animals destroyed for welfare reasons by decision of the owner, with or without advice of a veterinary surgeon.

The import of animals that transit infected areas or originate within infected areas is a risk for which the cost should be borne completely by the importer as it represents a considerable threat to the local livestock population.

Carcasses and contaminated materials must be disposed of in accordance with statutory requirements. There is no BTV disease risk associated with carcasses. Normal cleansing should be performed. There is no BTV disease risk associated with contamination of housing, equipment or fomites.

Information must be provided to all livestock owners, veterinary surgeons and other stakeholders, particularly within the Restricted Zone. This information must explain the signs of BTV and action to take if the disease is suspected. Information about movement restrictions and licensing procedures must be made widely available.

Additional information setting out clearly the responsibilities and restrictions applicable to infected premises and those within the designated area must be provided to these owners. Information must be provided on:

- Recording of animal movements, illness, deaths and births and any authorised introduction
- Measures to limit exposure of susceptible animals to vectors
- Vector control methods
- Safe use of insecticides and any with-holding periods after treatment before animals or products can be used for human consumption
- Results and interpretation of tests.

Owners must be advised of the results of any BTV tests performed on their animals and what the results mean.

The general public will be kept informed about the disease, the outbreak and control measures being implemented. The public will be re-assured that Bluetongue does not affect humans and has no public health implications. The public also needs to be informed that BTV is not spread in carcasses or fomites.

SERO-SURVEILLANCE

This will be required in the years following an outbreak in areas where BTV had been circulating the previous year with the objective to determine the following:

- Has BTV persisted over winter?
- Has it been reintroduced?
- Confirmation that BTV is no longer present.

Appropriate sampling should begin when vector numbers are increasing, usually from May onwards, and should continue on a monthly basis until vectors are unlikely to still be capable of spreading BTV, usually November although this may vary with geographical and climatic variations across the country.

If BTV is circulating, an appropriate response program will have to be implemented. The surveillance programme will be designed according to the circumstances of the previous outbreak and in accordance with the EU Regulation requirements.

VECTOR MONITORING

Vector sampling using light traps may also be undertaken to determine their geographical and seasonal distribution and prevalence in risk areas.

The World Organisation for Animal Health (OIE) International Animal Health Code, Chapter 2.2.13.2. Bluetongue specifies as below. Any Member State wishing to obtain disease free status would also need to seek agreement at EU SCoFCAH Committee.

BTV FREE COUNTRY OR ZONE

A country or a *zone* may be considered free from BTV when bluetongue is notifiable in the whole country and either:

- The country or *zone* lies wholly north of 53°N or south of 34°S, and is not adjacent to a country or *zone* not having a free status; or

- A surveillance programme has demonstrated no evidence of BTV in the country or *zone* during the past 2 years; or

- A surveillance programme has demonstrated no evidence of *Culicoides* likely to be competent BTV vectors in the country or *zone*.

A BTV free country or *zone* in which surveillance has found no evidence that *Culicoides* likely to be competent BTV vectors are present will not lose its free status through the importation of vaccinated, seropositive or infective animals, or semen or embryos/ova from infected countries or *zones*.

A BTV free country or *zone* in which surveillance has found evidence that *Culicoides* likely to be competent BTV vectors are present will not lose its free status through the importation of vaccinated or seropositive animals from infected countries or *zones*, provided:

- The animals have been vaccinated in accordance with the *Terrestrial Manual* at least 60 days prior to dispatch with a vaccine which covers all serotypes whose presence in the source population has been demonstrated through a surveillance programme and that the animals are identified in accompanying certification as having been vaccinated; or
- The animals are not vaccinated, and a surveillance programme has been in place in the source population for a period of 60 days immediately prior to dispatch, and no evidence of BTV transmission has been detected.

A BTV free country or *zone* adjacent to an infected country or *zone* should include a *zone* in which surveillance is conducted. Animals within this *zone* must be subjected to continuing surveillance. The boundaries of this *zone* must be clearly defined, and must take account of geographical and epidemiological factors that are relevant to BTV transmission

The Infected Area (Protection Zone and Surveillance Zone) will remain in place and these measures will continue to be implemented until amended or repealed by an Order of the Secretary of State or devolved government with the approval of the SCoFCAH. This may require demonstration that vector activity has ceased for at least 60 days and that BTV circulation is no longer occurring.

Surveillance may be required to demonstrate that BTV transmission is no longer occurring. The period may be no less than 12 months where vaccination has been carried out.

In summary

Raised awareness of the risk of entry of the disease and a paramount concern to identify the primary incursion of disease are major priorities in present control.

Surveillance of susceptible imports is important but, as *Culicoides* spp travel as the "plankton of the air", a credible and cost effective active surveillance at potential landfall sites would be useful.

The implementation of a vaccination strategy aimed at eradicating the disease is a possibility now, but will not remain so for long. Through a concerted drive, the goals we seek are to ensure that we reduce the risk to the livestock population and to regain BTV free status. To do less would allow the entry of yet another potentially endemic disease to establish and further erode our livestock industry's confidence and ability to compete in the global market.

Sharing responsibility as well as cost, and the ability of core stakeholder groups to challenge policy and expert advice in the development of contingency plans, are part of the exciting process of facing these threats.

The challenges that the development of inclusive solutions to animal health problems raise can be resolved by a concerted effort from these groups.

Acknowledgements

The considerable input from other members of the BVA, the BVA Ruminant specialists group, Core stakeholders including the NFU and NSA, Veterinary colleagues in the VLA, IAH and DEFRA has been invaluable in the preparation of this paper.

References and bibliography

Buschmann, A., Hoffmann, C., Eiden, M., Groschup, M.H. and Doherr, M.G. (2007) Scrapie – update on the European Situation with special emphasis on small ruminant TSE diagnosis in Germany Paper given at the Spring meeting of the Sheep Veterinary Society in Hannover. *SHEEP Vet Soc Proc* (in Press)

Darpel, K.E., Batten, C.A., Veronesi, E., Shaw, AE., Anthony, S., Bachanek-Bankowska, K., Kgosana, L., Bin-Tarif, A., Carpenter, S., Muller-Doblies, U.U., Takamatsu, H-H., Mellor, P.S., Mertens, P.P.C. and Oura, C.A.L. (2007) Clinical signs and pathology shown by British sheep and cattle infected with bluetongue virus serotype 8 derived from the 2006 outbreak in northern Europe. *Veterinary Record* 161 253-261.

Defra (2007) Bluetongue control strategy. via website www.defra.gov.uk

Defra (2007) Notifiable diseases of livestock. via website www.defra.gov.uk

Defra (2007) TSE Review 2007 Final Report (chief reviewers Bostock, C. and Perler, L.). Defra, London.

Dercksen, D., Lewis, C.J. (2007) Bluetongue virus serotype 8 in sheep and cattle: a clinical update   *In Practice* 29 (6) 314-318.

Jeffrey, M. and Gonzalez, L. (2007) Scrapie pp 241-250 in Diseases of Sheep 4th Ed. I.D. Aitken (ed)   Blackwell Publishing, Oxford.

Osburn, B.I. (2007) Bluetongue pp 455-459 in Diseases of Sheep 4th Ed.   I.D. Aitken (ed)   Blackwell Publishing, Oxford.

Takamatsu, H-H., Mellor, P.S., Mertens, P.P.C., Kirkham, P.A., Burroughs, J.N. and Parkhouse, R.M.E. (2003) A possible overwintering mechanism for bluetongue virus in the absence of the insect vector.   *J Gen Virol* 84 227-235

Savini, G., Maclachlan, N.J., Calistri, P., Sanchez-Vizcaino, J-M. and Zientara, S. (2007) Vaccines against bluetongue in Europe. *Comparat. Immunol. Microbiol. Infect. Dis* (in press).

Sheep Veterinary Society/ Defra/State Veterinary Service joint CPD meeting (2007) Bluetongue science and policy.

7

PLANT EXTRACTS AS ANTIMICROBIALS IN RUMINANTS

R. JOHN WALLACE

Rowett Research Institute, Aberdeen, AB21 9SB, UK

Introduction

Growth-promoting antibiotics in animal feeds were banned by the EC from the end of 2005. This decision was based on public and political concerns that the heavy use of antibiotics in general can give rise to transmissible resistance factors that compromise the potency of therapeutic antibiotics in man. Growth promotion was a clearly avoidable use. Other international legislators may soon follow suit. Thus, livestock producers in many countries must face a future without antibiotic growth promoters. Problems may be more acute in pig and poultry production, but ruminants will also be affected in the sense that existing and potential new strategies for manipulating rumen fermentation must avoid selective antimicrobials. Organically produced meat and milk are increasing in demand by consumers, and organic farmers therefore face the same problems. Thus, there is increasing interest in exploiting natural products, which have no similar public health hazard, as feed additives to solve problems in animal nutrition and livestock production. The 'natural' products include probiotics, prebiotics, enzymes, organic acids, and secondary plant compounds or their nature-identical chemicals. This chapter describes plants and their constituent phytochemicals in relation to manipulating ruminal fermentation, and reports progress in EC research projects that investigate the broader potential of plants and their extracts: 'Rumen-up' and its successor, 'REPLACE'.

Research projects screening for antimicrobial effects of plants: 'Rumen-up' and REPLACE

The potential of a range of plant materials to modify rumen fermentation was investigated in an EC-sponsored shared-cost action under Framework Programme 5, 'Rumen-up' [Contract number: QLK5-CT-2001-00992]. Partners in the project were the Rowett Research Institute, Aberdeen (coordinator); University of Reading; University of Hohenheim, Stuttgart, Germany; University of León, Spain; Alltech Inc., Ireland; Crina S.A., Switzerland.

The aim of the overall project was to develop new plants or plant extracts as dietary supplements for ruminants to replace chemical additives and growth-promoting antibiotics (Figure 1). Plant materials were collected from botanical and industrial collections, and evaluated for their ability to prevent lactic acidosis and bloat, and to decrease pollution by preventing methane formation and decreasing nitrogen excretions. Bloat and acidosis are distressing disorders that result from malfunction of microbial digestion in the rumen. Methane, a potent greenhouse gas, and ammonia, which forms urinary urea, arise from normal rumen fermentation. The project was intended to deliver plant-based, sustainable solutions to these problems, thereby benefiting European biotechnological and agricultural industries, and the new plants increasing the diversity of crops used in agriculture.

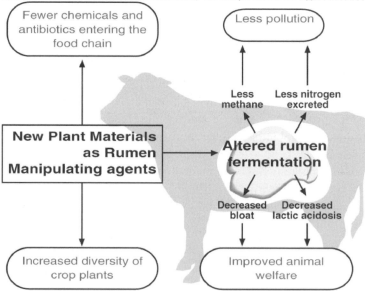

Figure 1. The EC Framework 5 project, 'Rumen-up'

The plants that were collected were not chosen randomly, rather they were selected on (a) the basis of known traditional uses in herbal medicine or for other purposes, (b) their known or suspected phytochemical content, or (c) botanical novelty as assessed by an expert botanist. All plants had to be cultivable in Europe. The composition of the 500-strong collection can be found at the project's website, www.rowett.ac.uk/rumen_up.

All samples were screened for their effectiveness in inhibiting rumen ciliate protozoa, rumen proteolysis, methane formation, microbial protein synthesis, lactic acidosis and bloat. The samples were also investigated to ensure that potentially useful samples had no detrimental effect on other basic functions of rumen fermentation, such as fibre digestion and volatile fatty acid production. The results for methane formation (Figure 2) illustrate the range of responses obtained. Once this evaluation was complete, an assessment was made of published information on traditional uses, known toxicity and palatability of samples that had been found to be positive in one or more categories, A select number of samples was taken forward for more detailed experimentation, with the aim of producing a short list of samples to be tested in animal production trials. Twenty-three samples were taken forward for patent protection (Becker *et al.*, 2005), fulfilling the criterion that they hit at least one of the target areas. Several samples had multiple hits: protozoa & methane, 5 samples; proteolysis & protozoa, 2 samples; protozoa & acidosis, 3 samples; methane & acidosis, 5 samples. The connection between protozoa and methane is known, because methanogenic archaea are known to attach to the surface of protozoa, and furthermore appear to live in the cytoplasm of the protozoa as intracellular commensal or symbiotic organisms (Finlay *et al.*, 1994). Protozoa are proteolytic (Lockwood *et al.*, 1988), which may explain the second connection. However, the relation between protozoa and acidosis is usually thought to be that protozoa protect against acidosis by engulfing starch and protecting it from bacterial attack (Williams and Coleman, 1992), not the opposite which seems to be the case here. Why methane and acidosis should be connected is unclear also, although both might result from an alteration in the stoichiometry of fermentation (Van Nevel and Demeyer, 1996).

Due to the terms of the Consortium Agreement drawn up by the partners, the full data will not be available publicly until August 2008. However, some of the results on inhibitors of ruminal proteolysis have been published (Selje *et al.*, 2007) and can be described here.

The sample collection was screened for inhibition of proteolysis *in vitro* using ^{14}C-labelled casein in a 1-h incubation with ruminal digesta and a 12-h batch fermentation system with soya protein and bovine serum albumin as proteolysis substrates. *Peltiphyllum peltatum*, *Helianthemum canum*, *Arbutus unedo* and *Arctostaphylos uva-ursi* inhibited proteolysis in both assays. These samples were rich in phenolics, and inhibition was reversed by polyethyleneglycol; thus, inhibition was likely to be caused by the formation of insoluble tannin-protein complexes. In contrast, *Knautia arvensis* (field scabious) contained low concentrations of phenolics and no tannins, had no effect in the 1-h assay, yet inhibited degradation rate of soluble protein and production of branched short chain fatty acids without precipitating protein in the 12-h batch fermentation. The effects resembled those obtained in parallel incubations containing 3 μM monensin, suggesting that *K.*

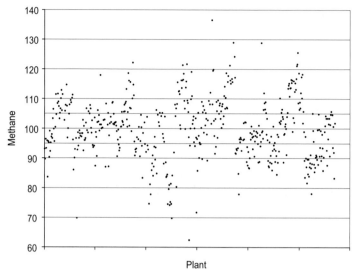

Figure 2. Frequency distribution of effect on methane production (as % of control) in response to the addition of each of 508 plant additives.

arvensis may be a plant-derived feed additive that can suppress growth and activity of key proteolytic ruminal micro-organisms in a manner similar to that already well known for monensin.

The Framework 6 programme, REPLACE, is a successor to Rumen-up in the sense that the same plant collection is being used to screen for properties that are useful in pig and poultry production and in aquaculture. Different targets from Rumen-up are being screened in ruminants, mainly the control of intestinal parasites and on using plants to create a healthier fatty acid profile in dairy products and meat. Several promising plants have been identified that may at least partially replace chemical anthelmintics. Among others, *Chrysanthemum coronarium* increases concentrations of PUFA in milk (Cabiddo *et al.*, 2006), an effect shown in the REPLACE project to be a direct inhibition of fatty acid metabolism by *Clostridium proteoclasticum*.

Essential oils

Essential oils are steam-volatile or organic-solvent extracts of plants, used traditionally by man for many centuries for the pleasant odour of the essence, or its flavour, or for its antiseptic and/or preservative properties (Greathead, 2003). Although commonly thought of as being derived from herbs and spices, they are present to some degree in many plants for their protective role against bacterial, fungal or insect attack. They comprise mainly cyclic hydrocarbons and their alcohol, aldehyde or ester derivatives (Table 1).

Table 1. Some common essential oil compounds

Hydrocarbon monoterpenes	Oxygenated monoterpenes
α-Pinene	Thymol
ß-Pinene	Eugenol
Limonene	Citronellol
Terpinene	Terpeneol
Cymene	Geranyl acetate
Myrcene	Linalool
Camphene	Fenchyl alcohol
Terpinolene	Citronellal

The use of essential oils as antimicrobials declined as the power of antibiotics became apparent. However, research interest has revived because essential oils are perceived to be natural alternatives to chemical biocides and, in some applications, antibiotics. Recently, for example, useful effects of essential oils have been demonstrated against food-borne pathogenic bacteria. *E. coli* O157:H7 was inhibited by oregano oil (Elgayyar *et al.*, 2001), peppermint oil (Imai *et al.*, 2001) and essential oils from other herbs (Marino *et al.*, 2001). In ruminal bacteria, essential oils were examined many years ago, in order to discover whether they contributed to poor palatability of some plant species (Oh *et al.*, 1968). General inhibitory activity was found across a range of plant materials. Oh *et al.* (1967) demonstrated that individual oils had different effects on mixed ruminal bacteria. Borchers (1965) and Broderick and Balthrop (1979) found that adding thymol, a prominent constituent of many essential oils, to ruminal fluid resulted in decreased amino acid deamination by ruminal bacteria. More recently, essential oils or their constituent individual compounds have been investigated for potential beneficial effects on ruminal fermentation.

A series of studies has been carried out at the Rowett Research Institute on a commercial mixture of nature-identical essential oil compounds that includes cresol, resorcinol, thymol, guaiacol and eugenol (McIntosh *et al.*, 2003; Newbold *et al.*, 2004). Both animal performance and effects on individual rumen microbial species *in vitro* and *in vivo* were measured. The breakdown sequence of protein to NH_3 was measured in ruminal digesta from sheep and cows receiving dietary essential oils by assaying rates of individual reactions in ruminal fluid *in vitro*. Ammonia formation was affected only at the last step, namely the deamination of amino acids (Figure 3), consistent with earlier observations with thymol. Addition of monensin to the *in vitro* incubations indicated that the essential oil mixture and monensin had overlapping modes of action, with monensin being more potent.

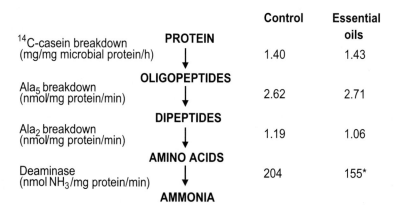

Figure 3. Influence of dietary essential oils on the catabolic reactions leading from proteolysis to NH_3 formation in ruminal digesta from sheep. From Newbold *et al.* (2004).

The bacteria most sensitive to essential oils were hyper-ammonia-producing HAP species, *Prevotella* spp. and *Ruminobacter amylophilus.* HAP bacteria have a high capability to generate NH_3 from amino acids (Russell *et al.*, 1991). *Prevotella* spp. are involved in all of the steps of protein catabolism (Wallace, 1996). *R. amylophilus* is a highly active starch and protein digester which proliferates on concentrate diets (Stewart *et al.*, 1997). Therefore, pure-culture results were consistent with observations *in vivo.*

Methane is an increasingly important target for manipulation in view of the global warming potential of methane from ruminants (Moss *et al.*, 2000). *In vitro* results for essential oils that affect methane formation, have been very positive, although care must be taken to ensure that the oils are not generally inhibitory to fermentation, which in itself would lead to decreased methane formation. Garlic oil and its constituent diallyl sulphide and related compounds seem to be particularly promising in that they inhibit methane formation specifically (Kamra *et al.*, 2005; Busquet *et al.*, 2005). Other plant extracts found to affect methane formation include cloves, fennel, onion, ginger and members of the *Rheum* genus (rhubarb) (Becker *et al.*, 2005; Kamra *et al.*, 2005; Patra *et al.*, 2005; García-González *et al.*, 2005).

Whether the effects of essential oils translate into improved productivity will depend on animal and dietary factors, such as the protein status of the animal and the composition of the diet. To date, production trials have been only partly convincing. Benchaar *et al.* (2006a) evaluated performance of beef cattle receiving and essential oil mixture; DM intake and average daily gain were unchanged, although feed efficiency increased. Benchaar *et al.* (2006b; 2007), fed an essential oil mixture to dairy cows and observed no change in DM intake, milk production, or milk constituents. Hosoda *et al.* (2005) fed peppermint (2% of DM) and found no production effect. Yang *et al.* (2006) found no effect of the addition of garlic (*Allium sativa*) and juniper berry (*Juniperus communis*). An interesting observation relating to product quality was made by Benchaar *et al.* (2007), who found that mixed essential oils increased the concentration of conjugated linoleic acid (CLA) in milk fat. CLA, which is believed to promote health in a number of ways (Wahle *et al.*, 2004), is formed by a small group of bacteria related to *Butyrivibrio fibrisolvens* (Wallace *et al.*, 2006). These bacteria are exceptionally sensitive to the toxic effects of PUFA (Maia *et al.*, 2007) and may also be sensitive to similar lipohilic properties of some essential oils.

The potential of essential oils as feed additives that will enhance ruminant nutrition is high. However, much work needs to be done in order to understand how different essential oil compounds work, how the mixtures work – there may well be synergy between different compounds in mixtures – and to explain how *in vivo* concentrations that are much lower than those found to inhibit any bacterial species *in vitro* can be effective (McIntosh *et al.*, 2003). Adaptation may be a key feature of the mode of action of essential oils. Adaptation of the microbial community may improve fermentation over time, for example by gradual diminution of the HAP population. On the other hand, the community structure may adapt to make the additives less effective over time. Effective doses of different essential oils have to be established. Dose effects must be considered along with the relatively low water solubility of many essential oil compounds. Do local concentrations, such as at the surface of plant fibres, increase to those that would be expected to suppress the growth of some bacteria? In this way, solids-associated microorganisms may be much more exposed to the selective effects of essential oils than species that exist predominantly in the planktonic form.

Saponins

Saponins are high-molecular-weight glycosides in which sugars are linked to a triterpene or steroidal aglycone moiety. Given the possible number of sugar moieties that could be added and the modifications that are possible in the ring structures, there is a huge number of possible structures that could be formed. The different classes of saponins are the triterpenes, the steroids and the steroid alkaloids (Hostettmann and Marston, 1995). Dietary saponins are poorly absorbed, so their biological effects occur in the digestive tract (Cheeke, 1996). Antimicrobial effects of saponins and saponin-containing plants are well known in other biological systems (Hostettmann and Marston, 1995), therefore saponins are potential feed additives that would be expected to alter the balance of the rumen microbial community and perhaps, therefore, to improve ruminal fermentation.

Most observations on the rumen suggest that saponins affect protozoa selectively. Valdez *et al.* (1986) found that sarsaponin, from *Yucca schidigera*, decreased protozoal numbers but not bacterial numbers in a 22-d semi-continuous system. Also *in vitro*, toxicity of *Y. schidigera* extract towards protozoa was noted from a fall in numbers in fermenters (Makkar *et al.*, 1998; Wang *et al.*, 1998) or in bacteriolytic activity (Wallace *et al.*, 1994). Butanol extraction of the *Y. schidigera* extract resulted in all antiprotozoal activity being located in the butanol fraction, consistent with the active component being saponins. Saponins from *Quillaja saponaria* and *Acacia auriculoformis* (Makkar *et al.*, 1998) and foliage from *Sesbania sesban* (Newbold *et al.*, 1997) were also antiprotozoal *in vitro*, the *S. sesban* active component again being extractable in butanol. *In vivo*, powdered *Y. shidigera* decreased rumen protozoal numbers in heifers (Hristov *et al.*, 1999). A decrease in protozoal numbers was reported in the rumen of sheep infused with pure alfalfa saponins (Lu and Jorgensen, 1987) or fed saponin-containing plants, including *S. sesban* (Newbold *et al.*, 1997; Odenyo *et al.*, 1997) and *Enterolobium cyclocarpum* (Navas-Camacho *et al.*, 1993). Agarwal *et al.* (2006) found that extracts of *Sapindus mukorossi* (soap nut) decreased protozoal numbers *in vitro*.

Bacterial numbers and activity can also be affected by dietary saponins. Partly this occurs indirectly, via effects on predation by ciliate protozoa – suppressing protozoa automatically leads to increased protozoal numbers. Newbold *et al.* (1997) found that bacterial numbers increased when foliage from *S. sesban* was introduced into the diet, presumably as a consequence of the suppression of protozoal numbers. Valdez *et al.* (1986) found a similar trend with *Y. schidigera* extract. In contrast, steroidal saponins from *Y. schidigera* had no effect on total or cellulolytic bacterial counts in Rusitec; however, inoculating fluid from the fermenter into medium containing saponins decreased the viable count (Wang *et al.*, 1998). Lu *et al.* (1987) discovered that alfalfa saponins appeared to suppress fermentation in continuous culture, the bacterial community changing from a morphologically diverse one in controls to one in which fewer morphotypes were present in vessels receiving alfalfa saponins. Subsequent *in vivo* investigation (Lu and Jorgensen, 1987) confirmed a general decrease in fermentative activity when alfalfa saponins were supplied to the sheep rumen, which decreased VFA concentrations and decreased cellulose digestion.

The danger of saponins inhibiting fibre digestion has been illustrated by a number of papers. Wina *et al.* (2005, 2006) demonstrated that *Sapindus rarak* saponins suppressed cellulolytic bacteria and fungi and therefore fibre digestion. *Y. schidigera* extract abolished growth of the fibre digester, *B. fibrisolvens* and inhibited cellulose digestion by *Ruminococcus* spp. and *Fibrobacter succinogenes* (Wallace *et al.*, 1994). The anaerobic ruminal fungi, *Neocallimastix frontalis* and *Piromyces rhizinflata*, were highly sensitive to *Y. schidigera* saponins (Wang *et al.*, 2000). Ruminal fungi appear to fill an important niche in the digestion of recalcitrant plant fibres, because they cause physical as well as enzymatic disruption of plant cell walls (Orpin and Joblin, 1997). Thus, any use of saponins to modify protozoal activity should ensure that fibre digestion is not affected.

Non-cellulolytic bacterial species may be affected also. *Y. schidigera* extract prolonged the lag phase of *Streptococcus bovis*, suggesting a possible role of saponins in controlling lactic acidosis, where *S. bovis* is thought to be a major contributor (Wallace *et al.*, 1994; Wang *et al.*, 2000). Agarwal *et al.* (2006) found that extracts of the saponins-rich *Sapindus mukorossi* (soap nut) inhibited methanogenesis, although it was unclear if a more general inhibition of fermentation also occurred. These papers illustrate that saponins might be used to control problematic aspects of ruminant production, namely acidosis and methanogenesis, which causes energy losses from the animal as well as environmental damage.

Ruminal microorganisms can metabolize saponins, which may or may not be useful depending on the circumstances. Makkar and Becker (1997) showed that saponins are degraded in batch cultures of rumen fluid *in vitro*. The resultant sapogenins are more resistant to degradation (Wang *et al.,* 1998), but much less toxic than the parent compounds (Teferedegne, 2000). A good example of the implications of this metabolism was when foliage from *S. sesban*, a multipurpose leguminous tree from sub-Saharan Africa, inhibited protozoal activity *in vitro* in ruminal fluid taken from sheep in the UK, but similar inhibition did not occur in ruminal fluid from Ethiopian sheep (Teferedegne *et al.*, 1999; Odenyo *et al.*, 1997). It was eventually established that ruminal fluid from the Ethiopian sheep converted the saponins to the less cytotoxic sapogenins, by cleaving sugar units from the saponins. The same activity could be induced in the UK sheep after a period of exposure to *S. sesban* (Figure 4). *F. succinogenes* apparently deglycosylated the saponins from *Y. schidigera* (Wang *et al.*, 2000), an interesting effect because of the importance of this bacterial species in cellulolysis. Thus, the implications of possible metabolism of saponins depends on the situation. If saponins in a feedstuff being consumed by the animal compromise fibre digestion by suppressing the cellulolytic flora, it may well be advantageous to promote the bacterial detoxification of saponins, for example in animals receiving poor quality forages or crop by-products. If, on the other hand, the saponins must remain intact to exert other effects, whether antiprotozoal, antimethanogenic, or against lactic acidosis, metabolism would be undesirable. Goetsch and Owens (1985) concluded that the benefits of sarsaponin would depend on the diet; sarsaponin increased digestion of sorghum silage and other fibrous feeds, but apparently decreased digestion of cereal and protein meals. To this should be added the nature of the saponin – whether easily metabolized or more stable to hydrolysis. Like essential oils, it is really too simplistic to regard saponins as a single or simple entity.

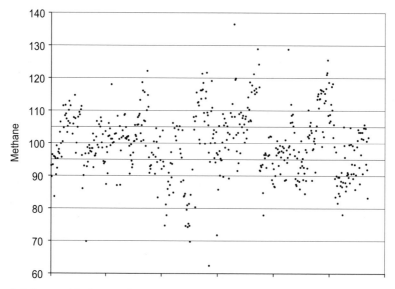

Figure 4. Influence of *Sesbania sesban* on protozoal numbers in the sheep rumen. Ground foliage from the leguminous shrub, *S. sesban*, was included at 250 g

Other plants and extracts

Research into plants as rumen-manipulating agents has barely scratched the surface of what might be achieved. The complexity of phytochemicals, or plant secondary compounds as they are often known, is bewildering (Crozier *et al.*, 2006). Tannins are abundant in many plants and have received much attention in ruminant nutrition (Barry, 1989), but they were not discussed here as the effects do not seem to be selectively antimicrobial. Alkaloids, glucosinolates and phytoestrogens are antinutritional, often poisonous to the animal (Dawson *et al.*, 1997). Other families of compounds have not been investigated at all, at least in a directed way. They may offer great value as feed additives that can be prepared at a subsistence farming level as well as industrially.

Conclusion

Research on plants and their extracts indicates a wealth of potential as manipulators of rumen fermentation for productivity and health benefits. Unfortunately, however, increasingly demanding regulatory hurdles can be a disincentive to developing these materials as truly novel feed additives.

Acknowledgements

The Rowett Research Institute receives most of its funding from the Scottish Executive Environment and Rural Affairs Department. 'Rumen-up' and 'REPLACE' were supported by the European Commission. Figure 2 was generated by Secundino López in 'Rumen-up'.

References

Agarwal, N., Kamra, D. N. Chaudhary, L. C. and Patra, A. K. (2006) Effect of *Sapindus mukorossi* extracts on in vitro methanogenesis and fermentation characteristics in buffalo rumen liquor. *Journal of Applied Animal Research*, **30**, 1-4.

Barry, T. N. (1989) Condensed tannins: their role in the ruminant protein and carbohydrate digestion and possible effects upon the rumen ecosystem. In *The Roles of Protozoa and Fungi in Ruminant Digestion* Edited by J. V. Nolan, R. A. Leng and D. I. Demeyer. pp. 153-169. Penambul Books, Armidale, New South Wales.

Becker, K., Duffy, C., Hoffmann, E., Losa, R., Mould, F.L., Muetzel, S., López, S., Selje, N. and Wallace, R.J. (2005) Use of plants and plant extracts as feed additive to affect the rumen fermentation. WO 2005/099729 A3.

Benchaar, C., Duynisveld, J.L. and Charmley, E. (2006a) Effects of monensin and increasing dose levels of a mixture of essential oil compounds on intake, digestion and growth performance of beef cattle. *Can. J. Anim. Sci.*, **86**, 91-96.

Benchaar, C., Petit, H.V., Berthiaume, R., Whyte, T.D. and Chouinard, P.Y. (2006b) Effects of addition of essential oils and monensin premix on digestion, ruminal fermentation, milk production and milk composition in dairy cows. *J. Dairy Sci.*, **89**, 4352-4364.

Benchaar, C., Petit, H.V., Berthiaume, R., Ouellet, D.R., Chiquette, J and Chouinard, P.Y. (2007) Effects of essential oils on digestion, ruminal fermentation, rumen microbial populations, milk production, and milk composition in dairy cows fed alfalfa silage or corn silage. *J. Dairy Sci.*, **90**, 886-897.

Borchers, R. (1965) Proteolytic activity of rumen fluid *in vitro*. *J. Anim. Sci.*, **24**,1033-1038.

Broderick, G.A. and Balthrop, J.E. (1979) Chemical inhibition of amino acid deamination by ruminal microbes *in vitro*. *J. Anim. Sci.*, **49**, 1101-1111.

Busquet, M., Calsamiglia, S., Ferret, A., Carro, M.D. and Kamel, C. (2005) Effect of garlic oil and four of its compounds on rumen microbial fermentation. *J. Dairy Sci.*, **88**, 4393–4404.

Cabiddo, A., Addis, M. Pinna, G. Spada, S. Fiori, M. Sitzia, M. Pirisi, A. Piredda, G. and Molle, G. (2006) The inclusion of a daisy plant (*Chrysanthemum coronarium*) in dairy sheep diet. 1: Effect on milk and cheese fatty acid composition with particular reference to C18:2 cis-9, trans-11. *Livestock Science*, **101**, 57-67.

Cheeke, P.R. (1996) Biological effects of feed and forage saponins and their impacts on animal production. In *Saponins Used in Food and Agriculture*, pp. 377-385. Edited by Waller, G.R. and K. Yamasaki. New York: Plenum Press.

Crozier, A., Clifford, M.N. and Ashihara, H. (2006) *Plant Secondary Metabolites. Occurrence, Structure and Role in the Human Diet.* Blackwell Publishing Limited, Oxford, UK.

Dawson, K.A., M.A. Rasmussen, and M.J. Allison (1997) Digestive disorders and nutritional toxicity. In *The Rumen Microbial Ecosystem*. Edited by C. S. Stewart and P. N. Hobson. pp. 633-660. Chapman & Hall, London.

Elgayyar, M., Draughon, F.A. Golden, D.A. and Mount, J.R. (2001) Antimicrobial activity of essential oils from plants against selected pathogenic and saprophytic microorganisms. *J. Food Prot.*, **64**, 1019-1024.

Finlay, B. J., Esteban, G. Clarke, K. J. Williams, A. G. Embley, T. M. and Hirt, R. P. (1994) Some rumen ciliates have endosymbiotic symbionts. *FEMS Microbiol. Lett.* **117**, 157-162.

García-González, R., López, S., Fernández, M. and González, J. S. (2005) Effects of the addition of some medicinal plants on methane production in a rumen stimulating fermentor (RUSITEC). In: *2nd International Conf. of Greenhouse Gases and Animal Agriculture* Edited by Soliva, C.R., Takahashi, J., Kreuzer, M. pp. 444-447. ETH Zurich, Zurich, Switzerland.

Greathead, H. (2003) Plants and plant extracts for improving animal productivity. *Proc. Nutr. Soc.* 62, 279-290.

Goetsch, A. L. and Owens, F. N. (1985) Effects of sarsaponin on digestion and passage rates in cattle fed medium to low concentrates. *J. Dairy Sci.* **68**, 2377-2384.

Hosoda, K., Nishida, T., Park, W.Y. and Eruden, B. (2005) Influence of *Menthaxpiperita* L. (peppermint) supplementation on nutrient digestibility and energy metabolism in lactating dairy cows. *Asian-Aust. J. Anim. Sci.* **18**, 1721-1726.

Hostettmann, K. and Marston, A. (1995) *Saponins*. Cambridge University Press, Cambridge.

Hristov, A. N., McAllister, T. A. Van Herk, F. H. Cheng, K. J. Newbold, C. J. and Cheeke, P. R. (1999) Effect of *Yucca schidigera* on ruminal fermentation and nutrient digestion in heifers. *J. Anim Sci.* **77**, 2554-2563.

Imai, H., Osawa, K., Yasuda, H., Hamashima, H., Arai, T. and Sasatsu, M. (2001)

Inhibition by the essential oils of peppermint and spearmint of the growth of pathogenic bacteria. *Microbios* **106** Suppl 1, 31-39.

Kamra, D.N., Agarwal, N. and Chaudhary, L.C. (2005) Inhibition of ruminal methanogenesis by tropical plants containing secondary plant compounds. In: *2nd International Conf. of Greenhouse Gases and Animal Agriculture* Edited by Soliva, C.R., Takahashi, J., Kreuzer, M. pp. 102-111. ETH Zurich, Zurich, Switzerland.

Lockwood, B. C., Coombs, G. H. and Williams, A. G. (1988) Proteinase activity in rumen ciliate protozoa. *J. Gen. Microbiol.* **134**, 2605-2614.

Lu, C. D. and Jorgensen, N. A. (1987) Alfalfa saponins affect site and extent of nutrient digestion in ruminants. *J. Nutr.* **117**, 919-927.

Lu, C. D., Tsai, L. S., Schaefer, D. M. and Jorgensen, N. A. (1987) Alteration of fermentation in continuous culture of mixed rumen bacteria. *J. Dairy Sci.* **70**, 799-805.

Maia, M. R. G., Chaudhary, L. C., Figueres, L. and Wallace, R. J. (2007) Metabolism of polyunsaturated fatty acids and their toxicity to the microflora of the rumen. *Antonie van Leeuwenhoek* **91**, 303-314.

Makkar, H. P. S., Sen, S., Blummel, M. and Becker, K. (1998) Effects of fractions containing saponins from *Yucca schidigera, Quillaja saponaria,* and *Acacia auriculoformis* on rumen fermentation. *J. Agric. Food Chem.* **46**, 4324-4328.

Marino, M., Bersani, C. and Comi, G. (2001) Impedance measurements to study the antimicrobial activity of essential oils from Lamiaceae and Compositae. *Int. J. Food Microbiol.* **67**, 187-195.

McIntosh, F. M., Williams, P., Losa, R., Wallace, R. J., Beever, D. A. and C. J. Newbold (2003) Effects of essential oils on ruminal microorganisms and their protein metabolism. *Appl. Environ. Microbiol.* **69**, 5011-5014.

Moss, A. R., Jouany, J.-P. and Newbold, C. J. (2000) Methane production by ruminants: its contribution to global warming. *Ann. Zootech.* **49**, 239-253.

Navas-Camacho, A., Laredo, M.A., Cuesta, A., Anzola, H. and Leon, J.C. (1993) Effect of supplementation with a tree legume forage on rumen function. *Livestock Res. Rural Develop.* **5**, 58-71.

Newbold, C.J., El Hassan, S.M., Wang, J., Ortega, M.E. and Wallace, R. J. (1997) Influence of foliage from African multipurpose trees on activity of rumen protozoa and bacteria. *Br. J. Nutr.* **78**, 237-249.

Newbold, C. J., McIntosh, F. M., Williams, P., Losa, R. and Wallace, R. J. (2004) Effects of a specific blend of essential oil compounds on rumen fermentation. *Anim. Feed Sci. and Technol.* **114**, 105-112.

Odenyo, A., Osuji, P.O. and Karanfil, O. (1997) Effect of multipurpose tree (MPT) supplements on ruminal ciliate protozoa. *Anim. Feed Sci. Technol.* **67**, 169-180.

Oh, H.K., Jones, M.B. and Longhurst, W.M. (1968) Comparison of rumen microbial inhibition resulting from various essential oils isolated from relatively unpalatable plant species. *Appl. Microbiol.* **16**, 39-44.

Oh, H.K., Sakai, T., Jones, M.B. and Longhurst, W.M. (1967) Effect of various essential oils isolated from Douglas fir needles upon sheep and deer rumen microbial activity. *Appl. Microbiol.* **15**, 777-784.

Orpin, C. G. and Joblin, K. N. (1997) The rumen anaerobic fungi. In *The Rumen Microbial Ecosystem* Edited by C. S. Stewart and P. N. Hobson. pp. 140-195. Chapman & Hall, London.

Patra, A. K., Kamra, D.N. and Agarwal, N. (2005) Effect of spices on rumen fermentation, methanogenesis and protozoa counts in *in vitro* gas production test. In: *2ⁿᵈ International Conf. of Greenhouse Gases and Animal Agriculture* Edited by Soliva, C.R., Takahashi, J., Kreuzer, M. pp. 115-118. ETH Zurich, Zurich, Switzerland.

Russell, J.B., Onodera, R. and Hino, T. (1991) Ruminal protein fermentation: new perspectives on previous contradictions. In: *Physiological Aspects of Digestion and Metabolism in Ruminants* Edited by Tsuda,T., Y.Sasaki, and R.Kawashima. pp. 681-697 Academic Press, San Diego,.

Selje, N., Hoffman, E. M., Muetzel, S., Ningrat, R., Wallace, R. J. and Becker, K. (2007) Results of a screening programme to identify plants or plant extracts that inhibit ruminal protein degradation. *Br. J. Nutr.* **98,** 45-53.

Stewart, C.S., Flint, H.J. and Bryant, M.P. (1997) The rumen bacteria. In: *The Rumen Microbial Ecosystem* Edited by Hobson, P.N. and C.S. Stewart. pp. 10-72 Chapman & Hall, London.

Teferedegne, B., Osuji, P. O., Odenyo, A. A., Wallace, R. J. and Newbold, C. J. (1999) Influence of foliage of different accessions of the sub-tropical leguminous tree, *Sesbania sesban*, on ruminal protozoa in Ethiopian and Scottish sheep. *Anim. Feed Sci. and Technol.* 78, 11-20.

Teferedegne, B. (2000) New perspectives on the use of tropical plants to improve ruminant nutrition. *Proc. Nutr. Soc.* **59**, 209-214.

Van Nevel, C. J. and Demeyer, D. I. (1996) Control of rumen methanogenesis. *Environ. Monit. Assess.* **42**, 73-97.

Valdez, F. R., Bush, L. J., Goetsch, A. L. and Owens, F. N. (1986) Effect of steroidal sapogenins on ruminal fermentation and on production of lactating dairy cows. *J. Dairy Sci.* **69**, 1568-1575.

Wahle, K. W., Heys, S. D. and Rotondo, D. (2004) Conjugated linoleic acids: are they beneficial or detrimental to health? *Prog. Lipid Res.* **43**, 553-587.

Wallace,R.J., Arthaud, L. and Newbold, C.J. (1994) Influence of *Yucca shidigera* extract on ruminal ammonia concentrations and ruminal microorganisms. *Appl. Environ. Microbiol.* **60**, 1762-1767.

Wallace, R. J. (1996) Rumen microbial metabolism of peptides and amino acids.

J. Nutr. **126,** 1326S-1334S.

Wallace, R. J., Chaudhary, L. C., McKain, N., McEwan, N. R., Richardson, A. J., Vercoe, P. E., Walker, N. D. and Paillard, D. (2006) *Clostridium proteoclasticum*: a ruminal bacterium that forms stearic acid from linoleic acid. *FEMS Microbiol. Lett.* **265**, 195-201.

Wang, Y., McAllister, T. A., Newbold, C. J., Rode, L. M., Cheeke, P. R. and Cheng, K.-J. (1998) Effects of *Yucca schidigera* extract on fermentation and degradation of steroidal saponins in the rumen simulation technique (RUSITEC). *Anim. Feed Sci. Technol.* **74**, 143-153.

Wang, Y., McAllister, T.A., Yanke, L.J. and Cheeke, P.R. (2000) Effect of steroidal saponin from *Yucca schidigera* extract on ruminal microbes. *J. Appl. Microbiol.* 88, 887-896.

Williams, A. G. and Coleman, A. G. (1992) *The Rumen Protozoa.* Springer-Verlag, New York.

Wina, E., S. Muetzel, E. Hoffmann, H. P. S. Makkar, and K. Becker (2005) Saponins containing methanol extract of *Sapindus rarak* affect microbial fermentation, microbial activity and microbial community structure in vitro. *Anim. Feed Sci. and Technol.* **121**, 159-174.

Wina, E., S. Muetzel, and K. Becker (2006) The dynamics of major fibrolytic microbes and enzyme activity in the rumen in response to short- and long-term feeding of *Sapindus rarak* saponins. *J. Appl. Microbiol.* 100, 114-122.

Yang, W.Z., Chaves, A.V., He, M.L., Benchaar, C. and McAllister, T.A. (2006) Effect of monensin and essential oil on feed intake, milk yield and composition of lactating dairy cows. *Can. J. Anim. Sci.* **86**, 598 (Abstr).

8

INDIAN ANIMAL PRODUCTION: IMPLICATIONS FOR UK LIVESTOCK

D. RAJEEVALOCHANA
Manager – International Business, Tetragon Chemie Pvt. Ltd., IS-40, KHB Industrial Area, Yelahanka New Town, Bangalore – 560064, India

Introduction

Livestock production worldwide is growing rapidly as a result of increasing demand for animal products. Livestock accounts for 40 per cent of the Agricultural GDP. It employs 1.3 million people and provides livelihood for one billion of the world's poor (FAO, 2006)

The livestock sector is undergoing massive changes in the global scenario in response to population growth, increased globalisation, and demand for food products of animal origin in developed and more so in developing countries. The trend in livestock production is towards a few of the developing countries emerging as large-scale producers in the global scenario.

A study by FAO, suggests that global meat production and consumption will rise from 233 million tonnes (2000) to 300 million tonnes (2020), and milk from 568 to 700 million tonnes over the same period (Delgado *et al.*, 1999).

Although the markets are gaining momentum, small producers will be dependent on bigger retailers and traders, which will reduce profit margins for the farming community. The demand for food, political scenarios and disease pattern are just a few of the factors that will drive production trends in the future.

The livestock sector in India plays an important role in the socio-economic development of rural households. It contributes about 6 per cent to the Gross Domestic Product and 25 per cent to the Agricultural Gross Domestic Product. Over the last two decades, the livestock sector has grown at an annual rate of 5.6 per cent, which is higher than the growth of the agricultural sector overall (3.3 per cent) (Jabir, 2007).

Livestock is likely to emerge as an engine of agricultural growth in the coming decades. It is also considered as one of the potential sectors for export earnings.

The importance of livestock goes far beyond its food production function (Birthal *et al.,* 2002). The country-wide GDP in 2006 and projected GDP in 2050 are given in Table 1.

Table 1. Top 10 GDP Countries 2000-2050 (GDP in billion dollars)

2050 Rank/ Country Name	*2000 GDP*	*2010 GDP*	*2020 GDP*	*2030 GDP*	*2040 GDP*	*2050 GDP*
1 China	1078	2998	7070	14312	26439	44453
2 United States	9825	13271	16415	20833	27229	35165
3 India	469	929	2104	4935	12367	27803
4 Japan	4176	4601	5221	5810	6039	6673
5 Brazil	762	668	1333	2189	3740	6074
6 Russia	391	847	1741	2980	4467	5870
7 United Kingdom	1437	1876	2285	2649	3201	3782
8 Germany	1875	2212	2524	2697	3147	3603
9 France	1311	1622	1930	2267	2668	3148
10 Italy	1078	1337	1553	1671	1788	2061

Source: Goldman Sachs

Several empirical studies indicate that livestock rearing has significant positive impacts on equity, in terms of income, employment and poverty-reduction in rural areas (Singh and Hazell 1993; Thornton *et al.,* 2002; Birthal and Ali, 2005). The distribution of livestock is more egalitarian compared to that of land (Taneja and Birthal, 2004).

India is emerging as a global player in livestock production with special reference to milk, poultry and egg production. Although livestock production is quite important in the United Kingdom (UK), environmental pressures, threat of diseases like Bovine Spongiform Encephalopathy (BSE) and increased cost of production are pushing the farming community to rethink future expansions. In this current situation, India has major potential to present a global stage for expansion and investments in the livestock sector in the future.

Population, GDP and demand for food

With the Indian population exceeding a billion, contributing to more than 17 per cent of the world population, the country demands the same share of the total world output of food grains and animal protein. Although more than 20 per cent of the Indian population is vegetarian, the other 80 per cent still demands significant amounts of food. The UK, in contrast, has a population just over 60 million and has less people to feed, ranking 22nd in the world (Table 2).

Table 2. World Population statistics

Rank/country / territory / entity	Popl(mil)	Per cent of world population
— World	6588.0	1
1 People's Republic of China	1318.0	20.03
2 India	1128.0	17.14
— European Union	494.9	7.52
3 United States of America	301.8	4.59
4 Indonesia	234.8	3.57
5 Brazil	186.3	2.83
6 Pakistan	160.0	2.43
7 Bangladesh	150.0	2.28
8 Russia	141.4	2.15
9 Nigeria	134.4	2.04
10 Japan	127.7	1.94
22 United Kingdom	60.2	0.91

Source: Wikepedia, WHO population statistics.

India is a low-income economy with a GDP per capita of US$ 493 (FAO, Livestock Information Sector Analysis Branch, 2005). The contribution of livestock to the total GDP is over 20 per cent (Table 1), with 72 per cent of the people living in rural areas and more than 40 per cent engaged in agriculture. The economy is growing towards double digit performance, but agriculture and livestock development has the slowest growth of around 4 per cent on average.

Contrary to the GDP growth of 9.4 per cent in India, the UK is growing by only 2.9 per cent (source: The Economist, Tables 3 and 4). Though the UK inflation rate is 2.5 per cent, compared to 4.03 per cent in India, there is a serious negative trade balance of 158.3 billion US$. The foreign exchange reserves of India have reached 229.34 billion US$ (Deccan Herald, Sunday August 12, 2007, page 13), which indicates positive industrial growth, purchasing power, increased foreign investments and also greater economic stability.

Indian livestock production compared to UK

Livestock is the backbone of the Indian economy. Not only looking at the contribution in value but also considering the number of people involved in

Table 3. India- economic track

	Latest period	One year ago
GDP Growth (per cent)	9.4 (FY07)	9.0 (FY06)
IIP Growth (per cent)	13.6 (Apr 07)	9.9 (Apr 06)
Inflation (per cent)	4.03 (16 jun 07)	5.5 (17 Jun 06)
Fiscal Deficit Growth (per cent)	(13.8) FY 08	51.4 (FY07)
Current A/c Bal (US$ Bn)	(3.04) Q3 FY 07	(4.78) Q3 FY06
BPO (US$ Bn)	7.5 (Q3 FY07)	(4.7) Q3 FY06
Forex Reserve (US$ Bn)	212.5 (22 Jun 07)	162 (23 Jun 06)

Source: India Trade Outlook, vol.4, Issue 11, July 2007

Table 4. Global economic scan

Country	GDP growth (per cent)	Inflation (per cent)	Industrial growth (per cent)	Trade balance (US$ Bn)
USA	3.4 (Q4 07)	2.5 (Dec 06)	3.0 (Dec 06)	(837.2) Nov 06
Euro Area	2.7 (Q3 06)	1.9 (Jan 07)	2.5 (Nov 06)	(15.7) Nov 06
UK	3.0 (Q4 07)	3.0 (Dec 06)	0.8 (Nov 06)	(152.2) Nov 06
Japan	1.6 (Q3 06)	0.3 (Dec 06)	4.6 (Dec 06)	79.6 (Nov 06)

Source: The Economist

agriculture and livestock production (Table 5). The commercial aspects of industrialization are driving the population more towards cities and less people are likely to be engaged in animal agriculture. This same relationship will also influence the contribution of livestock production to the GDP in the future.

Table 5. Agriculture and Livestock sector contribution to GDP

Year	GDP (Total)	GDP (Agri) US$	GDP (Livestock) per cent share
1999-00	440.45	105.6	23.98
2000-01	475.75	105.875	22.25
2001-02	522.75	115.775	22.15
2002-03	562.375	114.1	20.29
2003-04	629.925	130.375	20.7

Source : National Accounts Statistics-2005; Central Statistical Organisation; M/O Statistics and Programme Implementation

India has 57 per cent of the world's buffalo population and 16 per cent of the cattle population. India is largest milk producer in the world (Table 6). It ranks first in respect to cattle and buffalo population, third in sheep population and second in goat population in the world. The livestock population shows a high degree of diversity in its composition (Livestock Census, 2003).

Table 6. World Milk production (Mt)

	2004	*2005*	*Per cent growth*
World	625.2	640.2	2.4
EU 25	146.4	147.4	0.7
India	91.1	95.4	4.7
USA	77.5	80.6	4
Russian Fed	32.2	32.2	0
Pakistan	28.6	29.5	3.2
Brazil	23.7	24.6	3.8
China	27.1	32.5	20
New Zealand	15	14.6	-2.7
Ukraine	13.6	13.6	0
Mexico	10	10.1	1.2
Argentina	9.6	10.1	4.8

Source: Dairy India 2007

The livestock and agriculture industries are totally dependent on the land holding patterns in the country. The Land Reform Act of 1972 has changed the overall scenario of land holding in the country. This has led to many small farms in rural areas and multiple divisions when the land is distributed or inherited by children in the families. This has a major impact in turning the majority of people to very small or land-less families. Post the 1972 Act, many states which had the power to execute the law in their own fashion, abolished the Zamindari system and also imposed ceilings on the land holding pattern, which has led to severe fragmentation – average operational land holding is 1.41 ha, whereas the average holding in England was 55.4 ha in 2003 (Defra Statistics, 2007). This is one of the major determinants of growth or limitation of the livestock sector in Indian society (Table 6).

In the UK, contrary to the dramatic rise in profitability of the farming sector in the 1990s, the current euro/sterling exchange rate has reduced profitability. BSE and other diseases, such as Foot and Mouth Disease in 2001, have also played major roles in the economics of the UK livestock sector (Defra Statistics, 2007).

Many farmers in India depend on traditional methods of farming with very small holdings of animals. The sheer number of people involved in the business is so big, however, it has made India one of the largest producers of milk in the world (Table 7). Growth in the milk sector has been 4.2 per cent, and poultry 11.8 per cent, between 1990 and 2000; the trend is expected to continue without much increase in the population, leading to increased productivity both in terms of improved genetics and also better management practices. A majority of this effect can be attributed to the co-operative sector in the dairy industry and also to private organizations becoming more aggressive and promoting their concepts and products effectively in the market. The per capita consumption of milk and its products are increasing and with the population expected to grow to 1.3 billion by 2020, production is also expected to increase from 97 million tons (2006) to 165 million tons (2020) (Table 8).

Table 7. Average size of land holdings (ha)

No. classes	*Average size of holding (ha) during*						
	1970-71	*1976-77*	*1980-81*	*1985-86*	*1990-91*	*1995-96*	*per cent change (90-91/ 95-96)*
1 Marginal	0.4	0.39	0.39	0.39	0.39	0.4	1.9
2 Small	1.44	1.42	1.44	1.43	1.43	1.42	-1
3 Semi-medium	281	2.78	2.78	2.77	2.76	2.73	-1
4 Medium	6.08	6.04	6.02	5.96	5.9	5.84	-1.1
5 Large	18.1	17.57	17.41	17.2	17.33	17.21	-0.7
All Classes	2.28	2	1.84	1.69	1.35	1.41	4.4

Source : Agricultural Census —Dept. of Agri. and Cooperation. Ministry of Agriculture.

Even today, the principal players in the poultry farming industry are independent small farmers. This trend has been changing rapidly from small back yard activity to major commercial activity in the last decade and it has become the fastest growing sector in animal agriculture. The low cost labour situation has added to profitability of poultry farming in rural areas and makes India one of the top three low-cost producers of chicken meat in the world.

The need for more food has been ever pressing in recent years and per capita consumption of the food has also been increasing rapidly. As milk is the major protein source in the nation, driven by vegetarianism, it is ironically said that people who can afford meat do not want to eat it, but people who want to eat meat cannot afford it. This scenario has changed drastically in the last five years where middle class youth is taking a major share in the decision-making process in the family. With more education getting into rural India, the drift towards urbanization,

Table 8. Production and per capita consumption of milk

Year	Production Mt	Per capita availability g/day	kg/yr	Population million
1999-00	78.3	217	79.2	
2000-01	80.6	220	80.3	
2001-02	84.4	225	82.1	
2002-03	86.2	230	83.9	
2003-04	88.1	231	84.3	
2004-05	90.7	232	84.7	
2005-06(proj)	94.5	240	87.5	1080
Proj				
2006-07	97	243	88.6	1094
2007-08	100	247	90.1	1110
2008-09	103.5	252	91.8	1127
2009-10	107	256	93.5	1144
2015	134	296	108	1246
2020	165	240	124	1331

Source: Dairy India 2007

and economic freedom has pushed up the per capita consumption of meat. It is understood that demand for food from livestock production can be increased many folds if the consumption pattern continues to change in this way in the country (Delgado *et al.*, 1999).

Delgado *et al.*, 1999, have predicted that if there is a dramatic change in the meat consumption pattern in India, the consumption of meat products might increase by more than 500 per cent in poultry and pork, and by 154 per cent in milk consumption.

It is estimated that more than 2.6 million people are involved only in poultry production in India. An additional employment of 26,000 people would be necessary if the per capita consumption of eggs increases by one and poultry meat by 50g.

Analysis of current situation

India has lots to be proud of in terms of its livestock wealth and development. Being the largest milk producer in the world, India is totally self sufficient in providing milk to all those consumers in India. As an integral part of the culture and tradition of every household, milk has become part and parcel of human life.

Thus the prospects of augmented milk consumption are growing. The co-operative movement, which controls more than 50 per cent of milk production in India, has led India to self-sufficiency in milk production and has set an example in the global scenario.

Operation Flood, which was launched in 1970 by the Indian government, has been the largest and most successful dairy development program in the world. This has made Indian dairy production more scientifically based, profitable in terms of distribution, procurement, processing, value added products, and has been the key in increasing the profitability of the small farmer in India (Birthal and Taneja, 2006). With India's cattle population forecast to be 282 million in the year 2007, it is expected that there will be a 4 per cent increase in milk.

The growth in milk production can be attributed largely to increased milk consumption, although in milk marketing and distribution have also contributed. There is no country in the world with more variants of processed, and further-processed products (Fig. 1). This has further driven the increased consumption of milk as the majority of the vegetarian population depend on milk as the primary source of protein.

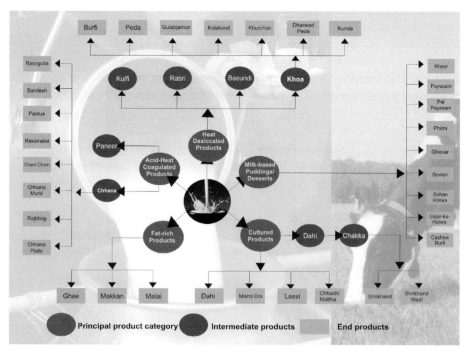

Figure 1. Conversion of milk into traditional dairy products.

The global market for animal-based foods has been expanding rapidly (Birthal and Taneja, 2006). Trends in India's exports and imports of livestock products for the last two decades are shown in Fig. 2 and Table 11. In value terms, exports of livestock products have increased remarkably, from US$ 90.8 million in 1980-82 to US$ 469.6 million in 2002-04, whereas imports declined from US$ 261.8 million to US$ 257.5 million during the same period.

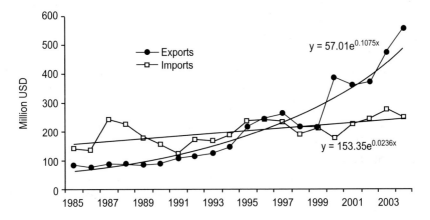

Figure 2. Trends in livestock sector trade in India.

Poultry production has seen its best situation in the year 2006 and early 2007, where market prices have been favourable to farmers. With a per capita consumption of 1.8 kg chicken meat, there is a big opportunity for significant growth in poultry production. With a per capita consumption of over 28 kg in UK, there is not much to expect in growth of consumption compared to India. The area where improvement is still needed in the poultry sector is in processing; post processing distribution, retail networking, sanitation and also awareness. India is today the second lowest-cost producer of broiler meat in the world, after Brazil, whereas the UK stands seventh (Table 9 and CLFMA, 2005).

Table 9. Cost of broiler meat production in the world

No.	Country	Cost US cents/ kg
1	Brazil	45
2	India	60
3	USA	62
4	Holland	98
5	Germany	98
6	France	99
7	England	105

Source: Industry estimates

Aquaculture in India consists of fish farming, fresh water prawn (Scampi) farming and brackish water shrimp farming. India is the second largest Scampi producer in the world with an annual production of 30,450 MT in 2002-03. With a 8,118 km coastline and abundant labour, India has the potential to meet the needs of domestic and overseas markets (CLFMA, 2005)

The UK has approximately 181 million poultry and exports a variety of poultry products, including live chickens and turkeys, various poultry meat, offal products, and eggs. UK exports of these products are sent to numerous countries worldwide. However, over half of the UK's poultry product exports are shipped to just four countries; Ireland, France, the Netherlands, and Germany. Poultry meat production in the UK totaled 1.52 million metric tons during 2004. (CEI, 2005)

With more open extensive land, sheep and goat production is gaining importance, which can be a very interesting feature for the UK when it looks at India as an opportunity. Low technology production without any stall-feeding, with low-cost labour has improved the profitability in this sector. The total sheep and goat population was 61.47 million and 124 million respectively in 2003 and is expected to grow at a rate of 1.12 per cent. With improved working practices and interventions, this can definitely be improved and potentially can be a good export market for India.

UK has a sheep population of 17 million and a pig population of over 4.731 million (Defra statistics, 2007), which contribute 3 per cent of the EU's pig meat production. There has, however, been negative growth in both species in 2005 compared to 2004 (Table 9). There is a substantial pressure on commercial farming in the UK and the trend is regressive. The total crossbred pig population is now just 2.1 million in India, where it may be possible to apply modern pig production technology to improve the genetics and pork for export, with the added advantage of lower cost of production (Table 10).

Table 10. Changes in UK livestock numbers:

	2004	Thousand head 2005	per cent change
Dairy cows	2 131	2 065.3	-3.1
Beef cows	1 739	1 767.5	1.6
Heifers in calf	691	639.2	-7.4
Ewes and shearlings	17 665	16 990.4	-3.8
Lambs	17 275	17 532.0	1.5
Breeding sows and gilts	515	469.9	-8.7
Other pigs	4 646	4 393.7	-5.4

Courtesy of: Alison Wray, Defra Statistics. June Survey of Agriculture and Horticulture 2007.

Turkey production is totally ignored in India, and there are many things that India can learn from UK. The Central Poultry Development Organisation (CPDO), which has been set up by the Government of India, has been doing some work on Turkey development, but there is real scope for improvement. Commercial turkey farming is not popular, but it can be a profitable venture for exports from India.

Areas of mutual co-operation between India and UK

The impact of even a small increase in per capita consumption in India is enormous. With a 1kg increase in per capita consumption of poultry meat, India needs to produce more than 500 million additional chickens per year, which would further employ many more millions in the industry. The Indian poultry industry currently doesn't have the technology to grow in terms of genetics, infrastructure, marketing network, disease monitoring and surveillance, and cold storage. These areas could be of great interest for a country like UK where the systems are already in place.

The opportunities for exports from India are also immense as the export trade has grown progressively in recent years (Table 11). Total exports in 2004-05 exceeded 1.2 billion US$ and the leather sector itself contributed 50 per cent of exports. Mutually beneficial business can be worked between the two countries in this sector. Milk and dairy products have a great potential to be exported from India along with powdered egg, which has captured a sizeable market outside India.

Table 11. Exports and imports of livestock products in India

| 2004-05 | US$ millions | |
Categories	Imports	Exports
Livestock	1.0	6.0
Meat and edible meat offals	0.33	430
Dairy and poultry products	16.57	169
Honey	0.00	0.00
Animal fodder and feed	37.9	8.45
Leather	260	665
Raw wool and animal hair	209	1.3
All groups (total)	526	1280

Source: Dairy India 2007

Some areas that might be of interest for the UK to look into in the Indian Livestock scenario are: technology development; India as a distribution point or locus for expanding markets to the Far East; disease management; laboratories; and improvement in processing and further processing. A lot of emphasis has been given on retail chain marketing recently and there may be a lot of opportunity for any investor in India. Many global leaders are already into procurement and retailing in India, and the sector is poised for growth. The UK can take the advantage of India as a Specific Pathogen Free (SPF) egg production centre for vaccine production. This is one area that seeks attention for global players as the market provides the base to operate for bigger volumes.

Factors affecting the growth of livestock

INFRASTRUCTURE AND LAND PRICES

Due to the recent economic boom in the subcontinent, especially in India, land prices have soared. There have been recent moves by local state governments to convert some agricultural land to special economic zones (SEZs). Farmers are finding the real estate business more lucrative than mainstream farming. This might push livestock production in and around the cities towards villages as land prices have increased tremendously.

DISEASE PATTERN

In the broiler industry, the move from segmented and fragmented business to consolidation driven by integration has involved application of more education and better management practices, and this is improving the level of bio-security in the industry. Open borders with Nepal, Bangladesh and Pakistan have frequently helped disease spread from these countries to India, which is not the case in the UK.

India notified the outbreak of Highly Pathogenic Avian influenza (HPAI) virus subtype H5N1 in poultry birds in western India on February 18, 2006. Effective control measures were taken by the government of India, including culling of entire populations, destruction of eggs, and infected material in 10-km radius of the outbreak location, also restricting the movement of poultry and poultry products from the infected area. The price of broilers crashed in many markets from Rs. 32-35 per kg live weight to Rs. 2-15 per kg live weight. The government also offered compensation for farmers affected (Gain report Number: IN6083).

A similar outbreak of HPAI was confirmed in the North Eastern state of Manipur in July 2007, and effective control measures were taken to prevent the spread. The infection was supposed to have spread from Bangladesh, which had been affected by HPAI in June 2007 and has open borders with North East India. It is encouraging that the poultry industry reacted quickly and professionally after absorbing the impact of the Avian Influenza induced market slump.

TRADE BARRIERS

Although India has been a member of WTO since 1995, and a driving force in the South Asian Association for Regional Co-operation (SAARC), trade barriers and farm subsidies of many developed nations have prevented Indian products from being exported freely. Being a leader in the sub-continent, India has easy access to the neighbouring countries like Nepal, Bangladesh and Sri Lanka, although consumption patterns in these countries do not support the trade. Sri Lanka, a processed chicken market, is in total contrast to the live bird market in India that occupies more than 92 per cent of the market allowing only 8 per cent for processed and further processed chicken.

Lots of work is being directed both by the government and also by the big integrators to enhance the image of the poultry processing industry in India so that the country is better placed to be a net exporter of both processed and further processed chicken to western countries.

India does not put any quantitative restriction on imports of livestock and livestock products, but high tariffs, restrictive hygiene import regulations and lack of infrastructure are major constraints for imports (Table 12).

Table 12. Tariff for imports of poultry and feed ingredients

HTS Code	Commodity	Trade policy	Tariff
10511	Poultry Grand Parent Stock	Subject to Sanitary Import Permit	35.9
207	Poultry Meat (cuts and offal)	Subject to Sanitary Import Permit	100.0/3
407	Eggs (Table/Hatching)	Subject to Sanitary Import Permit	30.6
408	Egg Yolks	Subject to Sanitary Import Permit	35.9
100590	Corn for Feed	TRQ	15.3/ 51.0
100700	Sorghum	State Trading	51
230120	Fish Meal	Subject to Sanitary Import Permit	5.1
2306	Oil Meals	Free	15.3
2309 9020	Concentrates for Compound Feeds	Subject to Sanitary Import Permit	30.6
2309 9010	Compounded Poultry Feed	Subject to Sanitary Import Permit	30.6

Source: Gain report NO. 6083

MEAT TRADE

Improved hygienic standards and low-cost production are the major factors that have improved exports of table eggs and egg powder, which are the major poultry exports from India. Poultry meat exports are negligible compared to production capacity in India, due to inadequate processing facilities, limited marketing resources for the products outside the country, and infrastructure limitations. Integrators from South India are exporting some poultry meat products to Middle East and South East Asian markets. The recent bans on imports from India due to the Avian Influenza (AI) outbreaks have hampered these exports seriously.

There are no restrictions from the government on exports of any livestock based products. In fact, the government has, been providing subsidies on transportation to encourage exports from India (http://www.apeda.com/apeda/Ta06-07.pdf).

What has been exciting is the export of buffalo meat from India, which is increasing steadily. The trend is going to improve due to the religious constraints of cow slaughter in India, which will provide a platform for other meat-product exports from the country.

Implications for world markets

The use of antibiotic growth promoters in India is a regular feature of production due to disease prevalence and level of biosecurity in the poultry business. Foot and Mouth Disease, Tuberculosis and Brucellosis are still common in cattle. Bovine Spongiform Encephalopathy (BSE) cases have never been recorded in India, which is an advantage for exports of non-poultry meat exports. The fact that India is producing enough vaccines for FMD and other common diseases without depending on foreign countries should attract more investment in this region.

Opportunities for United Kingdom and the western world

With opening up of financial markets and liberalization, Foreign Direct Investments (FDI) are increasing in many industrial sectors of India. There are lots of opportunities for investment in the livestock sector, including genetic improvement, management practices, services, animal health products and development, processing industry and retailing. Many multinational companies have already started to invest in the Indian retailing sector, but the opportunities are immense due to predicted future consumption patterns.

The Indian Council of Medical Research (ICMR) recommends annual per capita consumption of 180 eggs and 10.8 kg meat; the current numbers are 43 eggs and 1.8 kg meat. To fill this gap, in a population of over 1 billion people, demands a lot of work in terms of production, infrastructure, development and marketing opportunities, and would create a lot of employment in the sector.

Drawing the world's attention to the Asian markets, India has been quite successful in harnessing its potential to grow livestock in recent years. With improved technology and better management practices, the same may be effectively utilized for synergy between India and United Kingdom.

References

Birthal, P. S and Ali, J. (2005) Potential of livestock sector in rural transformation, In: *Rural Transformation in India: The Role of Non-farm Sector* (Rohini Nayyar and A N Sharma editors) Institute for Human Development and Manohar, New Delhi, India.

Birthal, P. S and Taneja, V. K. (2006) Livestock sector in India: Opportunities and Challenges, presented at the ICAR-ILRI workshop on 'Smallholder livestock production in India' January 24-25, 2006 at NCAP, New Delhi, India.

Birthal, P. S. (2002) Technological Change in India's Livestock Sub-sector: Evidence and Issues, In: *Technology Options for Sustainable Livestock Production in India* (P S Birthal and P Parthasarathy Rao, editors). National Centre for Agricultural Economics and Policy Research, New Delhi, International Crops Research Institute for the Semi-Arid Tropics, Patancheru, Andhra Pradesh, and International Livestock Research Institute, Addis Ababa. http://www.icrisat.org/Text/pubs/digital_pubs/J144_2002.pdf

Center for Emerging Issues (2005) *Impact Worksheet, Newcastle Disease*, United Kingdom July 20, 2005.

CLFMA of India (2005) *Livestock Industry Report*, pp.5-47.

Defra statistics (2007) http://statistics.defra.gov.uk/esg/datasets/euplace.xls

Delgado, C., Rosegrant, M., Steinfeld, H., Ehui, S. and Courbois, C. (1999) *Livestock to 2020: The Next Food Revolution.* Food Agriculture and Discussion Paper No. 28. International Food Policy Research Institute, Food and Agriculture Organization, International Livestock research Institute. http://www.fao.org/ag/AGA/LSPA/lvst2020/Default.htm

Food and Agricultural Organization of the United Nations (2001) *Livestock in India - a Perspective 2000-2030.* Techno Economic Research Institute, New Delhi, India.

Food and Agricultural Organization of the United Nations (2005) *Livestock Information, Sector Analysis and Policy Branch*, pp. 1-21.

Food and Agricultural Organization of the United Nations (2006) *Livestock's long Shadow- Environmental Issues and Options*. pp.22-23.

Gold man sachs, http://www.gs.com

India Infoline (2001) *India Infoline Sector Reports: Poultry*. http://www.indiainfoline.com/sect/poul/ch04.html

Jabir A. (2007) Livestock sector development and implications for rural poverty alleviation in India, *Livestock Research for Rural Development* **19** (2).

Poultry Times of India. 2000. *CLFMA Symposium*. http://www.poultrytimes ofindia.com/issues/2000/september/clfma.html

Singh S. (2006) India Poultry and Products Annual 2006, *Gain report- Global Agricultural information network*. Pp. 1-7.

Singh, R. P and Hazell, P. B. R. (1993) Rural Poverty in the Semi-Arid Tropics of India: Identification, Determinants and Policy Interventions, *Economic and Political Weekly* (28)12 and 13. Pp A-9:A-15.

Taneja, V. K and Birthal, P. S. (2004) Role of Buffalo in Food Security in Asia. *Asian Buffalo Magazine* (**1**)**1**: 4-13.

Thornton, P. K, Kruska, R. L, Henninger, N, Kristjanson, P. M, Reid, R. S, Atieno. F, Odero, A. N and Ndegwa, T. (2002) Mapping poverty and livestock in the developing world, ILRI, Nairobi, Kenya. http://www.ilri.cgiar.org/InfoServ/Webpub/Fulldocs/Mappoverty/index.htm

Vaidya, S.V. (2001) *The Indian Feed Industry*. AGRIPPA, FAO Rome.

Wray, A. (2007) Defra Statistics. June Survey of Agriculture and Horticulture 2007. www.defra.gov.uk

9

ENVIRONMENTAL BURDENS OF LIVESTOCK PRODUCTION SYSTEMS DERIVED FROM LIFE CYCLE ASSESSMENT (LCA)

A.G. WILLIAMS, E. AUDSLEY AND D.L. SANDARS

Natural Resource Management Centre, Cranfield University, Bedford, UK

Introduction

Environmental life cycle assessment (LCA) is a holistic way of calculating the environmental burdens resulting from the production of a commodity. It provides a way of objectively comparing alterative methods of production and, to a lesser extent, comparing commodities themselves. The two general types of burdens on the environment are resource use (e.g. fossil fuels) and emissions of pollutants (e.g. nitrous oxide). A commonly discussed sub-set of LCA is carbon-footprinting. LCA is more embracing than carbon-footprinting alone.

The work described here is mainly from a Defra funded project (Williams *et al.*, 2006) in which ten agricultural and horticultural commodities were analysed. Methods are described there more fully than here, especially for the crops production part. The work was applied to England and Wales, but most is applicable in other parts of the UK.

This paper describes the main features of the approaches used for the LCA of animal production that were used to produce the life cycle inventories (LCI) of each commodity. The work was implemented in working models that were coded in Excel (www.agrilca.org). Examples of analyses are shown that illustrate features of contemporary animal production and alternative production systems.

Methods

OUTLINE OF LCA PRINCIPLES

LCA analyses production systems systematically to account for all inputs and outputs that cross a specified system boundary (Figure 1). The mass and energy flows at the system boundary must balance. The useful output is termed the functional unit, which must be of a defined quantity and quality, for example 1 t of edible carcass. There may be co-products or waste products like manure, together with emissions to the environment, for example nitrate (NO_3^-) to water and nitrous oxide (N_2O) to the air. All inputs are traced back to primary resources, for example electricity is generated from primary fuels like coal, oil and uranium. Ammonium based fertilisers use methane as a feedstock and source of energy. Phosphate (P) and potassium (K) fertilisers require energy for extraction from the ground, processing, packing and delivery. Tractors and other machinery require steel, plastic, and other materials for their manufacture, all of which incur energy costs, in addition to their direct use of diesel. The minerals, energy and other natural resources so used are all included in an LCA. Allowance is made also for making the plant used in industrial processes (factory or power station) as well as the energy used directly.

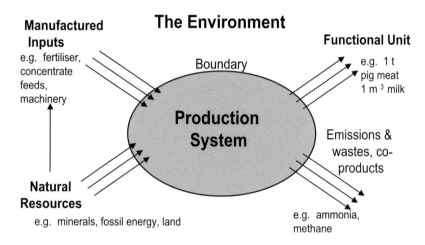

Figure 1. Example of the LCA approach showing the system boundary.

Agriculturally specific aspects of LCA

Agriculture has particular features that are not relevant to the LCA of industrial processes. The main one is land itself and the soil. Farming systems must be considered in the long term to avoid illusory benefits. LCA requires the soil nutritional status to remain the same (over the course of a crop rotation), so nitrogen (N), P and K inputs and outputs must balance. Omitting nitrogen fertiliser for one year may have a small effect on a conventional crop, but would have a much larger effect over many years as soil reserves are depleted. After one year, yields will be reduced only slightly owing to the soil fertility from previous seasons – the old system. The crop will, however, remove more nitrogen from the soil than enters the system as applied nitrogen. Over several years, the soil will reach a new steady state where input and output of nitrogen become equal – and the yield stabilises at a new lower level. This is the true yield of the new system, which must be used in the LCA. Estimating long term nitrogen balances requires simulation models to project how practices would cause leaching and denitrification without soil nitrogen accumulating or being depleted. One consequence of this is that the estimates of leaching are often higher than the current actual ones, as current practices often appear to cause increases in soil organic nitrogen, which may not get microbially degraded and hence reach the environment for many years. A similar process applies to straw incorporation and soil carbon. Also weed accumulation over a rotation must be prevented by sufficient herbicide or cultivation.

Agricultural land is of varying quality, for example soil texture, rainfall potential and altitude. Models are thus needed to adjust yields according to land type for both arable and grassland. These must also reflect emissions such as leaching and denitrification. Long term data are needed for major inputs, such as fertiliser and lime use, pesticide use and grain drying energy requirement to avoid the normal variability of weather from year to year on activities.

Although it is possible to consider arable crops in relative isolation, this is not true for animal production. In the simplest cases of eggs, pig and poultry meat production, there are typically breeding nuclei, from which secondary herds or flocks are derived, and these feed replacement genetic material into the commercial sector. Within the commercial sectors, several housing and rearing systems co-exist, each with its own characteristics. Changing the proportions of one part can have several interacting effects on other production areas. The situation with ruminant production (sheep meat and beef) is yet more complex. These may be reared in geographically diverse areas (such as hill, uplands and lowlands) and with a complex network of genetic flow. Beef animals are also derived partly from the dairy sector. Furthermore, ruminants interact with the grassland that supports them.

In addition, all livestock consume concentrates (e.g. wheat, soya, barley, maize, oil seed cake). These are grown on arable land and contribute to the total land requirements for livestock. Some are imported from overseas and their production and transport burdens must be estimated in addition to domestically produced feeds. Forages are conserved also as winter feed for ruminants (mainly grass and maize silages).

Livestock produce manure, which when it is applied to agricultural land promotes crop or grass growth. It contains plant nutrients that displace the burdens of manufacturing these nutrients, which is a benefit to animal production systems, making due allowances for the likely effectiveness of use. Manure storage and spreading, on the other hand, is a burden incurred by the animal production system.

Livestock, like crops, respond to different levels of nutrition. For many meat and egg production systems, a single level can be assumed, but for example in dairying, the diet (and associated management intensity) influences not only milk production but also longevity, fecundity and methane emissions. A model combining these factors allows exploration of production systems.

Product quality is an important consideration, especially when dealing with biological materials. At the simplest end, meat is quantified as edible carcass weight, as used in statistics produced by the Meat and Livestock Commission (MLC). This includes bones, fat, lean and skin in some cases. Milk is defined as the quantity of the 4% fat-corrected product.

The system boundary of this study was specified as *the farm gate*. Some assumptions were needed to handle this equitably. It was assumed that the burdens of grain drying occurred inside the farm. Egg packaging was assumed to be outside the gate, even though it may be economically linked to production, but it was considered to be part of distribution. The killing out percentage of carcasses is used to obtain edible carcass weights of animals, but slaughtering and transport to slaughterhouses are not included. Milk cooling on the farm is included, but not pasteurisation.

Allocation of burdens to arable co-products

Some crops and animals produce more than one useful output, for example grain and straw from cereals or oil and meal from rape. Although the latter are produced beyond the farm gate, we need to analyse them because rapeseed meal is used as an animal feed. Growing the crop incurs a set of burdens and these must be allocated equitably to the co-products. In some cases, a functional approach could be used, for example based on nitrogen or energy distribution between products, but the main approach we used was by economic value.

For example, milling wheat can be split into the high value product of flour and a variety of co-products (or by-products), collectively called wheatfeed, with weights and values as shown in Table 1.

Table 1. Parameters in example allocation of feed burdens.

Item	Weight	Value
Wheatfeed	M_W	V_W
Flour	M_F	V_F
Ratio: $\dfrac{Wheatfeed}{Flour}$		V_R

The burdens of growing 1 t wheat are B_G and milling 1 t wheat are B_P. The simple mass based allocations to wheatfeed (B_W) and flour (B_F) are thus

$$B_F = \frac{(B_G + B_P)M_F}{(M_F + M_W)}$$

Eqn 1

and

$$B_W = \frac{(B_G + B_P)M_W}{(M_F + M_W)} = B_G + B_P - B_F$$

Eqn 2

Including economic valuation in Eqn 1 gives:

$$B_F = \frac{(B_G + B_P)M_F}{(M_F + V_R M_W)}$$

Eqn 3

The economically allocated burdens per t wheatfeed ($B_{W,t}$) are thus:

$$B_{W,t} = \frac{(B_G + B_P - B_F)}{M_W}$$

Eqn 4

Separation of crops and animals

Although there are substantial interactions between animal and crop production, there is a need to separate them to determine the burdens of production of each commodity. Animals consume arable crops (and forages) and produce manure, which can fertilise grassland or arable land. Crops were analysed without manure. The benefits of the manure are credited to the animals in terms of displaced production and application of fertilisers. Summing a representative set of commodities will result in the same burdens as if the production systems were analysed as one integrated entity.

Organic production systems

The terms "conventional" and "non-organic" tend to be used synonymously. Non-organic is probably more descriptive, but "conventional" implies the aggregation of contemporary non-organic practices. The organic sector is currently relatively small (although parts are growing rapidly). The proportions of organically produced animal derived commodities analysed range from 0.006 (pig meat) to 0.025 (milk).

There may be many philosophical differences in outlook between organic and non-organic farmers, but there are only a few major differences that characterise the systems differently in LCA terms. The main one is fertilisation, in that organic farming does not use synthetically produced ammonium nitrate or urea (very energy intensive) or chemically processed P and K. Organic farming uses P and most K as directly extracted minerals, whereas P is commonly used as triple or single super-phosphate in the non-organic sector, because of the better availability of the nutrients in these forms. N is by far the biggest difference, however, with organic N being derived by N fixation through clover-grass leys. Cover crops are used much more in the organic sector between cash crops with a major aim of reducing N losses.

Pesticide use in the organic sector is minimal, with no herbicides used and fungicides effectively limited to a derogation to spray for potato blight using copper-based products. Organic farming places much more reliance on rotations and mechanical methods to control weeds. Ploughing is the dominant form of primary cultivation, although undersowing is often practised to provide control of weeds and other pests.

Livestock and manure are frequently an integral part of an organic cropping system. However the approach taken in the analysis was that the basic comparison between crops should be in stockless rotations because this determines the requirements of the crops and assesses their burdens more exactly and comparably. The fertiliser value of manure then becomes a reduction in fertility-building cropping required and hence land use of an organic arable crop, which is an environmental credit to the organic livestock. Note that the burdens of a whole farm, which are the sum of the burdens of the individual enterprises according to their proportions on the farm, are not affected by the choice of separation.

Aggregation of burdens

The use of resources and emissions to the environment are collectively termed environmental burdens. Environmental impacts are a consequence of particular burdens. For example nitrate leaching is a burden, while the consequent eutrophication is an impact. Emissions to the environment, whether from farms, industrial processes or transport, are initially quantified by individual chemical species. Several of these are aggregated into environmentally functional groups of which the major ones that we use are:

Global warming potential (GWP$_{100}$): GWP was calculated using timescales of 20, 100 and 500 years, but we report the 100 year one as being the most widely used standard. The main agricultural sources are nitrous oxide (N_2O) and methane (CH_4) together with carbon dioxide (CO_2) from fossil fuel. GWP is quantified in terms of CO_2 equivalents (Table 2).

Table 2. Global Warming Potential (GWP) factors for major gases using the IPCC (2001) climate change values.

Substance	GWP 20 years, [kg CO_2-equiv]	GWP 100 years, [kg CO_2-equiv]	GWP 500 years, [kg CO_2-equiv]
CO_2	1	1	1
CH_4	62	23	7
N_2O	275	296	156
N_2O-N	432	465	245

Eutrophication potential (EP): The main agricultural sources are nitrate (NO_3) and phosphate (PO_4) leaching to water and ammonia (NH_3) emissions to air. EP is quantified in terms of phosphate equivalents: 1 kg NO_3-N and NH_3-N are equivalent to 0.44 and 0.43 kg PO_4 respectively.

Acidification potential (AP): The main agricultural source is ammonia emissions, together with sulphur dioxide (SO_2) from fossil fuel combustion. Ammonia contributes despite being alkaline. When deposited or in the atmosphere, it is oxidised to nitric acid. AP is quantified in terms of SO_2 equivalents: 1 kg NH_3-N is equivalent to 2.3 kg SO_2.

Abiotic resource use (ARU): The use of natural resources was aggregated using the method of the Institute of Environmental Sciences (CML) at Leiden University (http://www.leidenuniv.nl/interfac/cml/ssp/index.html). Their data put many elements and natural resources onto a common scale that is related to scarcity of the resources. ARU is quantified in terms of the mass of the element antimony (Sb), which was an arbitrary choice. Their data include most metals, many minerals, fossil fuels and uranium for nuclear power.

Primary energy use: The major agricultural fuels include diesel, electricity and gas. These are all quantified in terms of the primary energy needed for extraction and supply of fuels (otherwise known as energy carriers). The primary fuels are coal, natural gas, oil and uranium (nuclear electricity). They are quantified as MJ primary energy which varies from about 1.1 MJ natural gas per MJ available process energy to 3.6 MJ primary energy per MJ of electricity. A proportion of electricity is produced by renewable sources such as wind and hydro-power, which account for 3.6% and 8% for UK and European electricity respectively.

Land use for crop production is reported assuming average yields for Grade 3a land (Bibby *et al.*, 1969). Yields were scaled up or down using linear coefficients derived from Moxey *et al.*, (1995) for other land grades (Table 3) and required land use per tonne of crop is one of these grades. However for animal grazing systems, owing to the network of rearing systems, land use is calculated as a proportion of each grade of land.

Table 3. Factors used to scale yields on different grades of agricultural land.

Grade	Scaling factor
2	0.88
3a	1.00
3b	1.08
4	1.12

DATA SOURCES

There are established inventories and factors for many industrial processes and impacts. These were used in the present study, together with some established agricultural ones and new ones that we developed. Although some values can be described satisfactorily by constants, many cannot and must be described by functional relationships. Typical examples are: yields in response to N in synthetic fertiliser or manure; leaching from soil in response to N application rate, crop yield, soil type and rainfall; milk yield and nutrients in the diet. Specific examples are included as needed.

Data were obtained from disparate sources (Williams *et al.*, 2006). These included the scientific literature, UK national inventories, annual surveys of pesticides and fertiliser use, levy board and Defra reports, farm management year books.

Emissions of N_2O from crops were essentially calculated using the 1997 IPCC method, as reported in the UK GHG emission inventory (Baggott *et al.*, 2004).

Apart from these standard sources, production data came from within the expertise of the project team. Commercial confidentiality precludes defining all such sources. We developed our own inventory of materials and processes for the project. This was based on some of the data sources above, together with inputs from an EU harmonisation study (Audsley *et al.*, 1997) and the *Ecoinvent* LCA data source (provided under the *SimaPro* platform). *Ecoinvent* is commercially sensitive so specific data have been masked in the working model.

CROP PRODUCTION

The full description of crop production is in Williams *et al.* (2006), but main features are summarised below. The main sources of agricultural burdens for field crop production are:

- Field diesel for cultivation, chemical and manure applications, irrigation and harvesting
- Machinery manufacture and maintenance
- Producing and delivering fertiliser and pesticides
- Energy for drying and cooling crops
- Direct soil-crop emissions to air and water (nitrate, nitrous oxide and ammonia)
- Construction of buildings
- Land use per t production

All except the last involve energy and abiotic resource use and involve some gaseous and aquatic emissions. These apply in general to all crops, whether produced non-organically or organically, but with clear differences between crops and systems. The same general set of activities applies to grassland management, but there is also a separate model for grazing productivity.

Crop nutrition and losses

Analysis of crop nutrient needs and losses to the environment is based on long term rotations. A fundamental rule of agricultural LCA is that soil nutrients are not allowed to build up or be mined. This can be summarised as:

$$\sum Inputs = \sum Useful\ offtake + \sum Losses$$

Rotations were analysed using Rothamsted's SUNDIAL soil-plant simulation model. This was run until steady state to ensure that there were no transient pools of soil N between the start and end of a rotation. SUNDIAL was used to calculate nitrate leaching and total denitrification; nitrous oxide emissions were calculated with the IPCC (1997) method. A small diffuse loss of P and K was assumed, but otherwise P and K were supplied to meet crop offtake. True long term yields in response to N were derived from long term experiments at Rothamsted's Broadbalk plots and were fitted with linear-exponential curves.

Methane oxidation by soil

A credit arises from agricultural land due to methane oxidation by methanotrophic soil bacteria. A value of 0.65 kg CH_4 / ha / year for all non-organic land was established after an extensive examination of the literature. This was arbitrarily increased by a factor of 1.25 for organically managed land on the basis that N fertiliser is not used and some work has shown inhibition of methane oxidation by N fertiliser.

CONCENTRATE FEEDSTUFFS

The precise mixture of ingredients varies for each concentrate fed to different classes of stock (Orr, 1995). Defra statistics (http://statistics.defra.gov.uk/esg/datasets/hstcomps.xls) show that wheat and derivatives dominate feeds blended by manufacturers (Table 4). Inclusion of six other main crops (and minerals) accounts for 0.84 of feed production. Diets were formulated using these feeds, assuming that the minor feeds provided similar nutritional properties for similar burdens and Orr's (1995) values were used as the basis for individual classes of stock.

We aimed to include most livestock concentrates, but originally set an arbitrary threshold for inclusion of 5%. We lowered this to enable inclusion of feeds already modelled, e.g. field beans and minerals, but minor feeds like oats and some by-products were omitted. The formulation of rations was thus based on the feeds in Table 4, with the nearest equivalent feeds substituted for minor ones.

Table 4. Mean distribution of main raw feeds used by feed blenders in 2000-2004.

Feed	Proportion of total, %	Burden calculation method
Wheat	25	Direct
Cereals by-products, wheat feed and other cereals by-products	21	Economic allocation from wheat and barley
Soya cake and meal	9	Direct for bean production and import plus economic allocation for oil extraction
Barley	6	Direct
Oilseed rape cake and meal	5	Direct for grain production plus economic allocation for oil extraction
Other oilseed cake and meal	8	Analogous to imported soya and rape
Whole and flaked maize, and maize gluten feed	5	Maize grain direct and derivatives by economic allocation from maize grains
Minerals	4	Direct
Field beans and peas	1	Direct (as beans)
Total accounted for	84	

Source: http://statistics.defra.gov.uk/esg/datasets/hstcomps.xls

Imported feed crops

Two main feed crops (maize grain and soya) are produced overseas. In these cases, production was modelled as closely as possible using local techniques, but transport burdens for importation were also included. Transport burdens were based on the ocean travel distances, together with assumptions about a split of terrestrial transport in the producing countries and in Britain (Table 5).

Table 5. Distances transported (km) and methods of calculating burdens for imported feeds.

Feed Ship	Country Proportion of	Road	Rail		
			soya imports		
Soya, Maize	USA	300	1,000	5,120	70%
Soya (*)	Brazil	300	1,000	8,320	20%
Soya	Argentina	300	500	10,080	10%
	Weighted mean	300	1,080	7,478	

(*) Organic soya assumed to come from Brazil only

CROP BY-PRODUCTS AND FEED PROCESSING

The main domestic by-product is straw for bedding (mainly from wheat) and feed (mainly from barley). Burdens for these were derived by economic allocation from the grain production burdens.

Major feeds are also produced from oil-bearing crops (e.g. rape, soya and maize) and cereals (e.g. fractions of milled wheat). Much animal feed is processed in mills, with the rest being home-fed, with little processing, except for crushing. Values for general feed processing on farms and in mills (rolling, flaking, pelleting etc) were derived from UKASTA data and the Ecoinvent database (Table 6).

Table 6. Energy consumption in general feed processing (not including oil extraction).

Type of feed	Primary energy, GJ/t
All feeds at mills	0.70
Domestic cereals ground on farms	0.30
Peas and beans ground on farms	0.45

Milled feeds are also transported from the point of production to the mill and out to receiving farms. For pigs and poultry, an eastern dominance was assumed with a mean 150 km back to farms; for cattle and sheep, a western dominance was assumed with a mean of 250 km to farms (by large lorries). Delivery to mills was assumed to be a mean of 100 km for wheat and barley and 260 km for rape (Elsayed *et al.*, 2003).

Separate terms were also evaluated for rape and soya oil extraction, wheat milling and maize fractionation. It was assumed that only whole soya beans are used in organic feed.

GRASSLAND PRODUCTION

Grass yield and nitrogen model

Grass yield was modelled using the grass site class system (Brockman and Gwynn, 1988). The dry matter (DM) yield (t/ha) of grass (Y_{GDM}) was related to site class (S) and N fertiliser applied (N_F, kg/ha) by regression to obtain the following expression for grazed pastures:

$$Y_{GDM} = \frac{c_S - a}{k} \ln(1 + b \cdot e^{-k(N-N_m)})$$

where c_s is a fitted parameter for each site class
$a = 0.01485 + 0.00112c_s$
$k = e^{(-5.302+0.594S)}$
$b = 1.5$
$N_m = 296/(1+e^{-0.836(cs-5.15)})$

The model takes into account the proportion of clover in a pasture, the N fertiliser applied, the type of animal grazing, and if the pasture is used for forage conservation or not. Long term excreted N is fully accounted for in forage yield, nitrate leaching and denitrification. Mechanisation needs for establishing, maintaining and harvesting pastures are also included (Williams *et al.*, 2006).

ANIMAL PRODUCTION MODELLING

Six animal commodities were studied: poultry meat, pig meat, sheep meat, beef, milk and eggs. Poultry meat was assumed to be a composite of chicken and turkey meat. The other commodities were all produced by one class or species of stock. Only milk from dairy cattle was considered. Similarly, all eggs are assumed to be produced by chickens.

In addition to field emissions, there are direct and indirect emissions from animals (indirect ones coming from manure). These are: methane (enteric and manure), nitrous oxide (manure in housing, storage and land application) and ammonia (same sources as nitrous oxide). Nitrate can also be leached from land-applied manure.

Modelling the structure of the animal production industries

In modelling the production of livestock commodities in England and Wales, account has to be taken of the structure and diversity of the national industry. Meat-producing animals are produced by mothers who themselves have to be produced. The components of the sheep industry are spread amongst different farm types. From a farm management perspective, the industry is thus studied and reported as a set of different enterprises. These enterprise descriptions provide the essential building blocks from which we have modelled the industry. Transport steps connect some of them. Enterprise descriptions also define different ways of doing the same job.

For example, piglets for finishing can be produced from indoor or outdoor breeding units. The non-organic sheep industry has a structure that maximises hybrid vigour in the terminal generation (Figure 2). Pure bred hill flocks produce draft ewes that are used in the kinder uplands to produce cross breeds, which in turn supply female breeding stock to lowland fat-lamb producers.

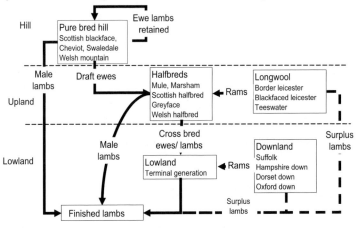

Figure 2. Simplified structure of the sheep industry.

These different ways co-exist, but the model can be used to examine the implications for the environment of changes in their proportions.

Animal production network structure

Changes in the proportion of any enterprise component must result in changes to the proportions of others in order to keep producing the desired amount of commodity. Establishing how much of each enterprise is required is found by solving simultaneous linear equations that describe relationships that link enterprises together.

The equations have the following structure. The solution is the amount, X, of each activity, i, that produces the desired mass of output Z,

$$Z = \sum_{i=1}^{n} z_i X_i$$

where z_i is the output (meat, milk or eggs) of activity i, and also satisfies the set of flows between activities:

$$\sum_{i=1}^{n} c_{ij} X_i = 0, \ j = 1 \ldots p$$

where c_{ij} is the supply or demand of j by activity i, which describes the relationship between enterprises. Demands are negative, supplies are positive, and total supply must equal total demand. For example, purebred lowland flocks produce rams, which are, in turn, demanded as terminal sires by lowland finishing flocks.

The total amount of material k flowing into the system is:

$$M_k = \sum_{i=1}^{n} m_{ik} X_i, \ k = 1 \ldots q$$

where m_{ik} is the flow of material k into activity i. The LCI for the system is the total of each burden l

$$B_l = \sum_{k=1}^{p} M_k b_{kl}, \ l = 1 \ldots r$$

where b_{kl} is the amount of burden l produced by the use or disposal of material k and M_k is the total amount of material. The LCI identifies the contribution of each material

$$B_{kl} = M_k b_{kl}$$

or activity

$$B_{il} = X_i \sum_{k=1}^{q} m_{ik} b_{kl}$$

which provides data to enable particular "hotspots" to be identified.

Note that one of the burdens from ruminant systems is the land use, which is a combination of different land classes, indicating the proportion of the production which is on hills, upland or lowland. This contrasts with the field crops where land use can be any one of the land classes, the amount required being dependent on the quality of the land.

Structures of sectors

All models include the overheads of breeding, such as rearing herd or flock replacements and maintaining dams between parturition as well as sires.

Pig and poultry models include a selection of main finishing and breeding systems (including indoor and outdoor types). For poultry this includes three generations of breeders that are required to produce the final generation. The beef industry is characterised by numerous finishing systems of various intensities, allowing for the different finishing characteristics of purebred dairy, crossbred dairy and suckler beef bred calves. A number of intermediate grass and indoor growing stages are modelled because beef take more than one season to finish. Milk production is modelled as self-contained herds at a series of three yield levels, each with defined characteristics. It was assumed that dairy cows must give birth to produce milk, so that the burdens of producing beef calves from dairy cows is debited to milk production. A credit is, however, given for beef from culled dairy cows.

The non-organic sheep industry is a network of pure and cross bred flocks that come down from the hills to produce the terminal generation of fat lambs in the lowlands. Each is linked by transfer steps in which adult or growing sheep may be transferred.

Emissions and manures from animal production

Direct emissions from livestock

Animals and their manures are the source of three important direct gaseous emissions: methane (CH_4), nitrous oxide (N_2O) and ammonia (NH_3). Methane is a consequence of fibre digestion in the rumen (and lower gut to a lesser extent).

Emissions from animals and from their excreta within housing systems are calculated following the methods of the national inventories for methane, ammonia and nitrous oxide.

Credit for displaced fertiliser and crops

Emissions from manure storage and land-spreading were quantified using an extension to the national inventory methods and data. Interactions between manures, soils and crops are complex. However, in the long term all of the nutrients that are applied to the soil as manure will be accounted for as either crop products or as losses to the environment (Sandars *et al.*, 2003).

Losses of N (mainly as ammonia) are calculated during housing, storage and land spreading, with specific emission terms for each system. The remaining N is partitioned into plant available N (ammoniacal N + 0.1 or organic N), which can be used by crops in the year of application, and residual organic N. Long term effects are then calculated to ensure that all applied N is accounted for in long term yield crop offtake or losses to the environment though leaching and denitrification. Account is taken for the effect of season and the crop to which the manure is applied. A factor is also used to allow for typical farmer valuation of manure N, which is higher for organic production.

With the routine use of soil testing it is safe to assume that all of the manurial P and K will, in time, be used as a source of fertility.

Ruminant manures are modelled as applied to grassland, whereas pig and poultry manure are modelled as applied to winter wheat. It is assumed that non-organically derived manures are applied to non-organic crop land. In the non-organic case the fertility in manure displaces the need for ammonium nitrate, triple super phosphate, and KCl fertiliser. In the organic case we assume that the equivalents are sacrificial legume N, Rock P from 25% Tunisian phosphate and Rock K.

In summary, animals are debited with the burdens of manure management and associated emissions, but are credited with fertiliser replacement value of manure.

Allocation of burdens to meats of different qualities

The focus of the meat production enterprises is prime meat, but meat also arises from culling breeding stock (ewes for mutton, sows, boars, dairy and beef cows, retired laying hens and broiler breeders). The quality of these meats is generally considered lower, but they are used in some catering and processed foods, which is reflected in lower prices, typically less than 25% of the value of prime meat. The basis of allocation is weight adjusted for the lower economic value. If the total meat production from a system consists of π kg prime meat with value χ £/kg and c kg culled meat with value c £/kg, then the weight adjusted meat output (w) is:

$$w = p + \frac{\chi}{\pi} c$$

This reduces the potential production of prime meat by less than 5% in most cases.

The interaction between milk and beef is complex. The primary purpose of pregnancy in dairying is to initiate lactation and the secondary purpose is to provide female herd replacements. A consequence is production of surplus calves that are often, but not always, taken into the beef industry. The bull used will be either a dairy or a beef bull and modern selection methods can increase the probability of a male or female calf. Purebred male dairy calves (e.g. Holstein-Friesian) are often killed just after birth, but the majority of crossbred (beef x dairy) male (and some female) calves enter the beef sector. The maintenance costs and burdens of lowland suckler cows are avoided when dairy bred calves enter the beef sector.

Organic livestock production

Differences between organic and non-organic animal production are much more apparent between dairying systems and poultry meat production, than production systems that are more extensive such as upland sheep and beef. All monogastric organic production is free range, and with greater land requirements per head than non-organic free range, while non-organic includes free range and fully housed systems. The non-organic sector uses slurry systems and bedded housing, while bedded is the norm in organic. Until September 2005, up to 20% of feed and bedding to organic could be sourced from the non-organic sector, if organic supplies were limited, with the bulk being organic. Now, feed and bedding should be all organic, with minor exceptions. These differences are accounted for in our analysis. Soya is used in both organic and non-organic sectors, but is used as whole beans in organic and mainly as meal, after oil extraction, in the non-organic sector. In terms of dietary composition, however, concentrations of energy and protein in compounded feeds are generally similar for both sectors.

Results

FEEDS

The burdens for producing the main feed crops are given in Tables 7 and 8. It is notable that the highest users of primary energy are the protein crops that fix their own nitrogen. This is because they have low yields and therefore the field work energy becomes more important per tonne.

Table 7. Main environmental burdens of non-organically produced feed crop (per t FW).

Impacts & resources used	Feed wheat	Winter barley	Spring barley	Field beans	Soya beans	Grain maize
Primary Energy used, GJ	2.3	2.4	2.4	2.5	3.0	2.0
GWP_{100}, t 100 year CO_2 equiv.	0.73	0.73	0.71	1.0	1.3	0.65
EP, kg PO_4^{3-} equiv.	3.0	2.5	2.3	5.9	7.3	2.8
AP, kg SO_2 equiv.	2.8	2.9	2.3	4.8	6.4	1.6
Pesticides used, dose ha	1.9	2.2	1.4	2.9	4.4	0.4
ARU, kg antimony equiv.	1.4	1.4	1.5	1.4	1.7	1.3
Land use grade 3a ha	0.13	0.16	0.18	0.30	0.42	0.14

Table 8. Main environmental burdens of organically produced feed crop (per t FW).

Impacts & resources used	Feed wheat	Winter barley	Spring barley	Field beans	Soya beans
Primary Energy used, GJ	2.0	2.2	2.4	2.3	2.7
GWP_{100}, t 100 year CO_2 Equiv.	0.70	0.61	0.74	0.82	1.0
EP, kg PO_4^{3-} Equiv.	8.3	5.6	7.9	5.5	7.0
AP, kg SO_2 Equiv.	3.3	2.5	2.7	3.7	4.4
Pesticides used, dose ha	0	0	0	0	0
ARU, kg antimony Equiv.	1.6	1.8	2.0	1.6	1.8
Land use, grade 3a, ha	0.32	0.40	0.48	0.34	0.44

Some major feeds are produced by extensive processing after the actual crop production. Total burdens of processed animal feeds include field production, processing, import and delivery transport (Table 9). Five were modelled, of which only wheatfeed was grown organically. There is a notable contrast between soya, which has its protein content increased by a relatively intensive process that also produces a high value product (oil), and wheatfeed where the feed is a cheap by-product of a relatively low-input process. Transport and processing burdens for soya are about the same, while wheatfeed milling incurs about nine times the burdens of transport.

Ruminants can graze or be fed on conserved grass. Energy requirements per unit DM fall as grassland becomes more extensive (Table 10) and silage takes more energy than grazed grass. Other burdens (mainly relating to ammonia emissions and nitrate leaching) increase with decreasing intensity and as the stock type moves from the more N-efficient dairy cow to sheep. Organic grass production takes less energy in the lowlands because of clover fixed N rather than synthetic N. Hill production, however, is considered to be identical.

Table 9. Total burdens of processed animal feeds, including field production, processing, import and delivery transport (per t FW).

Impacts & resources used	Wheat-feed (Non-organic)	Wheat-feed (Organic)	Maize gluten feed	Soya meal (no hulls)	Soya meal (with hulls)	Rape meal
Primary Energy used, GJ	0.80	0.58	3.8	6.6	6.0	3.5
GWP_{100}, t 100 year CO_2 equiv.	0.13	0.11	0.34	0.94	0.85	0.55
EP, kg PO_4^{3-} equiv.	0.9	1.9	1.1	7.5	6.8	3.9
AP, kg SO_2 equiv.	0.82	0.73	1.2	8.5	7.7	4.6
Pesticides used, dose ha	0.45	0.00	0.15	4.5	4.1	2.1
ARU, kg antimony equiv.	0.51	0.43	2.3	6.7	6.1	2.1
Land use grade 3a ha	0.032	0.083	0.055	0.42	0.38	0.14

Table 10. Burdens of producing 1 t DM of representative forages.

Item	Dairy				Beef		Sheep	
	Non-organic lowland grazing	Organic lowland grazing	Non-organic lowland silage	Organic lowland silage	Non-organic upland grazing	Organic upland grazing	Non-organic hill grazing	Organic hill grazing
Primary energy used, GJ	0.67	0.14	1.4	0.30	0.55	0.15	0.12	0.12
GWP_{100}, t CO_2 Equiv.	0.19	0.12	0.38	0.20	0.16	0.11	0.093	0.093
EP, kg PO_4 Equiv	4.8	5.7	1.3	0.6	5.6	6.8	9.5	9.5
AP., kg SO_2 Equiv.	12	13	1.2	1.6	14	15	19	19
Pesticides used, Dose-ha	0.0	0.0	0.0	0.0	0.0	0.0	0.0	0.0
Abiotic resource use, kg Sb Equiv.	0.45	0.16	0.88	0.27	0.38	0.16	0.13	0.13

STANDARD ANIMAL PRODUCTION BURDENS

The energy and GWP of meats (Table 11) are about an order of magnitude larger than for feeds. This reflects the concentration process in converting crops into highly concentrated sources of protein that are typical of animal products. The other main emissions of acidification and eutrophication potentials are about two orders of magnitude higher than feeds. This is almost all a result of surplus N being excreted and entering the environment directly as ammonia or after secondary processes as nitrate.

Table 11. Main burdens of animal products (from current national balance of systems) per functional unit produced (1 t edible carcass weight, 20,000 eggs or 1 m^3 milk). The assumed proportion of organic production (by volume) is shown in parenthesis.

Impacts & resources used	Beef (0.008)	Pig meat (0.006)	Poultry meat (0.009)	Sheep meat (0.01)	Eggs (0.02)	Milk (0.025)
Primary energy used, GJ	27	22	15	25	14	2.6
GWP$_{100}$, t 100 year CO_2 equiv.	14	5	4.0	14	4.2	1.0
EP, kg PO_4^{3-} equiv.	120	72	32	210	40	50
AP, kg SO_2 equiv.	300	270	96	500	140	140
Pesticides used, dose ha	1.2	2	1.5	0.9	1.2	0.8
ARU, kg antimony equiv.	34	41	27	29	35	31
Land use (*)						
Grade 2, ha	0.03	0	0	0.07	0	0.22
Grade 3a, ha	0.63	0.63	0.61	0.49	0.54	0.96
Grade 3b, ha	0.81	0	0	1.3	0	0
Grade 4, ha	0.65	0	0	1.1	0	0
Grade 5, ha	1.3	0	0	2.6	0	0

(*) Land use for grazing animals comprises a combination of land types from hill to lowland. Land use for arable feed crops consists of land of one of the types. In this table, arable land use is taken as all grade 3a.

The results also tend to show an effect of different genetic capacities for meat production, with highly selected broilers having a high feed conversion ratio and live-weight gain, together with low breeding overheads. These are in contrast to beef, where a calf also requires a cow to be fed. It should be remembered that the nutritional values of the meats will differ and cultural influences mean that they are not simply interchangeable. So a simple comparison of meat types may be misleading. Cattle and sheep are, of course, produced on land that is unsuitable for producing poultry or pig feed. One disadvantage is enteric methane and its contribution to GWP. This can be seen for example in the ratios of GWP / energy always being higher for ruminants than non-ruminants.

The differences in energy use between breeding overheads and finishing are clear (Figure 3) and reflect the low output of sucker beef cows compared with broiler-breeders. One feature in the figure is the high loading for beef calf production carried by milk production. Poultry (meat and eggs) and milk production are characterised by high efficiency in converting feed into produce. These are probably much closer to genetic limits than for pig, sheep or beef production.

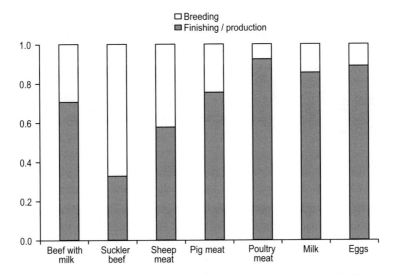

Figure 3. Distribution of energy between breeding overheads and production stages in animal production.

Feed clearly dominates the energy going into livestock (Figure 4). It ranges from 0.74 (milk) to 0.92 (beef) of energy use. Milk and poultry have relatively high direct energy inputs from features like milking and refrigeration, heating and cooling livestock. Most direct energy in sheep production is from vehicle use in stock management.

Although greenhouse gas emissions of arable production are dominated by N_2O (when weighted for GWP), methane and CO_2 have a larger role in animal production (Figure 5). N_2O is still the largest term for pigs and poultry, due to the large arable input. Enteric emissions (and manure storage) cause GWP by ruminant production to be dominated by methane. Methane from pig production is mainly from manure storage, both in and outside houses.

ALTERNATIVE PRODUCTION SYSTEMS

The main alternative production system considered for each commodity was organic. Comparisons show a considerable variety of outcomes (Table 12).

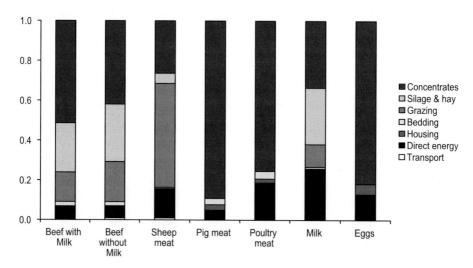

Figure 4. Distribution of energy going into livestock production.

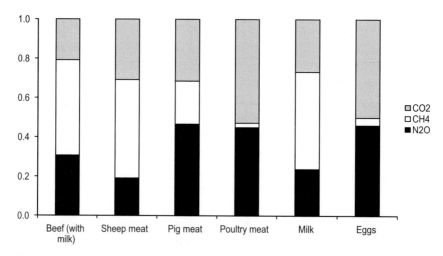

Figure 5. Distribution of gases causing global warming potential (weighted by impact).

Organic ruminant production takes less energy than non-organic, resulting from the lower energy needs of clover–based pasture. Organic pig production also takes less energy, mainly because outdoor production needs no electricity for ventilation. Organic poultry meat and egg production take more energy, mainly through lower productivity. For example, organic poultry meat is normally finished at a higher live weight than non-organic (3.0 and 2.5 kg), has a higher feed conversion ratio (2.71 and 1.85) and has a low killing out percentage (65% and 70%).

Table 12. Ratio of burdens of organic over non-organic production systems.

Item	Beef	Pig meat	Poultry	Sheep meat	Eggs	Milk
Primary energy	0.60	0.65	1.1	0.42	1.1	0.71
GWP_{100}	1.1	0.84	1.5	0.84	1.2	1.1
EP	1.6	0.63	1.7	0.91	1.3	0.95
AP	1.8	0.47	1.6	0.86	1.2	1.2
Pesticides used	0	0	0.07	0	0.01	0
ARU	0.79	0.79	1.5	0.60	1.1	1.1
Land use (*)						
Grade 2	2.6			0.75		1.9
Grade 3a	0.47	1.8	2.0	1.4	2.0	1.5
Grade 3b	1.7			0.63		1.7
Grade 4	1.7			0.63		1.7
Grade 5	2.1			1.7		2.1

(*) Land use for grazing animals comprises a combination of land types from hill to lowland. Land use for arable feed crops consists of land of one of the types. In this table, arable land use is taken as all grade 3a.

Other burdens vary between commodities, for differing reasons. The higher GWP from organic cattle is a consequence of increased enteric fermentation because of higher forage in organic diets, while the lower GWP from organic pigs stems mainly from not storing manure. Higher GWP, EP and AP from organic poultry result from higher feed requirements together with more excreta (hence ammonia) from organic systems. Pesticide use is zero in all but poultry, because (at the time of the analysis) organic production birds originate from non-organic breeding flocks. Organic production is intrinsically less intensive, so the land use is higher. Organically produced pigs and poultry need about twice the land of non-organic counterparts. Land use is more complex for organic cattle, with lower arable land (grade 3a) needed for concentrates, but about twice the amount of other grades for pasture.

The sheep comparison is limited because there were insufficient data to represent all possible land use for an organic flock, so that the organic system here is a set of self-contained flocks.

Beef

Beef production by alternative systems (Table 13) shows how the dairy industry reduces most burdens of beef production, particularly eutrophication and acidification potentials. Most burdens of suckler-based production are higher than the national mixture, although suckler breeding in the hills takes least energy. All sucker beef uses less pesticide owing to lower inclusion of arable-derived feeds. It should be noted that finishing enterprises are not necessarily in the same location as breeding herds.

Table 13. Ratios of burdens from alternative beef systems over the current national mixture (70% of calves from sucklers).

	Beef all dairy origin	All lowland sucklers	All upland sucklers	All hill sucklers
Primary energy	0.8	1.1	1.2	0.9
GWP$_{100}$	0.7	1.1	1.2	1.1
EP	0.4	1.3	1.3	1.5
AP	0.4	1.3	1.3	1.2
Pesticides used	1.7	0.7	0.7	0.7
Abiotic resource use	1.1	0.9	1.0	0.8

Pig meat

Finishing pigs at three weights was compared with the current balance (Table 14). Finishing pigs at higher weights tends to reduce burdens, although by relatively small amounts, mainly as a result of reducing the overheads of breeding piglets. Keeping the breeding herd (together with all weaner production) outdoors reduces most burdens by a larger amount than changing finishing weight. In contrast, pesticide use increases because outdoor sows eat more.

Table 14. Comparison burdens of production of some alternative pig meat systems. All values are the ratio of the alternative over the standard mixture. The current proportion of each system is shown in parenthesis.

	Finishing weight			Sow and weaner production	
Item	76 kg (0.75)	87 kg (0.25)	109 kg (0.05)	Indoor (0.67)	Outdoor (0.33)
Primary energy	1.0	0.97	0.95	1.0	0.87
GWP$_{100}$	1.0	0.97	0.95	1.0	0.92
EP	1.0	0.98	0.96	1.1	0.81
AP	1.0	0.98	1.0	1.1	0.74
Pesticides used	1.0	0.97	0.95	1.0	1.1
Abiotic resource use	1.0	0.97	0.95	1.1	0.84

Poultry meat

Increasing the proportion of free-range chickens and turkeys (in the non-organic sector) to 1 has no effect on energy use, but most burdens increased by 1.1 to 1.3 times (Table 15). In this case, there is an increase in environmental burdens through an alternative finishing system that is often perceived to have welfare benefits. The effects are, however, smaller than converting entirely to organic production. Improving technical efficiency by reducing feed conversion ratio (FCR) to 0.9 of its current values for chicken and turkey production reduces most burdens by a similar amount and the converse applies if FCR increases to 1.1 of current values. The mechanism for improving FCR has not been defined (and the same feed mixture is assumed), but it clearly indicates the benefits of improving technical performance.

Table 15. Comparison burdens of production of some alternative poultry meat systems showing the ratios of the alternative over standard values.

Item	100% free range	FCR 0.9 of normal	FCR 1.1 of normal
Primary energy	1.0	0.92	1.1
GWP100	1.2	0.93	1.1
EP	1.3	1.0	1.0
AP	1.3	1.0	1.0
Pesticides used	1.2	0.90	1.1
Abiotic resource use	1.1	0.93	1.1
Land use grade 3a	1.2	0.90	1.1

Eggs

The current mixture of non-organic egg production systems was assumed to be cage production (0.64), barn (0.06) and free range (0.30). These were compared by setting each system to represent all production (Table 16). The differences are generally not very large, but caged production tended to incur the lowest burdens. Barn production takes less energy, probably through using less ventilation energy than caged production, although needing more feed. Free range takes the 1.2 times the land and pesticide use of caged production by needing more feed. The land requirement for ranging is only 0.05 of that for feed production.

Milk

The current modelled distribution of milk yields is low (0.25), mid (0.55) and high (0.20). Setting any of these to represent all production shows that burdens

Table 16. Comparison burdens of production of some alternative egg production systems. The ratios of alternative of the current mixture of non-organic production are shown.

Item	All free range	All barn	All cage
Primary energy	1.0	0.94	1.0
GWP100	1.1	1.1	0.95
EP	1.1	1.1	1.0
AP	1.0	1.1	1.0
Pesticides used	1.2	1.1	0.91
Abiotic resource use	0.89	0.91	1.1
Land use grade 3a	1.2	1.1	0.90

tend to decrease as yield increases, although pesticide use increases as a result of more concentrate feed needed (Table 17). The differences are not very large, partly because higher yielding cows are heavier and thus have higher maintenance requirements. This partly offsets the reduced breeding requirement. An equal split of autumn and spring calving has been assumed as standard. Milk from autumn calving herds has higher burdens than from spring calving herds. This is mainly because more grass can be used with spring calvers and grazed grass has lower burdens than conserved grass or concentrates. Increasing the proportion of maize (as opposed to grass) silage used nationally from 0.2 to 1 reduces some burdens, especially energy and GWP. Of course, maize cannot be grown successfully everywhere and we have assumed good agricultural practice. Maize is sometimes treated as a dumping ground for manure rather than a crop with specific requirements. Such an approach would clearly increase environmental emissions.

Table 17. Comparison burdens of production of some alternative milk production systems. Ratios of burdens of alternatives over the standard vales are given.

Item	All high yielders	All mid yielders	All low yielders	All autumn calving	All spring calving	All maize silage
Primary energy	0.94	1.0	1.1	1.1	0.93	0.88
GWP100	1.0	1.0	1.0	1.0	1.0	0.89
EP	0.95	1.0	1.0	1.0	1.0	1.0
AP	1.0	1.0	0.92	1.0	1.0	1.0
Pesticides used	1.1	1.0	0.92	1.2	0.80	0.91
Abiotic resource use	0.94	1.0	1.05	1.11	0.89	0.72

Discussion

This study has quantified the burdens of animal production in England and Wales. It shows the high importance of feed supply and use in contributing to energy and resource use, together with emissions to the environment. The partitioning of energy use in different systems shows the areas where most attention is needed to reduce burdens, e.g. feed efficiency in poultry, increasing fecundity (and survival of offspring) in other species. Reducing FCR clearly reduces burdens through reducing feed requirements and manure outputs. There can be no question that improving technical efficiency reduces burdens.

Some aspects of burdens are outside the control of the animal farmer, depending on the species and system. Most arable feeds are produced by other farmers and major inputs are produced by other industries (e.g. synthetic N fertiliser). Some variations were explored (Table 18) and show how increasing urea use may decrease GWP (a specific manufacturing emission of N_2O is present with ammonium nitrate, but not urea), but increases acidification as urea emits more ammonia. Most burdens increase or decrease with N usage. Substituting direct drilling for ploughing (assuming the land type is suitable) has the biggest effect on energy at 0.95 of the standard. These influences are not arcane, but show the dependence of animal production on supply chains over which many farmers have no control. Several of the alternative systems investigated above had effects on burdens of similar magnitude to the agronomic ones in Table 18. This is of increasing significance in a world where retailers and other purchasers are expecting suppliers to provide carbon footprints or other measures of environmental performance. The knowledge needed of the supply chain that leads to the final product is very detailed.

Table 18. Effects of changes in agronomic practice on arable land of burdens of non-organic poultry production compared with standard practice.

Change in practice	Primary energy	GWP_{100}	Eutrophication potential	Acidification potential
Double urea use	1.00	0.98	1.00	1.02
N fertiliser use at 1.2 of current	1.02	1.04	1.05	1.00
N fertiliser use at 0.8 of current	0.99	0.96	0.96	1.00
Ploughing becomes direct drilling	0.95	0.99	1.00	0.99

The largest differences in emissions from crops and animal products relate to excreted N. This contributes to global warming, eutrophication and acidification potentials. The supply of N to crops also incurs huge effort both through synthetic fertilisation and rotational transfers from legumes. The supply and losses of N all reinforce the notion that agriculture has a C-N footprint rather than a C footprint, which is more appropriate for much industrial activity. Improving N utilisation in animal production must be a key target for research, although it must be undertaken with the holistic LCA view to ensure that other burdens are not increased.

The organic *vs* non-organic debate will no doubt continue for some years. This study has shown some environmental advantages in organic production over non-organic, but results were not uniform across commodities. The biggest energetic advantage comes from grass-clover leys in ruminant production. The non-organic ruminant sector could learn from this. One clear feature of organic production is the greater land requirement. It must be acknowledged that our work has been criticised by some in the organic movement. Some changes in modelling have already occurred and more will be implemented, but the lack of objective data in some critical areas has restricted progress.

Since this work was undertaken, the IPCC has issued new guidelines on reporting greenhouse gas emissions from industry and agriculture. The 2006 guidelines have re-interpreted a variety of N_2O emission factors from crops and grassland as well as CH_4 and N_2O from manure management. These will be implemented in our model and are likely to lead to lower apparent emissions of N_2O. It must be stressed that actual emissions have not changed, merely the interpretation of data and processes. It is problematic that N_2O contributes to high proportions of GWP from agriculture, but N_2O is very expensive to measure and it is the emission about which we have the least understanding.

Conclusions

- The burdens of six animal-derived commodities have been quantified at a national scale (England and Wales) in a model than can be interrogated.
- All burdens of meats are higher per t fresh weight than crops, resulting mainly from the concentration of feeds into high quality protein.
- Excretion of undigested N is the main contributor to eutrophication and acidification potentials in animal production.
- Excretion of undigested N also contributes to global warming potential, but enteric and manure emissions of methane are also major sources. Electricity for ventilation and heating is a main source for housed non-ruminants.
- The main use of energy in animal production is in the supply of feed.
- Partition of energy into production and breeding phases differs between species, with much higher overheads in ruminant meat production than the more fecund and feed efficient pigs and poultry.
- Improving technical efficiency reduces burdens.
- Alternative production systems have mixed effects on burdens and each

needs careful consideration.

- Ruminant production in the organic sector takes less energy than in the non-organic sector, owing mainly to N fixation by clover in pastures.
- The relative burdens of GWP, acidification and eutrophication between organic and non-organic animal commodities are more varied than energy in ruminant production.
- Organic pigs use less energy than non-organic counterparts, but poultry meat and eggs take more, resulting from the high overall efficiency of feed conversion in the non-organic sector.
- Organic production takes up to twice the land.
- Ruminant meats produce more burdens than pig or poultry meats, but ruminants can derive nutrition from land that is unsuitable for the arable crops that pigs and poultry must eat.
- Animal farmers often have limited control over production burdens owing to practices in the supply that can have substantial influences on overall animal production burdens.
- Future developments in the model, e.g. IPCC 2006 methods, may cause some values, and even conclusions, to change.

Acknowledgements

The authors are grateful to Defra for funding this work, especially the guidance and support of the Defra project officer, Dr Donal Murphy-Bokern.

References

Audsley, E., Alber, S., Clift, R., Cowell, S., Crettaz, P., Gaillard, G., Hausheer, J., Jolliett, O., Kleijn R., Mortensen, B., Pearce, D., Roger, E., Teulon, H., Weidema, B., and van Zeijts, H. (1997) *Harmonisation of environmental life cycle assessment for agriculture. Final Report, Concerted Action AIR3-CT94-2028*, European Commission, DG VI Agriculture, Brussels.

Baggott, S., Brown, L.M.R., Murrells, T., Passant, N., and Watterson, J. (2004) *UK Greenhouse Gas Inventory, 1990 to 2002. Annual Report for submission under the Framework Convention on Climate Change*, AEA Technology plc, Culham Science Centre, Abingdon, Oxon., OX14 3ED, UK.

Bibby J. S. and Mackney, D. (1969) *Land use capability classification.* Soil Survey technical monograph No 1, Soil Survey of England and Wales, Harpenden.

Brockman, J.S. and Gwynn, P.E.J. (1988) *Journal of the British Grassland Society,*

19, 169-155.

Elsayed, M.A., Matthews, R., and Mortimer, N.D. (2003) *Carbon and Energy Balances for a Range of Biofuels Options*, Project Number B/B6/00784/ REP, URN 03/836, DTI, Sheffield.

IPCC (1997), IPCC Revised 1996 *Guidelines for National Greenhouse Gas Inventories, Volumes 1 to 3, Greenhouse Gas Inventory Reporting Instructions*, IPCC WGI Technical Support Unit, Hadley Centre, Meteorological Office, Bracknell, UK.

Moxey, A.P., White B. and O'Callaghan J. R. (1995) The Economic Component of NELUP, *Journal of Environmental Planning and Management*, **38**, (1), 21-34.

Orr, R. M (1995) Livestock Feeds and Feeding, In Soffe, R.J. (eds) *Primrose McConnell's The Agricultural Notebook* (19th Edn), Blackwell Science, Oxford pp 394-420

Sandars, D.L., Audsley, E., Canete, C., Cumby, T.R., Scotford, I.M. and Williams, A.G. (2003) Environmental Benefits of Livestock Manure Management Practices and Technology by Life Cycle Assessment, *Biosystems Engineering*, **84**, (3), 267-281.

Williams, A.G., Audsley, E. and Sandars, D.L. (2006) *Determining the environmental burdens and resource use in the production of agricultural and horticultural commodities*. Main Report. Defra Research Project IS0205. Bedford: Cranfield University and Defra. Available on www.silsoe.cranfield.ac.uk, and www.defra.gov.uk

10

CO-PRODUCTS FROM BIODIESEL PRODUCTION

K.-H. SÜDEKUM
Institute of Animal Science, University of Bonn, Endenicher Allee 15, 53115 Bonn, Germany

Introduction

The move towards renewable energy sources has increased the production of biofuels, namely bioethanol and biodiesel. The previous Proceedings of the Nottingham Feed Conference discussed co-products from bioethanol production in detail (Gibson and Karges, 2007; Wilson, 2007). In general terms, biodiesel is a methyl-ester produced from vegetable oil, animal oil or recycled fats and oils. In Southeast Asia, biofuel is mainly produced from palm oil (Barnwal and Sharma, 2005), whereas biofuel production in the European Union is largely based on rapeseed oil, mainly in the form of rapeseed oil methylester (RME) or biodiesel, leaving glycerol (synonyms: glycerin and glycerine) as a co-product (see Körbitz *et al.*, 2003; Friedrich, 2004). The approximate proportions of the chemical reaction involved in the production of biodiesel are: (100 l of oil + 10 l of methanol) yield (100 l of biodiesel + 10 l of glycerol; review by Friedrich, 2004).

Starting more than 50 years ago, researchers have shown that glycerol may help to prevent keto-acidosis in the the high-yielding dairy cow by increasing glucose precursors (Forsyth, 1953; Johnson, 1955; Fisher *et al.*, 1971, 1973). Recent research on glycerol as a supplement fed to growing bulls (Pichler and Frickh, 1993) and dairy cows (Khalili *et al.*, 1997; DeFrain *et al.*, 2004; Bodarski *et al.*, 2005) has produced diverging results, thus demanding further research to elucidate the conditions under which glycerol may be used advantageously as a feedingstuff as opposed to the well-established use as feed additive.

In the first part of the chapter, a brief review and summary of data on glycerol for farm animals will be presented with emphasis on ruminants that will encompass the following topics: quality criteria for glycerol, rumen events, energy value and effects on feed intake and performance of dairy cows. In the second part, again putting an emphasis on ruminants, the feeding value of rapeseed products such as rapeseed meal (solvent-extracted) and rapeseed cake (mechanically extracted; synonym: rapeseed expeller) will be briefly treated, because further increases in the demand for and production of glycerol will also increase the amounts of rapeseed meal and cake. "Rumen-protected" protein feeds, which are also produced from solvent-extracted soybean and rapeseed meals and cakes applying physical, chemical and/ or biological treatments are not covered because this would go beyond the scope of the current chapter.

Glycerol

QUALITY

Glycerol of varying quality may be found in the marketplace depending on the extent of refinement of the crude glycerol that is obtained during biodiesel production. Table 1 shows data of glycerol of three different purities that were obtained from different stages of the processing of rapeseed oil. It is important to note that the impure quality with elevated methanol concentrations (267 g/kg dry matter (DM)) was not a commodity but an intermediary product that was used for experimental purposes only. Almost complete disappearance of methanol occurred when pelleted compound feeds were produced from the glycerols of varying quality at glycerol inclusion levels of 50, 100 and 150 g/kg concentrate DM (Südekum *et al.*, 2007). For the benefit of a fail-safe usage of glycerol in diets of all farm animals, methanol should be removed from the glycerol as far as technically possible. Lead and other heavy metals were low for all glycerols under investigation.

Table 1. Chemical composition of glycerol representing different stages of the rapeseed oil methylester production process (Schröder and Südekum, 2002).

Item	*Low*	*Purity of glycerol* *Medium*	*High*
Water (g/kg)	268	11	25
Dry matter composition (g/kg unless stated)			
Glycerol	633	853	998
Crude fat	7.1	4.4	NA[1]
Phosphorus	10.5	23.6	NA
Potassium	22.0	23.3	NA
Sodium	1.1	0.9	NA
Lead (mg/kg)	3	2	NA
Methanol	267	0.4	NA

[1]NA, not analysed; analyses were omitted because the glycerol content was close to 1000 g/kg and high purity glycerol is listed in the official European Union and United States pharmacopoeias.

Recently, and at least in part as a result of increasing biodiesel production and thus glycerol accumulation, glycerol was listed as feedingstuff in the "Positive List" of authorised feed materials in Germany (Normenkommission für Einzelfuttermittel im Zentralausschuss der Deutschen Landwirtschaft, 2006) that, among other objectives, was initiated to contribute to feed safety internationally (Anonymous, 1996) and nationally (Petersen and Flachowsky, 2004). The "Positive List" contains two different glycerols whose specifications are presented in Table 2. Crude glycerol is the quality currently used in farm animal feeding and it is strongly recommended that at least the specifications listed in Table 2 should be given in an instruction leaflet with each batch of crude glycerol. Due to legal restrictions as to the use of animal products in farm animal feeding and because crude glycerol may contain some residual fat, the source of the glycerol (vegetable versus animal) must also be known and stated.

Table 2. Standardized composition (g/kg) of two different glycerol qualities according to the German "Positive List" (Normenkommission für Einzelfuttermittel im Zentralausschuss der Deutschen Landwirtschaft, 2006)

Item	Glycerol	Glycerol, crude
Glycerol	Minimum 990	Minimum 800
Water	5 - 10	100 - 150
Ash	Maximum 1.0	Maximum 100
Methanol	0[1]	Maximum 5.0
Other	-	NaCl, K, P, S

[1]Number indicates concentrations below detection limit.
[2]German authority (Normenkommission für Einzelfuttermittel im Zentralausschuss der Deutschen Landwirtschaft) may change maximum content to 2.0 g/kg on short notice with the detection limit at 1.0 g/kg (W. Lüpping, pers. communication, August 2007).

In the experiment with pelleted compound feeds mentioned above (Südekum *et al.*, 2007) the effects of concentrates, in which glycerol plus soybean meal replaced wheat, on physical, chemical and hygienic pellet quality characteristics were investigated. The three glycerols were as in Table 1, thus reflecting different stages of the RME production process. Inclusion levels of glycerol in the concentrates were 50, 100 and 150 g/kg DM. The quality of the concentrates was assessed under two environmental conditions (good: 15 °C and 60% relative humidity; bad: 20 °C and 70% relative humidity) and two storage durations (four and eight weeks). In summary, chemical composition was only slightly affected by purity and concentration of glycerol or by storage condition or duration. Ergosterol, an indicator of fungal biomass, was used to evaluate the hygienic quality of the pellets and data indicated that glycerol of different purities had a preserving effect. Moreover, physical quality of the pellets was not affected by purity or concentrations of glycerol of up to 150 g/kg DM.

When glycerol, containing 200 g water/kg that was very similar to the water content of the glycerol of medium purity in the study of Südekum *et al.* (2007), was used for manufacturing high-fat broiler pellets and molassed pellets for fattening bulls at glycerol concentrations of 0, 30, 50, 80 and 100 g/kg, abrasion (i.e. proportion of fines of total pellet mass) also decreased with increasing glycerol proportion (Löwe, 1999). When pellets were produced with molasses, however, glycerol at concentrations greater than 50 g/kg resulted in a rough and scaly surface (Löwe, 1999). This author also noted that when feeds are stored in meal form, concentrations of greater than 50 g glycerol/kg may result in lump formation, and therefore suggested to restrict glycerol concentration in pelleted compound feeds to 60 - 70 g/kg based on general storage behaviour including storage in large silos.

In conclusion, glycerol of different purities as a by-product from RME production may help to stabilise the hygienic quality of pelleted compound feeds without compromising physical quality of the pellets.

ENERGY VALUE

Lebzien and Aulrich (1993), based on a digestibility trial on dairy cows, reported that glycerol contains 9.5 MJ net energy for lactation (NEL)/kg. Because theoretical considerations would suggest a higher value (11.1 MJ NEL/kg, based on 18.1 MJ gross energy/kg; H. Steingaß, pers. communication), a series of digestibility trials on sheep was conducted to study the effects of purity and concentration of glycerol on energy concentrations of glycerol and on nutrient digestibilities of mixed rations (Südekum and Schröder, 2002). In the study, concentrations of metabolizable energy (ME) and NEL of glycerols as related to purity of glycerol and glycerol content in the DM of mixed diets were derived from digestibility trials with wethers. Glycerol of varying purity (630, 850, > 995 g glycerol/kg in the product) was mixed with forage (wilted grass silage) and a high-starch concentrate. The mixed diets were formulated to contain (g/kg DM) 400 forage, 500 concentrate and 100 pure glycerol irrespective of the purity of the glycerol-containing product. A forage-only diet and a glycerol-free forage:concentrate diet (400:600 g/kg DM) served as controls. In addition, the glycerol of the highest purity (> 995 g/kg glycerol) was included in diets containing 400 g/kg DM forage and glycerol at 50, 100, 150 or 200 g/kg DM. The high-starch concentrate or a low-starch concentrate made up the balance of these diets (550 to 400 g/kg DM). The NEL concentrations were higher when glycerol was fed with the low-starch concentrate than when fed with the high-starch concentrate (Table 3).

Table 3. Concentrations of metabolisable energy (ME) and net energy for lactation (NEL) of pure glycerol estimated from different proportions of glycerol in the dry matter of rations containing high-starch or low-starch concentrates (Südekum and Schröder, 2002)

Glycerol	Concentrate type			
(g/kg of diet dry matter)	High-starch		Low-starch	
	ME	NEL	ME	NEL
50	14.4	9.6	11.1	6.9
100	13.1	8.4	14.6	9.7
150	12.6	8.0	14.9	9.9
200	13.2	8.5	14.4	9.5
SEM[1]	0.9	0.7	0.9	0.7

[1]SEM, standard error of the means

The estimated ME and NEL concentrations for glycerol derived from diets containing the low-starch concentrate and glycerol at 100, 150 or 200 g/kg DM were similar. When fed with the low-starch concentrate, either no or positive effects of glycerol on digestibilities (organic matter, starch, cell-wall components) were observed. When derived from diets containing the high-starch concentrate as opposed to the low-starch concentrate, glycerol of different purities and at different dietary inclusion levels (100, 150 or 200 g/kg DM) had markedly lower NEL concentrations (8.0 to 8.5 MJ/kg). Similarly, digestibilities of cell-wall components were depressed although without reducing organic matter digestibility. The observed interaction between glycerol and concentrate type are not well understood and require further investigation. It is interesting to note that the low NEL concentrations of glycerol observed with the combination of high-starch concentrate and glycerol are similar to estimates (8.0 MJ NEL/kg) calculated by the computer software package provided by National Research Council (2001).

In conclusion, glycerols of different purities can be included in mixed diets up to 100 g/kg diet DM without negatively influencing digestibilities. When fed with a low-starch concentrate, pure glycerol at dietary inclusion levels up to 200 g/kg DM had either no or even positive effects on digestibilities. When included in diets containing high-starch concentrates, however, glycerol reduced cell-wall digestibility but had no obvious effect on organic matter digestibility.

In summary, the net energy value for ruminants of glycerol was similar to previously published values for dairy cows (9.5 MJ NEL/kg; Lebzien and Aulrich 1993) but considerably lower than derived from theoretical considerations (11.1 MJ NEL/kg, based on 18.1 MJ GE/kg; H. Steingaß, pers. communication). The difference between the two values may be due to ruminal fermentation, post-absorptive metabolism and (or) limitations of standard digestibility trials to estimate ME and NEL values. It is noteworthy that poultry and pig data for ME values (17.5 to 17.6 MJ/kg; Bartelt and Schneider, 2002) better match theoretical considerations for ruminants (16.3 MJ/kg; H. Steingaß, pers. communication) than the ruminant data itself. For a more comprehensive and detailed appraisal of the value of glycerol for non-ruminant farm animals, the reader is referred to Bartelt and Schneider (2002) and conference proceedings on biofuels and co-products (van der Aar, 2007).

RUMEN EVENTS

Previous studies on ruminal metabolism of glycerol have indicated that glycerol is rapidly and extensively fermented in the rumen, and that propionic acid is the major product of glycerol fermentation (Bergner *et al.*, 1995; Kijora *et al.*, 1998). Khalili *et al.* (1997) and Schröder and Südekum (1999) also found increased ruminal butyrate concentrations when glycerol replaced a proportion barley- or wheat-based concentrates. In an *in vivo* study using ruminally-cannulated steers, evidence was provided that small but significant amounts of glycerol can be absorbed directly from the rumen (Südekum *et al.*, unpublished). To elucidate further the fate of glycerol in the rumen, a recent study evaluated effects of glycerol in compound feeds on nutrient turnover in the rumen and digestibilities in the total tract of cattle (Schröder and Südekum, 2002). Four ruminally cannulated steers were used in a 4× 4 Latin square design. They were fed on mixed diets (g/kg DM, 400 forage and 600 concentrate). The concentrate pellets were isonitrogenous and contained no glycerol or 150 g/kg DM of glycerol from glycerol commodities of different purities (630, 850 or > 995 g/kg glycerol in the product). Glycerol intake of the steers was > 1 kg/day.

   Total tract digestibilities of organic matter, cell-wall fractions and starch were similar for all dietary treatments. Irrespective of dietary treatment, postprandial pH values in ruminal fluid were always greater than 6.2. The postprandial decline in pH was more pronounced when the diets contained glycerol. Feeding glycerol resulted in a slight shift towards a reduced ratio of acetic acid to propionic acid. Rumen fill (kg) was slightly higher with the diets containing glycerol. The proportion of bailable liquids of total ruminal contents was also higher for the diets containing glycerol of either quality. Obviously, glycerol had an impact on ruminal water turnover. Estimated ruminal *in vivo* fermentation of fibre components was not impaired when glycerol was substituted for starch in the concentrate portion of the diet. However, when glycerol was supplemented (50 g/kg) *in vitro* to a medium containing cellobiose as the sole energy source (Roger *et al.*, 1992), it inhibited the growth and cellulolytic activity of two rumen cellulolytic bacterial species, *Ruminococcus flavefaciens* and *Fibrobacter succinogenes* subsp. *succinogenes*. At the same level of glycerol supplementation, the growth of an anaerobic fungal species, *Neocallimastix frontalis*, was inhibited and its cellulolytic activity had almost completely disappeared. The *in vitro* data do not allow a conclusion to be drawn on whether the strong inhibition of bacterial and fungal growth and cellulolytic activity was a supplementation effect or caused by specific *in vitro* conditions such as the single species and sole substrate combination, or both.

The *in vivo* data indicate that, when glycerol is substituted in ruminant diets for rapidly-fermentable starch sources, e.g. wheat, it should not exert negative effects on ruminal nutrient turnover and digestibilities of organic matter constituents in the total tract. These findings would suggest that glycerol should replace rapidly fermentable carbohydrates and thus, is not a direct competitor of propylene glycol. Further, it may be speculated that the sweet taste of glycerol may improve intake of diets with inferior palatability (containing, for example, extensively fermented silages) but this still needs to be investigated.

Further, possible effects of glycerol on rumen microbial protein metabolism may warrant more detailed investigations. Paggi *et al.* (1999) studied the effect of increasing concentrations of glycerol (50, 100, 200 and 300 mM) on the proteolytic activity of bovine rumen fluid *in vitro* and reported that glycerol reduced the proteoloytic activity by about 20% with all the concentration increases tested. Kijora *et al.* (1998) infused glycerol (400 g/day, corresponding to 100 g/kg DM intake) into the rumen of growing bulls fed on a hay-grain diet and observed lower concentrations of isobutyric and isovaleric acid in the rumen, indicating that fewer branched-chain amino acids had been degraded. A lower or slower rumen microbial crude protein and amino acid degradation would particularly increase the protein value of fermented forages which would also often benefit from the presumed better palatability of glycerol-containing rations.

FEED INTAKE AND PERFORMANCE OF DAIRY COWS

Early studies have shown that glycerol may help to prevent ketoacidosis in the high-yielding dairy cow by increasing glucose precursors (Forsyth, 1953; Johnson, 1955; Fisher *et al.*, 1971; Fisher *et al.*, 1973; Sauer *et al.*, 1973). In the majority of these experiments glycerol was delivered as an oral drench and, thus, similar to the route that is often used for propylene glycol. Recent research has focused on using glycerol as either a dietary supplement or as partial replacement of starchy dietary ingredients.

Khalili *et al.* (1997) fed grass silage for *ad libitum* consumption and 7 kg/day of a barley-based concentrate (600 g barley/kg) to mid-lactating Friesian cows. Barley was partially replaced (36 g barley/kg) with either glycerol or a fractioned vegetable fatty acid blend or a 1:1 mixture of glycerol and free fatty acids (72 g barley/kg) such that total glycerol intakes amounted to 0.150 kg/day with total DM intakes of around 16 kg/day. Glycerol alone had no effects on intake or performance but slightly decreased ruminal acetate concentrations and slightly increased ruminal propionate and butyrate concentrations. When given in combination, glycerol and free fatty acids tended to increase milk yield. DeFrain *et al.* (2004) fed complete diets to Holstein cows from 14 days prepartum to 21 days postpartum that were top-dressed with either 0.86 kg maize starch (control), 0.43 kg maize starch + 0.43 kg glycerol or 0.86 kg glycerol. Thus, rapidly fermentable glycerol replaced a slowly and incompletely fermentable carbohydrate source. Prepartum DM intake was greater for cows fed the control diet compared with the two glycerol-supplemented diets (13.3, 10.8, and 11.3 ± 0.50 kg/day, respectively). Rumen fluid collected postpartum from cows fed the glycerol-supplemented diets had greater total volatile fatty acids, greater molar proportions of propionate, and a decreased ratio of acetate to propionate. Furthermore, concentrations of butyrate tended to be greater in rumens of cows fed glycerol-supplemented diets. Postpartum DM intake was not affected by treatments. Yield of energy-corrected milk (ECM) during the first 70 days postpartum tended to be greatest for cows fed the control diet. Based upon prepartum DM intake and concentrations of glucose and ß-hydroxybutyrate in blood postpartum, feeding glycerol to dairy cows at the levels used in this experiment increased indicators used to gauge the degree of ketosis in dairy cattle. Bodarski *et al.* (2005) also found that glycerol added to complete diets of dairy cows at 500 mL/day for the first 70 days postpartum, increased ß-hydroxybutyrate in blood serum yet both glycerol supplementation levels decreased total non-esterified fatty acid levels compared with the non-supplemented control. Other than DeFrain *et al.* (2004), Bodarski *et al.* (2005) observed that glycerol-supplemented cows consumed more DM and gave more 13 to 15% more milk than the non-supplemented controls.

Recently, two German studies investigated glycerol in diets for dairy cows in direct comparison with propylene glycol. Engelhard *et al.* (2006) supplemented propylene glycol or glycerol to pre- and postpartum dairy cows using the same calculated amounts per cow of both compounds prepartum (150 g/day) and postpartum (250 g/day). Energy-corrected milk yields (average 38.9 kg/day) and concentrations of milk fat (average 39.0 g/kg) and protein (average 32.4 g/kg) were not different between cows fed propylene glycol or glycerol. Glycerol-supplemented older (≥ second lactation) cows consumed more DM and thus energy than cows receiving propylene glycol (weeks 2 to 8 postpartum: 22.2 versus 21.0 kg/day; weeks 9 to 15 postpartum: 25.2 versus 23.8 kg/day). Blood levels of indices of ketosis such as ß-hydroxybutyrate and non-esterified fatty acids were not different between groups. Results of this study would indicate that effects – not mode of action – of propylene glycol and glycerol were similar and the decision for either of the two supplements should be made based on the balance between greater feed intake and higher feed costs for glycerol and the lower product price of glycerol. Mahlkow-Nerge (2006), in designing the study, followed the rationale that glycerol should replace rapidly fermentable carbohydrates in the diet; a complete ration was supplemented with either 250 g/day of propylene glycol or replaced part of the concentrate with 800 g/day of glycerol. Total intakes (kg DM/day) of concentrate plus propylene glycol or concentrate plus glycerol were the same for all cows. Energy-corrected milk yields (average, 36.1 kg/day) and milk composition (fat, average 42.0 g/kg; protein, average 33.3 g/kg) were the same for both groups. In the trial, first-lactation cows receiving glycerol consumed more (1.2 kg) DM than those fed propylene glycol.

Data of Engelhard *et al.* (2006) and Mahlkow-Nerge (2006) indicates that complete diets containing glycerol may be (slightly) more palatable than diets supplemented with propylene glycol, thus stimulating DM intake. As greater intakes by cows did not result in an increased milk or milk component yield, processes of energy and nutrient conversion in the propylene glycol groups of these two trials likely were more efficient than those in the glycerol groups. Further research is thus required to explore fully the potential of glycerol in dairy cow diets, but type of diet and route of glycerol administration seem to play important roles.

(Other) Rapeseed products – rapeseed meal and rapeseed cake

The protein values of soybean (SBM) and rapeseed (RSM) meals published in feeding value tables differed significantly. The concentration (g/kg) of the crude protein (CP) that is ruminally undegraded (RUP) was 350 for SBM, significantly higher than the 250 stated for RSM (Universität Hohenheim – Dokumentationsstelle, 1997). Similar mean values and, consequently, the same magnitude of difference between the two protein feeds could be calculated from data reported in the feed composition table (Appendix 1) of the Agricultural and Food Research Council (1993), namely 280 g RUP/kg CP for RSM and 370 g for SBM at a rumen outflow rate of 5%/h. More recent experiments indicated that, above all, the considerable differences between the tabulated ruminal degradability values of the two meals in favour of SBM no longer reflect the current situation. Data on *in situ* ruminal degradation rate are shown in Table 4 and indicate that the CP of SBM is degraded even more rapidly than that of RSM. These data are based on a cross-sectional study conducted in Germany covering all oil mills processing rapeseed and soybeans and in addition encompassing some imported SBM commodities. Table 5 provides comparative values for RUP and the utilisable crude protein (uCP) at the duodenum, derived from a comparison of *in situ* and several *in vitro*

Table 4. Rates (%/h) of *in situ* ruminal degradation of crude protein of solvent-extracted rapeseed (RSM) and soybean (SBM) meals[1] (Südekum *et al.*, 2003)

	RSM	SBM
Mean	12	16
RSM vs. SBM	P < 0.001	
Maximum	19	19
Minimum	3	10

[1] 10 RSM (German oil mills) and 7 SBM (German (n = 4), Dutch, Argentine and Brazilian oil mills).

methods on the 17 SBM and RSM of the crosss-sectional study. An overall view of the findings presented in Table 5 and those published by others results in the following conclusions:

(1)   RSM contains more and SBM less RUP than previously stated.
(2)   The smaller difference (by comparison with the values in the tables) in uCP content between SBM and RSM is attributable to the changes in the proportion of RUP.

Table 5. Protein value of contemporary qualities of rapeseed (RSM) and soybean (SBM) meals as compared with feeding table values (Südekum *et al.*, 2003)

	RSM	SBM
Mean RUP[1], g crude protein/kg; DLG Table	300	300
(Universität Hohenheim – Dokumentationsstelle, 1997)	250	350
Mean uCP[1], g/kg dry matter	231	288
DLG Table (Universität Hohenheim – Dokumentationsstelle, 1997)	219	298 – 308

[a] RUP, ruminally-undegraded crude protein.
[b] uCP, utilisable crude protein at the duodenum (sum of microbial and ruminally undegraded crude protein).

Since the reference values determined *in vivo* on duodenally-cannulated dairy cows from selected meals largely, but not completely, confirm the very clear findings from other methods, a literature survey was undertaken in order to check the plausibility of findings reported in Table 5. Studies were considered only when direct comparisons of commercial SBM and RSM (including "canola" qualities but excluding specifically-treated "rumen-protected" feeds) were available and, within the same study, identical methods were used for the two meal types. A total of 15 studies published between 1983 and 1997 could be identified (Rooke *et al*, 1983; Mir *et al*., 1984; Voigt *et al*, 1990; Kendall *et al*., 1991; Tuori, 1992; Zinn, 1993; Khorasani *et al*, 1994; Liu *et al*., 1994; Moss and Givens, 1994; Vanhatalo *et al*., 1995; Stanford *et al*., 1995; Stanford *et al*., 1996; Gralak *et al*., 1997; Mustafa *et al*., 1997; Żebrowska *et al*., 1997) and the following observations were made: Nine studies reported greater RUP values (g/kg CP) for SBM than RES, three studies observed the opposite and three studies found no difference between RUP values of SBM and RSM. Both protein feeds had largely varying RUP contents ranging from 200 to 550 g/kg for SBM and from 120 to 560 g/kg for RSM. Thus, data reported by Südekum *et al*. (2003) appear acceptable and may more closely mimic recent or current SBM and RSM qualities than tabular values.

In conclusion, it is currently recommended that, currently, for RSM and SBM a mean RUP concentration of CP of 300 g/kg should be stated and the uCP values should be correspondingly adjusted. The DLG (Deutsche Landwirtschaftsgesellschaft), the German body responsible for documenting feeding values, accepted this proposal and published it on the internet under http://www.dlg.org/de/landwirtschaft/futtermittelnet/index.html.

At the same time when studies evaluated the fate of CP of SBM and RSM during ruminal degradation, other researchers in a number of applied research stations throughout Germany tested the hypothesis that RSM can fully replace SBM in dairy cow diets when fed on an approximate isonitrogenous and isocaloric basis, i.e. without considering differences in ruminal degradation and (or) amino acid pattern. Data summarized in Table 6 indicate that in the four trials, milk yield and milk component concentrations were similar for diets containing SBM or RSM and thus, the hypothesis can still be sustained.

In conclusion, it should be pointed out that the overall quality of RSM and rapeseed cake depends also on the concentrations of glucosinolates and, in the case of rapeseed cake, the content and quality of the lipid portion. Table 7 would indicate that the average glucosinolate concentrations of RSM are low and that of rapeseed cake are considerably higher and that both feedstuff types show a considerable variation for this item. In addition, crude fat in rapeseed cake varies considerably, making ration formulation a difficult task without having analytical data of specific batches at hand. Increasing crude fat contents lowers crude protein concentration and vice versa. Grouping of rapeseed cakes according to crude fat concentration (g/kg) appears necessary, e.g., 70 to 100, 120 to 150, other (greater values are often found in small-scale enterprises). Additionally, storage stability

Table 6. Comparative evaluation of rapeseed (RSM) and soybean (SBM) meals in diets for high-producing dairy cows - summary of German trials (Spiekers and Südekum, 2004)

Location, duration of trials and diets	Protein supplement kg/(day x cow)	Milk kg/day	Fat g/kg milk	Protein g/kg milk
LWZ Haus Riswick: lactation weeks 5 - 35				
Basal diet	SBM 2.3 kg	31.1	39	31
1/3 MS[1] + 2/3 GS[2]	RSM 3.1 kg	31.3	39	32
LWZ Haus Riswick: lactation weeks 2 – 44				
TMR[3] with	SBM 1.6 kg	25.2	42	34
500g MS + 250g GS/kg	RSM 2.2 kg	25.8	41	34
LVA Iden: until lactation week 17				
TMR with 400g (MS +	SBM 4.0 kg	40.0	38	33
EMS[4]) + 250g GS/kg	RSM 4.3 kg	40.5	39	33
LVA Köllitsch: 17 weeks				
Basal diet	SBM 1.6 kg	31.2	39	34
500g MS + 500 gGS/kg	RSM 2.0 kg	32.7	40	34

[1]MS, maize silage.
[2]GS, grass silage.
[3]TMR, totally mixed ration.
[4]EMS, ear-maize silage.

Table 7. Quality of rapeseed cake and rapeseed meal – survey data from Germany (miscellaneous sources; Weiß, 2007)

Type and source of feed	n =	GSL[1] (mmol/kg DM[2]) (Min - Max)	Crude fat (g/kg DM) (Min - Max)
Rapeseed meal (solvent-extracted)			
10 German oil mills	637	8.3 (1 - 20)	
Monitoring 2006 (UFOP)	68	8.2 (4.4 - 11.2)	
Rapeseed cake (mechanically extracted)			
6 plants	85	22.1 (15 - 29)	126 (90 – 170)
31 local plants	94	15.9 (7 - 28)	151 (90 - 280)
22 local plants	22	13.5 (5 - 22.4)	169 (129 - 243)

[1]GSL, glucosinolates
[2]DM, dry matter

should be considered because the fat is in a non-protected form after mechanical extraction of the seed. It has also been reported by farmers and consultants that physical characteristics resulting from plaque forming during oil extraction make rapeseed cake difficult to handle and that a homogenous distribution in complete diets or silage mixtures is difficult to achieve.

It also becomes evident from these data that a more widespread use of RSM and rapeseed cake in diets for pigs and poultry requires further reduction of glucosinolate levels, particularly for the cake, and smaller variations would also be helpful in this respect. The crude fat content of the cakes should also be more standardized to make use of the commodities easier and more reliable.

Table 8 summarizes current German recommendations for rapeseed products in diets of cattle and pigs. Pigs would particularly benefit from progress in further reduction of glucosinolate levels whereas, in cattle, a safer quality assessment of the rapeseed cake is needed from which also pigs would benefit.

Table 8. Practical recommendations for daily amounts or dietary concentrations (as fed basis for dry diets) of rapeseed products for cattle and pigs (Weiß, 2007)

Animal category	Rapeseed meal, solvent-extracted	Rapeseed cake, mechanically extracted
Dairy cow	Maximum 4 kg	1.5 - 2.0 kg
Beef cattle	Maximum 1.2 kg	1 kg
Fattening pigs	Maximum 100 g/kg	70 – 100 g/kg
Sows	50 – 100 g/kg	50 – 100 g/kg
Piglets	-	50 – 100 g/kg

Summary and conclusions

The current chapter reviews utilization of glycerol as a by-product from biodiesel production and that of other rapeseed products such as rapeseed meal and cake in diets for farm animals with a focus on ruminants. For the benefit of a fail-safe usage of glycerol in diets of all farm animals, methanol should be removed from the glycerol as far as technically possible. Glycerol inclusion levels of 50, 100 and 150 g/kg concentrate dry matter (DM) and storage of concentrates under good (15 °C and 60% relative humidity) or bad (20 °C and 70% relative humidity) environmental conditions for four or eight weeks revealed that physical quality of pellets was not affected by purity of glycerol or by glycerol concentrations of up to 150 g/kg DM. Glycerol at different purities may help to stabilise the hygienic quality of pelleted compound feeds without compromising physical quality of pellets. Glycerol is a versatile feedingstuff in particular for ruminants but is different from propylene glycol. Data on ruminal turnover of glycerol would suggest that it should replace rapidly fermentable carbohydrates and, thus, is not a direct competitor of propylene glycol. Mature cattle can consume considerable quantities of glycerol (1 kg/d). Further, it may be speculated that the sweet taste of glycerol may improve intake of diets with inferior palatability (containing, e.g., extensively fermented silages) but this still needs to be investigated.

The NEL concentration for ruminants is approximately 9.5 MJ/kg of glycerol. Conflicting results from trials on dairy cows indicate that more research is necessary to define conditions that allow glycerol to be used advantageously. The most recent data indicate that complete diets containing glycerol may be (slightly) more palatable than diets supplemented with propylene glycol, thus stimulating DM intake. As greater intakes by cows did not result in an increased milk or milk component yield, processes of energy and nutrient conversion in the propylene glycol groups of these two trials likely were more efficient than those in the glycerol groups. Further research is thus required to explore fully the potential of glycerol in dairy cow diets but type of diet and route of glycerol administration seem to play important roles.

Other rapeseed products for ruminants, such as rapeseed meal, compare well with soybean meal for dairy cows if fed on an isonitrogenous basis. Recent research on rapeseed meal has shown that it can fully replace soybean meal in dairy cow diets when fed on an approximate isonitrogenous and isocaloric basis, i.e. without considering differences in ruminal degradation and (or) amino acid pattern. Milk and milk component yields were similar for diets containing soybean meal or rapeseed meal. Rapeseed cake needs further consideration and more reliable data because variations in the processing conditions result in varying chemical composition, particularly regarding the crude fat content and this currently hampers the prediction of its feeding value for all categories of farm animals. The value of rapeseed cake would benefit from a standardization of the composition, because varying crude fat and crude protein concentrations makes the feeding value difficult to predict and could also affect storage stability of the cake.

References

Agricultural and Food Research Council (1993). *Energy and Protein Requirements of Ruminants*. CAB International, Wallingford.

Anonymous (1996) Council Directive 96/25/EC of 29 April 1996 on the circulation of feed materials, amending Directives 70/524/EEC, 74/63/EEC, 82/471/EEC and 93/74/EEC and repealing Directive 77/101/EEC. *Official Journal of the European Union* L **125**, 35-58.

Barnwal, B.K. and Sharma, M.P. (2005) Prospects of biodiesel production from vegetable oils in India. *Renewable and Sustainable Energy Reviews* **9**, 363-378.

Bartelt, J. and Schneider, D. (2002) Untersuchungen zum energetischen Futterwert von Glycerol in der Fütterung von Geflügel und Schweinen. *UFOP-Schriften* **17**, 15-36.

Bergner, H., Kijora, C., Ceresnakova, Z., and Szakács, J., (1995) In vitro Untersuchungen zum Glycerinumsatz durch Pansenmikroorganismen. *Archives of Animal Nutrition* **48**, 245-256.

Bodarski, R., Wertelecki, T., Bommer, F. and Gosiewski, S. (2005) The changes of metabolic status and lactation performance in dairy cows under feeding TMR with glycerin (glycerol) supplement at periparturient period. *Electronic Journal of Polish Agricultural Universities* **8** (4), 9 pp. Accessible online at: http://www.ejpau.media.pl/volume8/issue4/art-22.html.

DeFrain, J.M., Hippen, A.R., Kalscheur, K.F. and Jardon, P.W. (2004) Feeding glycerol to transition dairy cows: Effects on blood metabolites and lactation performance. *Journal of Dairy Science* **87**, 4195-4206.

Doppenberg, J. amd van der Aar. P. (Editors) (2007) *Biofuels: Implications for the Feed Industry*. Wageningen Academic Publishers, Wageningen.

Engelhard, T., Meyer, A., Staufenbiel, R. and Kanitz, W. (2006) Vergleich des Einsatzes von Propylenglykol und Glyzerin in Rationen für Hochleistungskühe. In *Forum angewandte Forschung in der Rinder- und Schweinefütterung*, pp 26-29. Verband der Landwirtschaftskammern, Bonn.

Fisher, L.J., Erfle, J.D., Lodge, G.A. and Sauer, F.D. (1973) Effects of propylene glycol or glycerol supplementation of the diet of dairy cows on feed intake, milk yield and composition, and incidence of ketosis. *Canadian Journal of Animal Science* **53**, 289-296.

Fisher, L.J., Erfle, J.D. and Sauer, F.D. (1971) Preliminary evaluation of the addition of glucogenic materials to the rations of lactating cows. *Canadian Journal of Animal Science* **51**, 721-727.

Forsyth, H. (1953) Glycerol in the treatment of (1) bovine acetonemia, (2) pregnancy toxaemia in ewes. *Veterinary Records* **65**, 198.

Friedrich, S. (2004) A world wide review of the commercial production of biodiesel – a technological, economic and ecological investigation based on case studies. *Schriftenreihe Umweltschutz und Ressourcenökonomie*, 41. Institut für Technologie und nachhaltiges Produktmanagement, Wirtschaftsuniversität Wien, Austria.

Gibson, M.L. and Karges, K. (2007) By-products from non-food agriculture: Technicalities of nutrition and quality. In *Recent Advances in Animal Nutrition – 2006*, pp 209-227. Edited by P.C. Garnsworthy and J. Wiseman. Nottingham University Press, Nottingham.

Gralak, M.A., Kamalu, T., von Keyserlingk, M.A.G and Kulasek, G.W. (1997) Rumen dry matter and crude protein degradability of extracted or untreated oilseeds and *Leucaena leucocephala* leaves. *Archives of Animal Nutrition* **50**, 173-185.

Johnson, R.B (1955) The treatment of ketosis with glycerol and propylene glycol. *Cornell Veterinarian* **44**, 6-21.

Kendall, E.M., Ingalls, J.R. and Boila, R.J. (1991) Variability in the rumen degradability and postruminal digestion of the dry matter, nitrogen and amino acids of canola meal. *Canadian Journal of Animal Science* **71**, 739-754.

Khalili, H., Varvikko, T., Toivonen, V., Hissa, K. and Suvitie, M. (1997) The effects of added glycerol or unprotected free fatty acids or a combination of the two on silage intake, milk production, rumen fermentation and diet digestibility in cows given grass silage based diets. *Agricultural and Food Science in Finland* **6**, 349-362.

Khorasani, G.R., Robinson, P.H. and Kennelly, J.J. (1994) Evaluation of solvent and expeller linseed meals as protein sources for dairy cattle. *Canadian Journal of Animal Science* **74**, 479-485.

Kijora, C., Bergner, H., Götz, K.-P., Bartelt, J., Szakács, J. and Sommer, A. (1998) Research note: Investigation on the metabolism of glycerol in the rumen of bulls. *Archives of Animal Nutrition* **51**, 341-348.

Körbitz, W., Friedrich, S., Waginger, E. and Wörgetter, M. (2003) *Worldwide Review on Biodiesel Production*. Austrian Biofuels Institute, Wieselburg.

Lebzien, P. and Aulrich, K. (1993) Zum Einfluss von Glycerin auf die Rohnährstoffverdaulichkeit und einige Pansenparameter bei Milchkühen. *VDLUFA-Schriftenreihe* **37**, 361-364.

Liu, Y.-G., Steg, A. and Hindle, V. (1994) Rumen degradation and intestinal digestion of crambe and other oilseed by-products in dairy cows. *Animal Feed Science and Technology* **45**, 397-409.

Löwe, R. (1999) Processing-specific consequences of the use of glycerine. *Kraftfutter/Feed Magazine* **82**, 394-402.

Mahlkow-Nerge, K. (2006) Vergleich des Einsatzes von Propylenglykol und Glyzerin in Rationen für Hochleistungskühe. In *Forum angewandte Forschung in der Rinder- und Schweinefütterung*, pp 30-34. Verband der Landwirtschaftskammern, Bonn.

Mir, Z., MacLeod, G.K., Buchanan-Smith, J.G., Grieve, D.G. and Grovum, W.L. (1984) Methods for protecting soybean and canola proteins from degradation in the rumen. *Canadian Journal of Animal Science* 64, 853-865.

Moss, A.R. and Givens, D.I. (1994) The chemical composition, digestibility, metabolisable energy content and nitrogen degradability of some protein concentrates. *Animal Feed Science and Technology* **47**, 335-351.

Mustafa, A.F., McKinnon, J.J., Thacker, P.A. and Christensen, D.A. (1997) Effect of borage meal on nutrient digestibility and performance of ruminants and pigs. *Animal Feed Science and Technology* **64**, 273-285.

National Research Council (2001) *Nutrient Requirements of Dairy Cattle*. 7th revised Edition. National Academy of Science, Washington, DC.

Normenkommission für Einzelfuttermittel im Zentralausschuss der Deutschen Landwirtschaft (2006). *Positivliste für Einzelfuttermittel (Futtermittel-Ausgangserzeugnisse)*. 5th Edition. Zentralausschuss der Deutschen Landwirtschaft, Berlin, Germany. Available online at: http://www.futtermittel.net/pdf/positivliste_5.pdf.

Paggi, R.A., Fay, J.P. and Fernández, H.M. (1999) Effect of short-chain fatty acids and glycerol on the proteolytic activity of rumen fluid. *Animal Feed Science and Technology* **78**, 341-347.

Petersen, U. and Flachowsky, G. (Editors) (2004). Workshop Positivliste für Futtermittel als Beitrag zur Futtermittelsicherheit – Erwartungen, Konzepte und Lösungen. *Landbauforschung Völkenrode Sonderheft* **271**, 158 pp

Pichler, W.A. and Frickh, J.J. (1993) Der Einsatz von Glycerin aus der Rapsölmethylestererzeugung in der Jungstiermast. *Förderungsdienst* **41** (4), 25-28.

Roger, V., Fonty, G., Andre, C., Gouet, P. (1992) Effects of glycerol on the growth, adhesion, and cellulolytic activity of rumen cellulolytic bacteria and anaerobic fungi. *Current Microbiology* **25**, 197-201.

Rooke, J.A., Brookes, I.M. and Armstrong, D.G. (1983) The digestion of untreated and formaldehyde-treated soya-bean and rapeseed meals by cattle fed a basal silage diet. *Journal of Agricultural Science (Cambridge)* **100**, 329-342.

Sauer, F.D., Erfle, J.D. and Fisher, L.J. (1973) Propylene glycol and glycerol as a feed additive for lactating dairy cows: An evaluation of blood metabolite parameters. *Canadian Journal of Animal Science* **53**, 265-271.

Schröder, A. and Südekum, K.-H. (1999) Glycerol as a by-product of biodiesel production in diets for ruminants. In *New Horizons for an Old Crop*, Paper No. 241. Edited by N. Wratten and P. A. Salisbury. Proc. 10th Int. Rapeseed Congr., Canberra, Australia.

Schröder, A. and Südekum, K.-H. (2002) Effekte von Glycerin unterschiedlicher Reinheit auf die Pansenfermentation und Nährstoffverdaulichkeiten bei Rindern. *UFOP-Schriften* **17**, 51-67.

Spiekers, H. and Südekum, K.-H. (2004) *Einsatz von 00-Rapsextraktionsschrot beim Wiederkäuer*. UFOP-Praxisinformation. UFOP, Berlin.

Stanford, K., McAllister, T.A., Lees, B.M., Xu Z.J. and Cheng, K.-J. (1996) Comparison of sweet white lupin seed, canola meal and soybean meal as protein supplements for lambs. *Canadian Journal of Animal Science* **76**, 215-219.

Stanford, K., McAllister, T.A., Xu Z.J., Pickard M., and Cheng, K.-J. (1995)

Comparison of lignosulfonate-treated canola meal and soybean meal as rumen undegradable protein supplements for lambs. *Canadian Journal of Animal Science* **75**, 371-377.

Südekum, K.-H., Nibbe, D., Lebzien, P., Steingaß, H. and Spiekers, H. (2003) Comparative evaluation of the protein values of soybean and rapeseed meals by *in vivo, in situ* and laboratory methods. In: *Towards enhanced value of cruciferous oilseed crops by optimal production and use of the high quality seed components*, pp 1241-1243. Proc. 11th Int. Rapeseed Congr., Copenhagen, Denmark.

Südekum, K.-H. and Schröder, A. (2002) Einfluß der Reinheit und Konzentration von Glycerin auf die Energiegehalte von Glycerin und die Nährstoffver-daulichkeiten gemischter Rationen für Wiederkäuer. *UFOP-Schriften* **17**, 37-50.

Südekum, K.-H., Schröder, A., Fiebelkorn, S., Schwer, R. and Thalmann, A. (2007) Quality characteristics of pelleted compound feeds under varying storage conditions as influenced by purity and concentration of glycerol from biodiesel production. *Journal of Animal and Feed Sciences* (in press).

Tuori, M. (1992) Rapeseed meal as a supplementary protein for dairy cows on grass-silage based diet, with the emphasis on the Nordic AAT-PBV feed protein evaluation system. *Agricultural Science in Finland* **1**, 367-439.

Universität Hohenheim – Dokumentationsstelle (Editor) (1997). *DLG-Futterwerttabellen Wiederkäuer*. 7th Edition. DLG, Frankfurt/Main.

Vanhatalo, A., Aronen, I. and Varvikko, T. (1995) Intestinal nitrogen digestibility of heat-moisture treated rapeseed meals as assessed by the mobile-bag method in cows. *Animal Feed Science and Technology* **55**, 139-152.

Voigt, J., Piatkowski, B., Schönhusen, U., Kreienbring, F., Krawielitzki R. and Nagel, S. (1990) Studies on the evaluation of feed protein for ruminants. 1. Passage of nitrogen fractions to the duodenum of dairy cows fed different protein and carbohydrate sources. *Archives of Animal Nutrition* **40**, 245-257.

Weiß, J., 2007. Futtermittel aus der Rapsverarbeitung. In *Winterraps - Das Handbuch für Profis*, pp 277-289. Edited by O. Christen and W. Friedt. DLG, Frankfurt/Main.

Wilson, T. (2007) By-products from non-food agriculture: Implications for the feed supply industry. In *Recent Advances in Animal Nutrition – 2006*, pp 199-207. Edited by P.C. Garnsworthy and J. Wiseman. Nottingham University Press, Nottingham.

Żebrowska, T., Długołęcka, Z., Pajak, J.J. and Korczyński, W. (1997) Rumen degradability of concentrate protein, amino acids and starch, and their digestibility in the small intestine of cows. *Journal of Animal and Feed Sciences* **6**, 451-470.

Zinn, R.A. (1993) Characteristics of ruminant and total tract digestion of canola meal and soybean meal in a high-energy diet for feedlot cattle. *Journal of Animal Science* **71**, 796-801.

11

MYCOTOXINS IN ANIMAL FEED: IS THERE REALLY A PROBLEM?

E.M. BINDER[a*], E. PICHLER[b], M. KAINZ[b], V. STARKL[c]
[a]Biomin Research Center, Technopark 1, 3430 Tulln, Austria; [b]Quantas Analytik GmbH, Technopark 1, 3430 Tulln, Austria; [c]Biomin, 11 de Septiembre, No 2628, Piso 12, Dpto 4, Ciudad de Buenos Aires, ZIP 1428, Argentina

Summary

A three-year survey program was initiated by feed additive producer Biomin® in order to evaluate the incidence of mycotoxins in feed and feed raw materials in some of the major European animal production regions. Mycotoxins tested for were those known for their impact on feed industry and animal husbandry: deoxynivalenol (DON), T-2 toxin, zearalenone (ZON), ochratoxin A (OTA), and aflatoxin B1 (AfB1). A total of 1838 samples sourced from European and Mediterranean markets was tested, with 3231 single analyses performed (1838 tests for DON, 943 ZON, 270 T-2 toxin, 109 OTA, and 71 AfB1, respectively). All tested commodities were affected by DON, which had high incidence particularly in maize, wheat and wheat bran, oat and finished feed, with more than two thirds of all tested samples contaminated. ZON was also frequently found in maize, wheat and wheat bran, and finished feeds, though at a somewhat lower incidence than DON.

Introduction

Mycotoxins are secondary metabolites produced by filamentous fungi that can cause a toxic response (mycotoxicosis) when ingested by higher animals. Due to modern analytical methods and thanks to a growing interest in this field of research, more than 300 different mycotoxins have currently been differentiated. However for a practical consideration in the feed manufacturing process only a small number of toxins is of relevance, with aflatoxins, trichothecenes, zearalenone, ochratoxins and fumonisins being of particular interest, though it has to be mentioned that the extent of harm each toxin (group) can cause is highly species-dependant (Binder *et al.*, 2007).

Cereal plants may be contaminated by mycotoxins in two ways: fungi growing as pathogens on plants or growing saprophytically on stored plants, whereas it has to be pointed out that not all fungal growth may result in mycotoxin formation and detection of fungi does not imply necessarily the presence of mycotoxins. Consumption of a mycotoxin-contaminated diet may induce acute and long-term chronic effects resulting in teratogenic, carcinogenic, and oestrogenic or immune-suppressive effects. Direct consequences of consumption of mycotoxin-contaminated animal feed include: reduced feed intake, feed refusal, poor feed conversion, diminished body weight gain, increased disease incidence (due to immune-suppression), and reduced reproductive capacities, which leads to economic losses (Huwig *et al.*, 2001).

Although scientific literature and research offer substantial information on the effects of individual mycotoxins in selected animal species, concurrent exposure to multiple mycotoxins is rarely investigated. In field outbreaks, naturally-contaminated feeds may contain multiple mycotoxins, not only because some fungi are able to produce different types of toxins but also due to cross contamination during the feed manufacturing process, where different raw materials are combined, being a source for a variety of fungal toxins.

The aim of the current chapter is to summarize the results of a three-year mycotoxin survey conducted in regions relevant to the European feed industry. Grain and feed samples were sourced directly at feed mills or animal production sites and sent for analysis to Quantas Analytik in Austria, where all analyses were performed by means of high performance liquid chromatography.

Materials and methods

ANALYTICAL SAMPLES

Grain and feed samples were sourced directly at animal feed production sites and sent for analysis to the former Romer® laboratory in Tulln, Austria, now Quantas. Sample providers could choose between "full toxin screens", which covered major A- and B-trichothecenes, zearalenone, fumonisins, aflatoxins, and ochratoxin A, and analyses of selected mycotoxins. The origin (name and location of submitter) of samples was kept strictly confidentially; analytical certificates were submitted only to the originators of samples. The current chapter summarises the occurrence of mycotoxins with regard to regions of their sourcing and commodities. Data on fumonisins are not presented as the overall number of tests performed was quite small, with only 20 samples submitted for fumonisin analysis, and thus not at all representative.

REAGENTS

Mycotoxin standards were purchased from Biopure® Referenzsubstanzen GmbH, Austria. Organic solvents, HPLC-grade water, salts and other chemicals were purchased from Merck AG, Germany.

SAMPLE PREPARATION AND CLEAN-UP PROCEDURES

Sample clean-up and reverse-phase high performance liquid chromatographic (HPLC) analyses were undertaken as described earlier (Binder *et al.*, 2007). In brief 25g of sample material were extracted with 100ml of acetonitrile water mixture, and purified by solid phase extraction (Mycosep® or Multisep® cartridges, Romer Labs, MO) or immunoaffinity columns (OchraStar®, ZearaStar®, AflaStar® Fit, Romer Labs Diagnostic GmbH, Austria). HPLC was performed using equipment of the HPLC series 1100 from Agilent® technologies, Germany, comprising a micro vacuum degasser, a binary capillary pump, a micro autosampler, column oven as well as a mass spectrometer (single quadrupole) connected via an API-ES interface in case of T-2 toxin and fumonisin analysis, a variable wavelength detector for DON, or a fluorescence detector for zeralenone, aflatoxin and ochratoxin A determination. For method validation uncontaminated grains were spiked at seven different concentration levels using toxin standards dissolved in acetonitrile. Three replicates of blanks and each fortified level were analysed. Control samples were analysed with each series of routine samples, results plotted using a CCPro Plus computer program (Chem SW, USA).

Limits of quantification (LOQ) and recoveries are summarized in table 1.

Table 1. Recoveries and Limits of Quantification (LOQ) of methods applied

	Recovery (%)	*Limit of quantification (µg/kg)*
Deoxynivalenol	72	50
T-2 toxin (LC-MS)	103	30
Zearalenone	100	10
Fumonisins (LC-MS)	80	25
Ochratoxin A	83	1
Aflatoxin B1	87	0.5

Results

All analysed samples were part of an initiative with the aim of surveying animal feed and raw materials in Europe and Mediterranean regions for occurrence and levels of mycotoxins, which account for major problems in the animal feed industry. Samples of raw materials and finished feed were taken directly at animal farms or animal feed production sites, and analysed in the period from January 2004 to December 2006.

In order to get a better overview about toxin occurrence in certain regions, data were grouped as follows:

- *Northern Europe* (Denmark, Belgium, Finland, UK, Norway, Lithuania, the Netherlands, Latvia),
- *Central Europe* (Romania, Poland, Slovakia, Ukraine, Hungary, Switzerland, Austria, Germany, Czech Republic), and
- *Southern Europe and the Mediterranean* region (Slovenia, Bulgaria, Portugal, France, Croatia, Spain, Greece, Turkey, Cyprus, Italy).

DON

A total of 1838 samples were tested for DON contamination, 0.63 of these were positive (mean level 380μg/kg; median 300μg/kg). Slight differences were observed in the course of years: highest incidence was observed in 2006, when 0.73 of all samples detected positive for DON, followed by 2005 with 0.63 positives and 2004 with 0.59 positives. Average levels were also highest in 2006, with a mean contamination of all samples of 622 μg/kg and a median, which was calculated of all positives, of 431 μg/kg (mean and median levels were 375 and 329μg/kg in 2005, and 277 and 230μg/kg in 2004, respectively).

In 2004 0.72 of Northern European samples were contaminated with DON (mean 277μg/kg, median 229μg/kg), 0.53 of those from Central Europe, which had similar levels (260 and 240μg/kg, respectively), and 0.52 of Southern European samples at somewhat lower levels (196 and 171μg/kg). The picture changed in the year after, when 0.68 of Northern European samples, 0.62 of Central European samples and 0.57 of samples sourced in Southern Europe and the Mediterranean region tested positive. Average levels were highest in the south (mean of 653 and median of 380μg/kg), followed by commodities sourced in the north (445 and 306). The mean level of central European samples was 308μg/kg and the median 320μg/kg.

Only a small number of Northern European samples was obtained in 2006; out of a total of 12, five tested positive for DON, but at very low levels (mean of 66μg/kg, median of 140μg/kg). The majority of samples were received from Central Europe, and 0.75 (i.e. 229) out of 306 samples were positive, mean levels amounted to 667μg/kg, the median was 456μg/kg. Of 26 samples received from the south, 16 were positive; the average level was 349μg/kg, the median 273μg/kg.

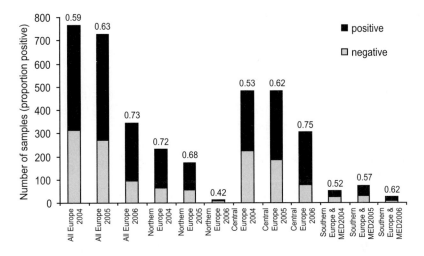

Figure 1. Occurrence of DON.

Commodities mostly affected by DON were maize (0.59 positives in 2004, 0.79 in 2005, and 0.90 in 2006, respectively) and wheat (0.79 in 2004, 0.66 in 2005; only 6 samples were tested in 2006, half of them were positive). Alhough only 28 analyses were performed on wheat bran in total, it is important to mention the remarkably high DON incidence, which was 0.93, with a mean of 678µg/kg, and a median of 584µg/kg. The average contamination level of barley was 0.28, at relatively low levels (108 and 210µg/kg).

The analysis included 394 finished feed samples over the years, 0.62 of them were positive, with again a higher incidence in the year 2006 at 0.79 and also highest levels observed (mean 676 µg/kg, median 368µg/kg; in 2004: 0.56 contamination rate, mean of 145µg/kg, median of 167µg/kg; in 2005: 0.57, 199 and 214µg/kg, respectively). The category "other feed ingredients" covers commodities that were not specified by clients and which could not be attributable definitively. The number tested was 468, 0.66 were positive, the highest contamination rate was found in 2004 (0.70), followed by 0.64 in 2006, and 0.56 in 2005. Levels observed were similar in all three years: means ranged from 334 to 359µg/kg, median levels from 223 to 253µg/kg.

Only a small number of soy samples was tested (56); about one third was contaminated (mean 78µg/kg, median 279µg/kg). 8 out of a total of 14 triticale samples were positive, the mean level was 227µg/kg, the median 435.

Detailed information of DON contamination with regard to commodities is given in table 2.

Table 2. Incidence of mycotoxin DON in feed grain and animal feed sourced in Europe and the Mediterranean Region 2004-2006 data.

	DON - 2004		DON - 2005		DON - 2006		DON 2004-2006	
	Total number[a] Mean/ median[c]	*Num, positive[b] Max. level[d]*	*Total number[a] Mean/ median[c]*	*Num, positive[b] Max. level[d]*	*Total number[a] Mean/ median[c]*	*Num, positive[b] Max. level[d]*	*Total number[a] Mean/ median[c]*	*Num, positive[b] Max. level[d]*
Corn	152	90 (59%)	196	155 (79%)	128	115 (90%)	476	355 (76%)
	246/290	5000	528/360	3870	927/604	7530	546/425	7530
Wheat	96	76 (79%)	53	35 (66%)	6	3 (50%)	155	115 (74%)
	600/284	ca. 10 000	452/370	2230	72/161	202	530/280	ca. 10 000
Wheat bran	6	6 (100%)	20	18 (90)	2	2 (100%)	28	26 (93%)
	768/707	1099	616/486	2500	1037/1037	1547	678/584	2500
Barley	107	33 (31%)	76	20 (26%)	20	4 (20%)	203	57 (28%)
	96/150	1550	135/450	2350	70/358	612	108/210	2350
Oat	12	8 (67%)	29	29 (97%)	3	1 (33%)	44	37 (84%)
	476/490	2600	859/772	3021	48/143	143	700/630	3021
Finished feed	136	76 (56%)	164	94 (57%)	94	74 (79%)	394	244 (62%)
	145/167	2226	199/214	3340	676/368	6057	295/235	6057
Other feed ingredients	227	160 (70%)	168	100 (59%)	73	47 (64%)	468	307 (66%)
	334/223	3800	354/225	5510	359/253	6572	345/232	6572
Soy	24	3 (13%)	14	7 (50%)	15	2 (13%)	53	12 (23%)
	12/96	131	192/370	780	94/708	960	78/279	960

[a] Total number of samples analysed
[b] Number of samples tested positive
[c] Arithmetic mean of all samples tested/median of positives in µg/kg
[d] Maximum level detected in µg/kg

ZON

During the survey a total of 943 samples were tested for ZON, indicating an overall contamination rate of 0.34. While in 2004 only 0.17 of 312 samples were positive for ZON, 0.33 positives out of 409 samples analysed in 2005 were found. In 2006 only 222 samples were tested, the contamination rate was at 0.58, with Central and Southern Europe contributing most to this high incidence level. While ZON contamination incidence decreased from 0.38 (in 2004) to 0.23 (in 2005), and to 0.17 (in 2006) in northern European samples, Southern and Central Europe showed a contrary trend: the ZON contamination rate in the south was 0.20 in 2004, 0.42 in 2005, and 0.64 in 2006; in Central Europe data were 0.09 (2004), 0.38 (2005), and 0.60 (2006), respectively. The same tendency, i.e. increase of contamination rate from 2004 to 2006 in commodities sourced in Central and Southern Europe, was also monitored with DON, with rates increasing from 0.53 to 0.62 and 0.75 (Central Europe) and 0.52, 0.57, and 0.62 (Southern Europe), respectively, indicating favourable growth conditions for *Fusarium sp.*, which are capable of producing both toxins.

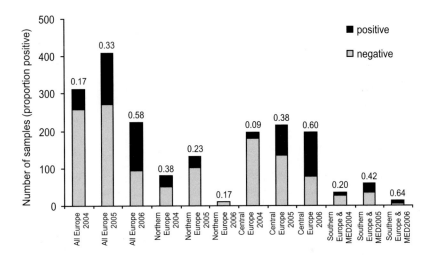

Figure 2. Occurrence of ZON.

Major commodities affected were maize, with 0.13 testing positive in 2004, 0.60 in 2005, and 0.84 in 2006. The year 2006 also entailed the highest contamination levels, with an overall mean of 213µg/kg, and the median of positives at 132µg/kg. Wheat and wheat bran were also substantially affected (0.44 and 0.55, respectively), though the number of samples tested in each year would not allow a clear conclusion on tendencies. With regard to finished feed an increasing contamination level was found over the years similar to maize, i.e. in 2004 0.13 of samples tested positive for ZON, in 2005 0.57 were positive and in 2006 the rate was 0.74. The category "other feed ingredients", i.e. samples that were not specified by customers, showed – in comparison to DON incidence, which was 0.64 – a relatively low contamination rate, i.e. 0.20 over the full testing period.

Sample numbers of other commodities tested were too low to give a conclusive interpretation of data.

Table 3 displays ZON occurrence according to commodities affected in detail.

Table 3. Incidence of ZON contamination in feed grain and animal feed sourced in Europe and the Mediterranean Region 2004-2006 data

	ZON - 2004 Total number[a] Mean/ median[c]	Num, positive[b] Max. level[d]	ZON - 2005 Total number[a] Mean/ median[c]	Num, positive[b] Max. level[d]	ZON - 2006 Total number[a] Mean/ median[c]	Num, positive[b] Max. level[d]	ZON 2004-2006 Total number[a] Mean/ median[c]	Num, positive[b] Max. level[d]
Corn	60 20/101	8 (13%) 491	75 79/61	45 (60%) 960	67 213/132	56 (84%) 2857	202 106/98	109 (54%) 2857
Wheat	41 68/66	19 (46%) 9210	36 78/88	16 (44%) 528	4 7/29	1 (25%) 29	81 183/94	36 (44%) 9210
Wheat bran	4 16/62	1 (25%) 62	16 34/44	9 (56%) 207	2 46/46	2 (100%) 48	22 32/46	12 (55%) 207
Barley	67 21/324	3 (4%) 970	46 16/34	11 (24%) 242	13 3/18	2 (15%) 22	126 17/36	16 (13%) 970
Finished feed	63 16/86	8 (13%) 287	82 25/55	32 (57%) 217	72 450/113	53 (74%) 2770	217 16/60	93 (43%) 2770
Other feed ingredients	57 43/107	14 (25%) 632	141 18/73	21 (15%) 454	52 39/36	14 (27%) 844	250 28/73	49 (20%) 844
Soy	14 n.a.	0 n.a.	7 7/50	1 (14%) 50	7 n.a.	0 n.a.	28 50/50	1 (4%) 50

Triticale: only 7 samples in total, 2 positive, mean 9, median 32, max 46 µg/kg
Oats: only 10 samples in total, 1 positive, 19ppb

[a] Total number of samples analysed
[b] Number of samples tested positive
[c] Arithmetic mean of all samples tested/median of positives in µg/kg
[d] Maximum level detected in µg/kg
n.d. = non detect according to LOQ as indicated in table 1.
n.a. = non applicable

T-2 TOXIN

In 2004 165 samples were tested for T-2 toxin; the contamination rate was 0.40 with most of the positive samples originating from Northern Europe (64 positive of 152 tested). In the subsequent year 0.32 of 59 tested samples were positive, again also primarily derived from the North (18 out of 32 samples). In 2006 only 46 samples were tested for T-2 toxin, all of them were negative. In contrast to earlier years only five samples were sourced in Northern Europe while the majority, i.e. 34 samples, came from Central Europe, which also did not account for relevant T-2 contamination in previous years, so the result is not surprising at all. T-2 toxin occurrence on different commodities is summarized in table 4.

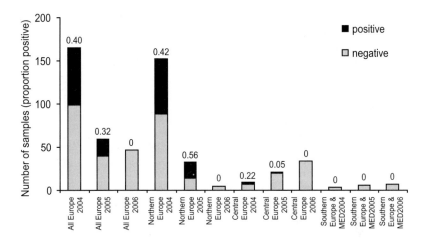

Figure 3. Occurrence of T-2 toxin.

Table 4. Incidence of T-2 toxin contamination in feed grain and animal feed sourced in Europe and the Mediterranean Region 2004-2006 data.

	T-2 toxin- 2004		T-2 toxin - 2005		T-2 toxin - 2006		T-2 toxin 2004-2006	
	Total number[a]	*Num, positive[b]*	*Total number[a]*	*Num, positive[b]*	*Total number[a]*	*Num, positive[b]*	*Total number[a]*	*Num, positive[b]*
	Mean/ median[c]	*Max. level[d]*	*Mean/ median[c]*	*Max. level[d]*	*Mean/ median[c]*	*Max. level[d]*	*Mean/ median[c]*	*Max. level[d]*
Oat	0	n.a.	24	13 (54%)	0	n.a.	24	13 (54%)
	n.a.	n.a.	45/60	194	n.a.	n.a.	45/69	194
Finished feed	18	4 (22%)	11	4 (36%)	12	0	41	8 (20%)
	37/66	492	52/133	230	n.a.	n.a.	30/84	492
Other feed	139	62 (45%)	7	2 (29%)	15	0	161	64 (40%)
ingredients	66/111	524	9/33	35	n.a.	n.a.	58/109	524

All samples tested for T-2 toxin contamination in corn (20), wheat (13), soy (3), and barley (4) were negative

OTA

Throughout the three year survey 109 samples were tested for Ochratoxin A, indicating an average contamination rate of 0.30. In 2004 11 out of 42 samples tested positive, in 2005 15 out of 32, and in 2006 7 out of 35, respectively. No clear geographic allocation of contamination could be made, though it can be stated that the overall contamination rate was higher in 2005 (0.47), and samples from Central Europe and the South contributed primarily to this high incidence.

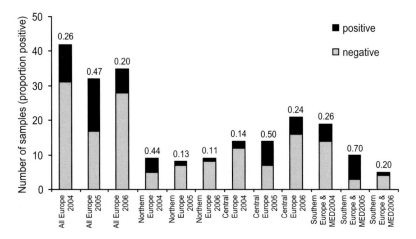

Figure 4. Occurrence of OTA.

AFB1

Out of 71 analyses performed over the full project period, which included nine corn samples, 8 soy samples, one wheat and barley, each, as well as 18 finished feeds and 34 unspecified feed ingredients, only 5 samples were positive, the highest level identified at 14µg/kg in an unspecified feed ingredient. Thus the aflatoxin sample population cannot be considered representative at all but is reported here in order to give a comprehensive picture of the full survey.

Conclusions and discussion of strategies to prevent and counteract mycotoxins

INCIDENCE AND IMPACTS OF MYCOTOXINS

In summary 0.50 of all mycotoxin analyses performed indicated contamination with one of the fungal toxins tested for; incidence was highest for DON, with 0.63 of all samples tested being positive at a quantification limit of 50µg/kg. Approximately 0.11 of samples (i.e. 195 out of 1838 tested), contained more than 1000µg DON/ kg. 65 samples tested higher than 2000µg/kg, six of them were labelled as finished feed. 12 samples (0.05) had levels exceeding 5000µg/kg, with three of them being finished feed.

About one third of samples tested positive for ZON, T-2 toxin or ochratoxin A; only AfB1 contamination did not seem to be substantial at all. With regard to

ZON, only 27 out of 943 samples exceeded 500µg/kg, 17 grains contained more than 1000µg/kg, 11 samples more than 2000µg/kg.

Thus it can be concluded that the incidence of mycotoxins relevant for animal production is quite high in animal feed, though the assessment of the relevance of levels occurring is difficult to undertake. Diagnosis of animal mycotoxicosis is based on experimental studies with specific toxins and specific animals, very often under well-defined toxicological laboratory conditions, so that the results of such studies can be far from real-life or natural situations. Furthermore factors such as breed, sex, environment, nutritional status, as well as other toxic entities can affect the symptoms of intoxication and may contribute to the significance of mycotoxin damage on economic output and animal health. Diagnosis is very much dependent on receiving a sample of feed that was ingested prior to intoxication, but also on data from another representative group of animals of the facility and the results of a post-mortem examination (CAST, 2003).

Another aspect is that research of mycotoxin occurrence in animal feed has concentrated primarily on commodities such as grains and cereals. As ruminant diets contain a high proportion of ingredients like grass silage, hay and stray, it is important also to pay attention to these raw materials, which have been rather poorly researched so far. The mould flora found on forage crops may lead to a significantly different spectrum of toxins and has to be considered. The potentially large number of fungal toxins, which have been found in forage crops, and their diverse chemical structure pose the largest problem in identification and classification of mycotoxicoses due to forage contamination. In contrast to the determination of commonly occurring mycotoxins in cereals and grain, where methods have become simple, reliable, rapid and sensitive, analysis of forages has not thus far been developed and methods available often lack sensitivity or validation. Grass-associated mycotoxins were recently reported for New Zealand, the US, and Europe, and involves symptoms facial eczema, infertility, tremorgenic diseases as rye grass staggers, fescue toxicosis related livestock losses, ergotism, suspected immunosuppression, abomasal ulceration (Scudamore and Livesey, 1998). In a study reported earlier (Binder *et al.*, 2007) straw and straw silage samples sourced in Australia were surveyed and surprisingly high contamination levels and incidence was found: 0.44 were contaminated by zearalenone (median 208µg/kg, maximum 4738µg/kg), 0.41 by deoxynivalenol (median 250 µg/kg, maximum 1860µg/kg), and 0.24 by aflatoxin B1 (median 9 µg/kg, maximum 17 µg/kg). As only 6 samples of straw/silage were analysed for ochratoxin A the high rate of contamination (0.50) may not reflect the actual situation. No similar studies are known to survey the current European situation in this respect.

While mycotoxin-associated losses in industrial countries are typically market losses as a result of rejected crops, necessary redirection of their use or even disposal in cases of severe contamination, developing countries suffer additionally from health impacts. Chronic exposure to high levels of mycotoxins, often combined with malnourishment, cause different levels of toxicosis up to casualties (Wu, 2004). The economic costs of mycotoxins are impossible to be accurately determined, but the US Food and Drug Administration (FDA) give estimations based on a computer model: in the US only the mean economic annual costs of crop losses from the mycotoxins aflatoxins, fumonisins, and deoxynivalenol, are estimated to be USD 932million (CAST, 2003).

PREHARVEST STRATEGIES

Preharvest management practices to maximize plant performance and decrease plant stress can decrease mycotoxin contamination substantially. This includes planting adapted varieties, proper fertilization and fungicide treatment, weed control, necessary irrigation, and proper crop rotation. However even the best management strategies cannot eliminate mycotoxin contamination in years favourable for fungal development (CAST 2003).

Plant breeding for improvement of host-plant resistance to fungal infection has shown promising results for wheat, maize, and peanuts. Besides conventional breeding strategies, molecular-marker-assisted-breeding is also applied currently in field crops, e.g. when chromosomal regions are identified by their statistical association with a measurable trait in a segregating population. Traits such as *Fusarium* head blight in wheat and barley or resistance to aflatoxin accumulation in maize rely on more than a few genes for optimal expression; these traits can be mapped as quantitative trait loci (QTL) using large segregating populations. Molecular markers linked to these QTL could potentially provide an aid to conventional breeding (Varga and Toth, 2005; Miedaner *et al.*, 2006).

Biological control of aflatoxin-producing *Aspergillus* isolates by applying non-toxigenic *A. flavus* isolates in peanut fields showed promising results recently. Biocompetitive exclusion proved also effective in lowering fumonisin contents in corn and deoxynivalenol levels in wheat, while *Bacillus subtilis* or *Cryptococcus isolates* were successfully used as antagonists to *Fusarium graminearum* (Varga and Toth, 2005).

Genetic engineering allows two possible approaches to mycotoxin prevention: on the one hand plant genes can be modified so that they become less susceptible to fungal infection, on the other hand genes responsible for detoxification can be introduced to the plant. Thus fumonisin esterase enzymes were expressed in transgenic maize plants, which resulted in lower manifestation of fumonisin B1 as compared to conventional maize plants (Varga and Toth, 2005).

Transgenic approaches to mould/mycotoxin resistance have been followed as well and include genetically-enhanced resistance to insect feeding, increased fungal resistance and detoxification/prevention of mycotoxins in the grain. An example of the first of these approaches is the transgenic maize expressing *Bacillus thuringiensis* (Bt) toxin, targeted to the European corn borer. Some Bt maize hybrids have the potential to reduce fumonisin levels in field-harvested grain, presumably through reduced feeding of Bt-susceptible insects in ear tissues (Hammond *et al.*, 2004). Another strategy is the over-expression of specific antifungal proteins and metabolites, or enhancement of the plant's own defence systems in kernel tissues. In a third approach, transgene strategies aimed at preventing mycotoxin biosynthesis, or detoxifying mycotoxins in plants have recently shown promising results with regards to fumonisin and zearalenone prevention: enzymes capable of degrading fumonisins have been identified in a filamentous saprophytic fungus isolated from maize, and corresponding genes have been cloned and are currently being tested in transgenic maize (Duvick, 2001; Blackwell *et al.*, 1999). Zearalenone was detoxified by a lactonohydrolase from *Clonostachys rosea*, expressed in leaves of rice. When protein extract from leaves was incubated with zearalenone, the amount of the toxin decreased significantly as measured by HPLC. Zearalenone degradation activity was also detected *in vivo* in transgenic seeds (Higa-Nishiyama *et al.*, 2005)

POSTHARVEST STRATEGIES

The first step in postharvest mycotoxin control is the prevention of conditions that favour fungal growth and subsequent toxin production, including factors such as water activity of stored products, temperature, and presence of chemical or biological preservatives.

Where mycotoxin contamination became evident, the most practical approach thus far has been the blending of low or non- contaminated material with material above the limits, thus lowering the average contamination levels to the accepted standards. In case that is not possible, or even prohibited by law (as in Europe), other methods need to be applied.

Some common physical methods employed are mechanical separation of broken kernels, density segregation, colour sorting, and screening. Electronic and hand sorting, density segregation and combinations thereof have been reported for removal of aflatoxin contamination in peanuts (CAST, 2003). Simple washing procedures using water or sodium carbonate solution resulted also in some reduction of mycotoxins in corn or grains.

A wide variety of chemical compounds have been found to be effective against mycotoxins, including acids, bases, oxidizing or reducing reagents, gases, aldehydes, and others. Although many proposed treatments may successfully destroy aflatoxin, they may be impractical or potentially harmful due to generation of toxic byproducts and/or significant alteration of product quality. Ammoniation, ozoniation, and reaction with sodium bisulphite proved effective for aflatoxin alleviation, while other toxins seem to be more stable (CAST, 2003).

The most commonly used detoxification strategy for feed involves the use of adsorbent materials capable of binding mycotoxins within the gastrointestinal tract of animals and thus reducing bioavailability of these hazards, which leads to a reduction of mycotoxin uptake and distribution to the blood and target organs. Various substance groups have been tested and used for this purpose with aluminium silicates, in particular clay and zeolitic minerals, as the most commonly-applied groups. Important criteria for the evaluation of adsorbent materials are their effectiveness within a broad pH range, as occurring within the gastrointestinal tract, and a high stability of the sorbent-toxin bond, in order to prevent desorption of the latter. In particular hydrated sodium alumino silicates (HSCAS) have been extensively studied because of their good aflatoxin-binding capacity. Although HSCAS were demonstrated to be very effective with regard to preventing aflatoxicosis in a variety of animals, their efficacy against other mycotoxins relevant in animal husbandry seems to be limited (Ramos *et al.*, 1996; Huwig *et al.*, 2001). The extensive use of adsorbents in the livestock industry has led to the introduction of a wide range of new products on the market, most of them claiming high *in vitro* mycotoxin adsorption capacity. However, adsorbents that may appear effective *in vitro* do not necessarily retain their efficacy when tested *in vivo* (Avantaggaito *et al.*, 2005).

In particular the elimination of mycotoxins other than aflatoxins (e.g. trichothecenes, ochratoxins or fumonisins) from contaminated feedstuffs by the use of adsorbents did not lead to any satisfactory results so far, as most of the tested adsorbing agents – with the exception of activated carbon - bind them only to a low extent *in vitro* (Döll *et al.*, 2004) and prove often ineffective *in vivo* (Diaz *et al.*, 2005). *In vitro* experiments with natural and modified clay minerals showed little or no binding of DON and other trichothecenes, in contrast to the extensive binding of aflatoxins (Avantaggaito *et al.*, 2004; Döll *et al.*, 2004). Cholestyramine, a resin used for pharmaceutical purposes, proved efficient in adsorbing zearalenone, aflatoxins, ochratoxin A and fumonisins, but might be too expensive to be used in animal husbandry (Varga and Toth, 2005). Zearalenone was adsorbed by some products tested *in vitro* (Döll *et al.*, 2004), while piglet *in vivo* trials using a modified aluminosilicate as detoxifying agent for Fusarium toxins deoxynivalenol and zearalenone did not prevent or alleviate any of the tested experimental parameters like feed intake, live weight gain, and blood parameters (Döll *et al.*, 2005).

The variety of different *in vitro* test models applied for evaluation of adsorbent agents as well as different feeding trial designs indicate the difficulties to compare *in vitro* and *in vivo* trial results of different studies and underline the need for standardized trial protocols for the evaluation of detoxifying feed additives (Döll and Dänicke, 2004).

In recent years efforts to counteract mycotoxins by microbiological and/or enzymatic approaches increased. Several authors described a de-epoxidation of trichthecenes by ruminal or intestinal flora (Kollarczik *et al.*, 1994, He *et al.*, 1992). Binder *et al.* (2001) isolated a bacterial strain of the genus Eubacterium out of bovine rumen fluid, which was able to bio-transform the epoxide group of trichothecenes into a diene, thus detoxifying all relevant trichothecene toxins by this reaction.

A yeast strain of the genus Trichosporon was isolated and characterized which has the capability of degrading ochratoxin A and zeralenone. On the basis of the yeast's affiliation to the genus of *Trichosporon* and to its main property to degrade OTA and ZON to non-toxic metabolites (*lat. vorare = degrade*), this strain was named *Trichosporon mycotoxinivorans* (*MTV*) (Schatzmayr *et al.*, 2003; Molnar *et al.*, 2004).

References

Avantaggaito, G., Havenaar, R., Visconti, A. (2004) Evaluation of the intestinal adsorption of deoxynivalenol and nivalenol by an in vitro gastrointestinal model, and the binding efficacy of activated carbon and other adsorbent materials. *Food Chem. Toxicol.* **42**, 817-824.

Avantaggaito, G., Solfrizzo, M., Visconti, A. (2005) Recent advances on the use of adsorbent materials for detoxification of Fusarium mycotoxins. *Food Addit. Contam.*, **22 (4)**, 379-388.

Binder, E., Tan, L., Chin, J.L., Handl, J. Richard, J. (2007) Worldwide occurrence of mycotoxins in commodities, feeds and feed ingredients. *Animal Feed Science and Technology*, **Vol. 137**, Issue 3-4, 265-282.

Binder, E.M., Heidler, D., Schatzmayr, G., Thimm, N. Fuchs, E., Schuh, M., Krska, R. and Binder, J. (2001) Microbial detoxification of mycotoxins in animal feed. In: Willem J. de Koe, R.A. Samson, H.P. van Egmond, J. Gilbert, M. Sabino (Eds) Mycotoxins and Phycotoxins in perspective at the turn of the Millennium. Proceedings of the 10th International IUPAC Symposium on Mycotoxins and Phycotoxins, 21-25 May, 2000. Guarujá, Brazil, 271 - 277.

Blackwell, B.A., Gilliam, J.T., Savard, M.E., Miller, J.D., Duvick, J.P. (1999) Oxidative deamination of hydrolyzed fumonisin B_1 (AP_1) by cultures of Exophiala spinifera. *Nat. Toxins,* **7 (1)**, 31-38.

CAST Report (2003) Mycotoxins: Risks in Plant, Animal, and Human Systems. In: J.L. Richard, G.A. Payne (Eds). Council for Agricultural Science and Technology Task Force Report No. 139, Ames, Iowa, USA. ISBN 1-887383-22-0.

Diaz, G.J., Cortés, A., Roldán, L. (2005) Evaluation of the Efficacy of Four Feed Additives Against the Adverse Effects of T-2 Toxin in Growing Broiler Chickens. *J. Appl. Poult. Res.* **14**: 226-231.

Döll, S., Dänicke, S. (2004) In Vivo detoxification of Fusarium toxins. *Archives of Animal Nutrition,* **58 (6)**, 419-441.

Döll, S., Dänicke, S., Valenta, H., Flachowsky, G. (2004) In vitro studies on the evaluation of mycotoxin detoxifying agents for their efficacy on deoxynivalenol and zearalenone. *Arch Anim. Nutr.,* **58 (4)**, 311-324.

Döll, S., Gericke, S., Dänicke, S., Raila, J., Ueberschär, K.-H., Valenta, H., Schnurrbusch, U., Schweigert, F.J., Flachowsky, G. (2005) The efficacy of a modified aluminosilicate as a detoxifying agent in Fusarium toxin contaminated maize containing diets for piglets. *J. Anim. Phys. Anim. Nutr.,* **89 (9-10)**, 342-358.

Duvick, J. (2001) Prospects for reducing fumonisin contamination of Maize through genetic modification. *Environmental Health Perspectives,* **109** (SUPPL. 2), 337-342.

Hammond, B.G., Campbell, K.W., Pilcher, C.D., Degooyer, T.A., Robinson, A.E., McMillen, B.L., Spangler, S.M., Riordan, S.G., Rice, L.G, Richard, J.L. (2004) Lower Fumonisin Mycotoxin Levels in the Grain of Bt Corn Grown in the United States in 2000-2002. *J. Agric. Food Chem.,* **52 (5)**, 1390-1397.

He, P., Young L.G., and Forsberg C. (1992) Microbial Transformation of Deoxynivalenol (Vomitoxin). *Appl. Environ. Microb.* **58, 12,** 3857-3863.

Higa-Nishiyama, A., Takahashi-Ando, N., Shimizu, T., Kudo, T., Yamaguchi, I., Kimura, M. (2005) A model transgenic cereal plant with detoxification activity for the estrogenic mycotoxin zearalenone. *Transgenic Res.,* **14 (5)**, 713-717.

Huwig, A., Freimund, S., Käppeli, O., Dutler, H. (2001) Mycotoxin detoxication of animal feed by different adsorbents. *Toxicol. Lett.,* **122 (2)**, 179-188.

Kollarczik, B., Gareis, M., Hanelt M. (1994) In Vitro Transformation of the Fusarium Mycotoxins Deoxynivalenol and Zearalenone by the Normal Gut Microflora of Pigs. *Natl. Toxins* **2**: 105-110.

Miedaner, T., Wilde, F., Steiner, B., Buerstmayr, H., Korzun, V., Ebmeyer, E. (2006) Stacking quantitative trait loci (QTL) for Fusarium head blight resistance from non-adapted sources in an European elite spring wheat background and assessing their effects on deoxynivalenol (DON) content and disease severity. *Theor. Appl. Gen.,* **112 (3)**, 562-569.

Molnar, O., Schatzmayr, G., Fuchs, E. and Prillinger H.J. (2004) Trichosporon mycotoxinivorans sp. nov., A New Yeast Species Useful in Biological Detoxification of Various Mycotoxins. *Appl. Syst. Microbiol.,* **27(6)**:

661-671(11).

Ramos, A.-J., Fink-Gremmels, J., Hernández, E. (1996) Prevention of toxic effects of mycotoxins by means of nonnutritive adsorbent compounds. *J. Food Protection,* **59 (6)**, 631-641.

Schatzmayr, G., Heidler D., Fuchs, E., Mohnl, M., Täubel. M., Loibner, A.P., Braun, R. and Binder E.M. (2003) Investigation of different yeast strains for the detoxification of Ochratoxin A. *Mycotoxin Res.,* **Vol. 19**, No. 2, 124-128.

Scudamore, K.A., and Livesey, C.T. (1998) Occurrence and Significance of Mycotoxins in Forage Crops and Silage: a Review. *J. Sci. Food Agric.* **77**, 1-17.

Varga, J., Tóth, B. (2005) Novel strategies to control mycotoxins in feeds: A review. *Acta Veterinaria Hungarica,* **53 (2)**, 189-203.

Wu, F. (2004) Mycotoxins Risk Assessment for the Purpose of Setting International Regulatory Standards. *Environ. Sci. Technol.,* **38, 15**, 4049-4055.

12

ORGANIC FARMING: CHALLENGES FOR FARMERS AND FEED SUPPLIERS

A. SUNDRUM[1], P. NICHOLAS[2] AND S. PADEL[2]

[1]Department of Animal Nutrition and Animal Health, Faculty of Organic Agricultural Sciences, University of Kassel, Nordbahnhofstr. 1a, D-37213 Witzenhausen, Germany; [2]Institute of Rural Sciences, University of Wales, Aberystwyth, SY233AL

Introduction

Organic agriculture has shown rapid growth and dynamic developments in recent years throughout Europe (Willer and Yussefi, 2007). This success is not only related to plant products but also includes organic products of animal origin. Consequently, there is an increasing demand for organic feedstuffs to meet the requirements of organically-reared farm animals. Whilst in conventional production, increasing demands for nutrients are covered mainly by increased importation of feedstuffs from outside the farm, the possibilities for such imports into the organic farm system are limited. High nutrient imports conflict with a principal idea of organic farming that is to establish a nearly complete nutrient cycle within a farm system or through cooperation with different types of farms using local resources (Köpke, 1995). By utilising renewable natural resources (livestock manure, legumes and fodder crops), the cropping/stock farming system and the pastoral farming system allow soil fertility to be maintained and improved in the long term. According to the new EU-Regulation (EC/834/2007) on organic agriculture, that is currently under revision (CEC, 2007), organic livestock farming is intended to contribute to the equilibrium of agricultural production systems; to establish and maintain interdependence between soils, plants and animals; to establish land-related and rule out landless production, and thereby support the development of a sustainable agriculture.

Taking these goals into account, the appropriate use of external feed is of high relevance for the integrity of organic production (Sundrum and Padel, 2006). However, not only farmers, but many other individuals and organisations such as policy makers, small agri-businesses, agri-food corporations, supermarkets and consumers, seek to influence the production process in accordance with their own goals and values. Thus, there are many different perspectives on organic agriculture with different understandings of what it is and what makes it develop (Alroe and Noel, 2007). The authors describe three significant perspectives on organic agriculture based on protest, meaning and market which cannot be merged to one but are helpful in understanding the previous and future development of organic agriculture.

Although the framework conditions of organic agriculture are defined by the EU-Regulation (CEC, 2007), the way the guidelines are implemented varies considerably between organic farms. Common ideas and guidelines exist only on a meta-level whilst implementation in farm practice results in a large variety of stocking densities, performance levels, or nutrient flows or efficiency in the use of home-grown and bought-in feedstuffs.

Both organic farmers and the feed milling sector are faced with a number of key issues in terms of the macro-nutrients in organic feed. They are required to follow the different goals that derive from the guidelines of organic farming and the internal processes within the farm. These issues have been identified through studies into the possibilities and limitations of protein supply in organic poultry and pig production (EU-project: EEC 2092/91 - (Organic) Revision), and through discussions with the organic feed industry. Although some of these issues are specific to farmers, many are common to both farmers and feeds millers alike. Key issues include balance of supply and demand, quality of supply, shortages in the supply of organic feed and suggestions for overcoming them. In order to understand better the goals and values of organic farming and the challenges that these pose, general differences between conventional and organic livestock production are now explained.

General differences between conventional and organic livestock production

Organic livestock production represents an alternative to progressive intensification in conventional animal production. In contrast to performance-oriented conventional production, the system-oriented approach of organic farming is based on voluntary self-limitation of the use of inputs in order to achieve an animal- and environmentally-compatible production of high-quality animal products in a largely closed farm system (Sundrum, 1998). The realization of this approach usually requires a complete re-organization of the farm, in which crop requirements have to be tailored to the concerns of animal husbandry and the extent and direction of animal husbandry adapted to home-grown feedstuffs. The aim is to achieve production of animal products principally through precautionary and avoidance strategies.

With respect to environmental compatibility, the avoidance strategy is based on a conscious limitation of external resources (including mineral nitrogen fertilizers and additional commercial feedstuffs) and avoiding risk-laden production means (including pesticides and GMOs). In addition, the presence of certain residues of synthetic chemicals from sources other than agriculture should be avoided. Consequently, the abandonment of specific means of production, which have been developed to increase productivity, will inevitably lead to increased production costs, which have to be passed on to the consumer in the form of higher prices.

In organic livestock production the objectives of land based systems, the avoidance of specific means of production and the priority of quality production rather than maximizing production are of overriding importance. To deal with a limited availability of resources is therefore a main feature of organic livestock production. In contrast to conventional production, maximization of performance is only a subordinate objective. Differences in the priorities between conventional and organic livestock production, and a comparison between the hierarchies related to objectives are presented in Table 1.

Table 1. Differences in priorities between conventional and organic livestock production.

	Conventional		*Organic*
i.	Minimizing production costs	i.	System-oriented production, based on land use and use of organic feedstuffs
ii.	Maximizing productivity of farm animals	ii.	Maximizing efficiency within the whole farm system
iii.	Maximizing performance (milk yield, carcass yield, number of eggs)	iii.	Optimising product and process quality (animal health and welfare, environmentally-friendly production, naturalness)
iiii.	Optimising single quality traits	iiii.	Reducing production costs

With regard to the different objectives, different priorities and different framework conditions, it has to be taken into account that organic and conventional livestock production represent different production systems. Therefore, the traditional approach, that often reduces agricultural problems to the level of single production traits or feeding strategies, is not directly comparable and compatible with the organic approach. In the same way, general conclusions derived from conventional production systems are not directly compatible and therefore have not the same validity in organic livestock production.

Feeding principles in organic farming

A main principle of organic farming is to establish a balanced production system and, as far as possible, have closed nutrient cycles, i.e. self-sufficiency in terms of resource use. To achieve this principle, non-organic and external inputs should be reduced to a minimum, and feed should be sourced preferentially from within the farm unit or through close co-operation with other units to which nutrients can be returned. The feeding principles are set out in the European Regulation (EEC) 2092/91 on organic agriculture. The detailed rules (Table 2) specify which organic, in-conversion or non-organic feed can be used. Conventionally-produced feedstuffs can only be used if organic or in-conversion feed (either grown within or outside the farm system) is not available in sufficient quantity and quality (Annex IB 4.8). Even then, only a set proportion of non-organic components can be used, and these feedstuffs have to be listed in Annex II. For herbivores (though not non-ruminant animals at present), there is an additional requirement that at least 0.50 of the feed must come from the farm unit itself or, if this is not feasible, has to be produced in cooperation with other organic farms.

Apart from the demands with respect to the external nutrient input, "feed is intended to ensure quality production rather than maximising production, while meeting the nutritional requirements of the livestock at the various stages of their development" (Annex IB 4.1). However, the preferable use of home-grown feedstuffs and limitations in the choice of bought-in feedstuffs can be the cause of considerable variation in the composition of the diets, and restrict the possibilities for the adaptation of the feed ration to the specific requirements of the farm animals and the production system. For biosynthesis, the organism requires energy and amino acids that need to be provided in a specific ratio. Strong deviations from this ratio can lead to malfunctions that, if they have a negative effect on growth, utilization, feed intake and other physiological parameters, are designated as imbalances (D'Mello, 2003). Due to the limited availability of high quality feed, there is concern that nutritional imbalances encountered might lead to deteriorating animal health and welfare. On the other hand, there is also the concern that allowing conventional feedstuffs to be fed in organic livestock production will result in a marked intensification of the production process. This intensification might cause the same problems in organic production as found in conventional production with regard to animal health (Rauw, Kanis, Noordhuizen-Stassen and Grommers, 1998; European Commission, 2000; Martens, 2007) and environmental pollution (Erisman and Monteny, 1998; European Environment Agency, 2003). Thus, the use of non-organic feedstuffs may have a damaging effect on consumer confidence in organic products of animal origin, because it increases the risk of residues in meat and milk products and reduces the integrity of an organic product (Hermansen, 2003).

Table 2. Summary of feed provisions in Regulation (EEC) 2092/91 on organic production.

Organic feed (Article 4.2)	Livestock must be fed on organic produced feed stuffs
In-conversion feed (Article 4.4) amended in March 2007, (not yet implemented by all certification bodies)	Until 31 December 2008, up to 0.50 of the feed formula of rations on average may comprise in-conversion feed stuffs. When the in conversion feed stuffs come from a unit of the holding itself, this percentage may be increased to 0.80. As from 1 January 2009, up to 0.30 of the feed formula of rations on average may comprise in-conversion feed stuffs. When the in conversion feed stuffs come from a unit of the holding itself, this proportion may be increased to 0.60. These figures shall be expressed as a proportion of the dry matter of feed stuffs of agricultural origin
Non-organic feed (Article 4.8 – as amended in August 2005)	The maximum proportion of conventional feed stuffs of agricultural origin authorised per period of 12 months is: (a) for herbivores: 0.05 during the period from 25 August 2005 to 31 December 2007; (b) for other species: - 0.15 during the period from 25 August 2005 to 31 December 2007, - 0.10 during the period from 1 January 2008 to 31 December 2009, - 0.05 during the period from 1 January 2010 to 31 December 2011. These proportions apply where the farmer can show that he/she is unable to obtain feed exclusively from organic origin. These figures shall be calculated annually as a percentage of the dry matter of feed stuffs from agricultural origin (Annex II). The maximum proportion authorised of conventional feed stuffs in the daily ration, except during the period each year when the animals are being moved, must be 0.25 calculated as a proportion of the dry matter.
Home grown feed (Article 4.3)	Livestock must be reared using feed from the unit or, when this is not possible, using feed from other units or enterprises subject to the provisions of this Regulation. Moreover, in the case of herbivores, except during the period each year when the animals are being moved, at least 0.50 of the feed shall come from the farm unit itself or in case this is not feasible, be produced in cooperation with other organic farms.

Demand for external nutrients

Home-grown feedstuffs alone often do not provide the nutrients needed to formulate balanced diets for farm animals in their different stages. The difference between diet requirements and the availability of nutrients from home-grown feedstuffs varies considerably between farms, regions and countries, depending among other things on the local conditions, portion of arable land, crop rotation, animal species and the performance level of the herd or flock. Therefore, it is necessary to use some external feed materials, even though this conflicts with the principle of closed nutrient cycles. Taking these different and partly conflicting objectives of organic farming into account, the principle in relation to the use of external and non-organic inputs should be: *to use as few external inputs as possible and as many as necessary* (Sundrum and Padel, 2006). There are, however, no clear criteria on how to assess at the farm level how many external nutrients are really needed and what might be seen as a high or a low amount of nutrient input.

From the perspective of an animal nutritionist, the demand for external feed results from what is needed to meet the specific requirements of the farms animals in their different stages and what cannot be covered by home-grown feedstuffs. In general, the need for external feed is expected to increase with an increase in the performance level, as the demands for high quality feed, especially with respect to the protein quality, increase and often can be covered to a lesser degree by home-grown feedstuffs.

From an economic point of view, quantity and quality of bought-in-feedstuffs depend primarily on the increase in productivity that is expected with the use of external nutrients and the price the farmer is willing or able to pay in relation to the development of the food markets. Correspondingly, the cost-benefit relationship with regard to the production costs is relevant in the first place while the aspects of environmental pollution, for instance in connection with the production and transport of external feedstuffs, are often neglected.

From an organic perspective, evaluating the need for external feed inputs is not only based on the nutrient requirements of the livestock and the possible impacts on the production costs, but has additionally to take into account the nutrient flow within the farm system as well as factors outside the farm gate, such as consumer expectations. According to the EU-Regulation (CEC, 2007), livestock must be fed on organically produced feedstuffs. By way of a derogation, for a transitional period expiring on December 2011, the use of a limited proportion of non-organic feedstuffs is authorised where farmers can show, to the satisfaction of the inspection body, that they are unable to obtain feed exclusively from organic production (for further detail see table 2). Ultimately, the organic industry wants to achieve systems that are sustainable, comply with the EU-Regulation on organic farming, and fulfil the broader principles of organic farming without compromising animal health and welfare. Due to the abandonment of conventionally-produced feedstuffs in the long run, the limited availability of nutrient resources is a characteristic of organic farming, and it is an on-going challenge for organic farmers to maintain a balance between nutrient demands for the farm animals and the organic resources available.

Shortages in the supply of organic feed in Europe

Shortages of organically-produced cereal and protein crops are a major problem facing several countries in the EU. The reasons for these shortages vary between countries. In the UK for instance, fewer crop-producing than livestock farms have converted to organic agriculture, resulting in an undersupply of organically-grown crops and hence a reliance on imported feed. According to Padel (2005) the EU would have produced enough cereal crops in 2002/2003 to feed all organic stock completely with organic diets. This was similar in 2004 and there appeared to be a surplus of organic cereals which would allow for further increases in stock numbers. A study by Padel and Sundrum (2006) indicates there could be sufficient organic cereal grown to feed all organic livestock, but that organic protein is currently in short supply. This has particular implications for organic pig and poultry producers who are reliant on adequate protein supply in the diet to ensure good production and high levels of animal health and welfare. Higher prices (particularly for protein-rich crops) are likely to stimulate higher production, but this would increase cost of production for organic livestock producers maybe above a level that consumers are willing to pay for. Regional imbalances occur, because the main countries producing feed materials are not necessarily those that also keep most organic livestock (Padel and Lowman, 2005). Hence, both the feed industry and organic farmers will need to make significant changes over the next years to meet the challenges.

Strategies at the farmers' disposal

Under organic farming conditions, it is much easier to meet the nutritional requirements of the ruminant than those of non-ruminant animals. While ruminants can utilise home-grown forages, and only limited inputs of energy and protein concentrate feeds are required, non-ruminant animals need certain quantities of essential amino acids in their diets for protein biosynthesis. They require feed materials with a relatively high concentration of energy and high biological quality of protein, and as such are directly competing with humans for feed sources. In order to bring nutrient supply and requirements for the farm animals into balance, there are several options available to farmers. In general, they can either increase the availability of nutrients by home-grown and external feed, or reduce the demand for nutrients by decreasing the stock size and/or the level of performance, or increase the efficiency in the use of those nutrients that are available or modify simultaneously various factors operating on the farm.

Concerning the cultivation of fodder crops, the organic farmer has to follow specific demands with respect to a balanced crop rotation including among others things nitrogen fixation via legumes, and weed and pest control via a high variability in the crop rotation (Köpke, 1998). On the other hand, the farmer has the option between a higher portion of cash crops or fodder crops, but often tends towards cash crops for economic reasons. The more an organic farmer strives for self-sufficiency by increasing the availability of various home-grown feedstuffs, the more they become independent from feed markets and price fluctuations, and are able to balance the nutrient flow within the farm system.

The total demands for feed on a farm are primarily a function of the number of farm animals and the performance levels expected by the farmer. In intensive production systems, expectations are focused primarily on high growth rates or milk yields, consequently resulting in various efforts to increase the availability of high quality feedstuffs and the use of synthetic amino acids for non-ruminant animals as essential production tools to meet the continually increasing demands (Flachowsky, 2002).

The restrictions in relation to external feedstuffs and the banning of synthetic amino acids in organic farming markedly limit the potential for maximising the performance level in comparison to conventional production. In contrast to the development in conventional production, the EU-Regulation (EEC No. 2092/91) even restricts the minimum slaughter ages of poultry. For instance, the minimum age at slaughter shall be 81 days for chickens and 140 days for turkeys (Annex IB, 6.19). Where producers do not apply these minimum slaughter ages, they must use slow-growing strains. Due to the demand of the market for heavy turkeys of around 20 kg live-weight it is possible to use conventional strains in organic livestock farming for a fattening period of 140 days (20 kg in 20 weeks), while in organic broiler production slow-growing strains are essential to produce a marketable product in a minimum of 81 days without excess weight (Sundrum, Schneider and Richter, 2005). Protein requirements are clearly reduced if slow growing strains like those in the 'label rouge' programme are used compared to conventional strains (Peter, Dänicke, Jeroch, Wicke and von Lengerken, 1997a,b). Health problems can arise when organic production relies on genetic strains bred for high performance in conventional production (Damme, 2000). However, examples of feed rations for broiler and turkeys based completely on organic feedstuffs indicate that, in general, it is possible to formulate diets without the use of non-organic feedstuffs (Bellof and Schmidt, 2005; Sundrum et al., 2005).

Nutrient supply for farm animals is a function of both the concentration of nutrients within the feed ration and the voluntary feed intake. Both variables can be modified by management. However, feed intake of farm animals (even when the same age) varies considerably within the herd and between farms, and the source of this variation is multi-factorial. Increasing feed intake by improving the living environment and management is an important option when there is a lack of high quality feedstuffs but other feedstuffs are available. For instance, an increase in feed intake by young pigs from 1.0 to 1.1 kg feed/day of a diet with 13.0 MJ ME and 50 g methionine per kg effects an improvement of the energy provision by 1.3 MJ ME and an improvement of methionine provision by 5 g per animal and day. Under the restrictions of the Regulation (EEC) 2092/91 it seems to be easier to achieve a 10% better energy and methionine supply through a higher feed intake than by increasing the energy content and the concentration of methionine in the feed ration.

Nutrition x environment interactions play an important role in regulating food intake and performance. Marked increases of feed intake by means of optimisation of feeding and housing conditions have been described in the case of sows (Black, Mullan, Lorschy and Giles, 1993), fattening pigs (Hyun, Ellis and Johnson, 1998; Ferguson, 1999), broilers (Parr and Summers, 1991; Bessei, 1993) and turkeys (Auckland and Morris, 1971; Günther, 2001). For pigs, differences of approximately 30% have been determined between different genotypes with otherwise equal feed rations and living conditions (Schinkel, Smith, Tokach, Dritz, Einstein, Nelssen and Goodband, 2002).

Efficiencies in feed usage, particularly of the scarce protein component, can be improved by tailoring diets to particular life stages. Implementation of a multiple phase feeding is an appropriate and well established measure to adapt the supply more closely to the requirements in the different stages of production and thereby economize the use of feedstuffs with high quality protein. In particular, the specification of starter rations for young and growing animals should be met to prevent risks in relation to animal health and welfare. The implementation of separate sex rearing can help to match the feed supply more closely to the different requirements of the sexes in different species (Fuller, Franklin, McWilliam and Pennie, 1995; Chamruspollert, Pesti and Bakalli, 2002; Frankenpohl, 2002).

By making use of compensatory growth effects, the demand for feedstuffs of high quality protein can be reduced, which is especially relevant in the case of pigs (Chiba, Hyun, Ellis and Johnson, 1999, Fabian, Chiba, Kuhlers, Frobish, Nadarajah, Kerth, McElhenney and Lewis, 2002). Schutte and Pack (1995) confirmed that broiler are able to compensate partially for a low content of essential amino acids in the diet by a higher feed intake. Auckland and Morris (1971) studied the compensatory effects in turkeys and Cherry and Siegel (1981) in laying hens.

The use of non-starch polysaccharides for pigs, especially in the case of dry sows and finishing pigs can be an appropriate instrument to reduce the amount of concentrate needed by an organic farm (Meunier-Salaun, 1999; Pluske, Pethick, Durmic, Hampson and Mullan, 1999). At the same time this feeding strategy follows the EU-Regulation (CEC, 2007), which requires that roughage, fresh or dried fodder, or silage must be added to the daily ration for pigs and poultry (Annex IB, 4.11).

It can be concluded that, on each farm, there are different ways for optimising the nutrient supply and the efficiency in the use of limited resources. However, there is a need for the development of feeding strategies that are closely related to the farm specific situation.

Shortages in availability of accurate information and suitable tools

While the recommendations in relation to the nutrient requirements show a high accuracy on the level of an individual organism (NRC, 1994, 1998, 2001), predictability is clearly reduced when the recommendations are transformed to the herd and the farm level as systems of a higher order. Different variables such as feed intake, genetic potential for performance, nutrient and energy need for immune function and locomotion etc. result in large system variation which are amplified when these variables interact with each other. Digestibility of organic matter can vary considerably between and within farms even when using the same diet. Studies of Elbers, Den Hartog, Verstegen and Zandstra (1989) and Schinkel et al. (2002) have shown that the variation in digestibility, live-weight gain and rates of protein and lipid accretion in pigs are much more associated with the differences between the farms than with the genetic background of the farm animals, resulting in considerably different amino acid requirements. This makes a prediction of the specific requirements at the farm level very complex and difficult.

To optimise the use of limited resources, the farmer is required to adapt the level of nutrient supply to the performance capacity of the animals and at the same time adapt the number of farm animals and their performance level to the availability of nutrients as suboptimal supply reduces the performance while excess supply with nutrients cannot further increase performance. In order to be able to formulate rations accurately and make most efficient use of nutrients available, it is very important to analyse the feed. Due to the large variation between different harvests of the same feed crops, the use of feed tables does not accurately enough describe the quality of the feed sufficiently accurately. Many farmers, however, formulate their rations without any feed analysis of single ingredients or feed mixtures and without detailed knowledge about the specific feed intake of the farm animals (Krutzinna, Boehncke and Herrmann, 1996; Sundrum and Ebke, 2004; Dietze, Werner and Sundrum, 2007). Whilst having home-grown feeds analysed is an additional cost for farmers, it can be expected to reduce feed costs in the long term by providing information required for more accurate formulation of rations, thereby improving feed conversion and increasing productivity. Simultaneously, farmers often do not have accurate information about the feed intake of the farm animals in the different stages, due to a lack of appropriate equipment or because farmers are unwilling to gather the information.

Multiple phase feeding is a suitable tool to meet efficiently the specific requirements of farm animals in the different stages. The recommendations are, however, often not implemented into practice. Feeding for different life stages increases the complexity of feed management and ration planning on farms. Different diets need to be mixed and stored separately, and the different groups of animals need to be fed separately. On many farms the number of silos available for home-grown and bought-in feed storage is a limiting factor. Farmers even tend to store different cereals or grain legumes in the same feed silo rather than investing in additional silos. This makes it nearly impossible to estimate how much feed of which quality is available to formulate an appropriate feed ration.

The farm manager is the most important regulator of the system to bring demand and supply of nutrients into balance. Feedback and control measures on different levels represent a way of monitoring and regulating the behaviour of sub-systems. Feedback mechanisms that have the potential to improve the balance between demand and supply are:

- Farm gate nutrient balance sheets to improve nutrient management and reduce nutrient losses,
- Farm specific feed balance sheets to improve the amount and the efficiency in the use of home-grown feedstuffs and to assess the necessity for supplementation (analysis of feed ingredients, assessment of feed intake and feed conversion etc.)
- Animal health plans to strengthen the efficiency of a range of preventive measures and to prevent the occurrence of nutritional and metabolic disorders.

The implementation of feed-back mechanisms is expected to improve significantly the production processes within the farm system. In particular, the efficiency in the use of nutrients and the level of animal health are expected to benefit from the feed-back mechanisms. If the need for the quantity and quality of external nutrient inputs can be identified more clearly, possible alternatives will be more obvious whilst at the same time efficiency and appropriateness of the external inputs will be improved. In order to increase efficiency, a high degree of accurate information and management skills as well as resources such as labour time and investments are required. However, the availability of these factors is often limited.

Impacts on environmentally friendly production

Organic farms not only have to match the need for energy and nutrients under the preconditions of a limited availability of nutrients without jeopardizing animal health and welfare but they also have to fulfil the demands with respect to an environmentally-friendly production. Due to the use of high proportions of home-grown feed and limitations in the availability of external feed, it is generally more difficult in organic than in conventional farming to provide balanced feed rations especially in relation to the protein supply (Sundrum et al., 2005). On the other hand, unbalanced feed rations are less efficient in the use of nutrients, resulting in a lower animal performance and lower feed conversion ratio, and simultaneously leading to a higher excretion of nutrients per edible protein of animal origin compared to a balanced diet. Taking the efficiency in the use of nutrients by the farm animals as an indicator for the degree of environmentally friendly production (Flachowsky, 2002, 2007), organic livestock production will not be able to compete with the conventional production, and may be assumed to be less environmentally friendly. What seems to be obvious when focussing on the metabolism of the farm animals can lead, however, to different results when the nutrient flow of the whole farm is taken into account.

One problem in comparing the performance of farming systems with respect to nutrient loss is that it is very difficult to measure directly. Therefore, such comparisons are often made on the basis of nutrient balance sheets (Dalgaard, Halberg, Kristensen, 1998; Hansen, Kristensen, Grant, Hogh-Jensen, Simmelsgaard and Olesen, 2000). Farm-scale balances are the outcome of a simple nutrient accounting process, which details all inputs to, and output from a farm over a fixed period of time. Nutrient input by mineral fertilizer and by feed, which are not matched by corresponding higher nitrogen outputs is by far the most relevant factor for high surpluses in nutrient balance sheets in conventional production (Hansen et al., 2000; Dalgaard, Heidmann, Mogensen, 2002; De Boer, 2003; Knudsen, Kristensen, Berntsen, Petersen and Kristensen, 2006). On the farm level, nutrient inputs and nutrient losses from the farm into the environment are clearly reduced in organic livestock systems compared to conventional production (Haas, Wetterich and Köpke, 2001; Scheringer, 2002; Knudsen et al., 2006). Other studies have also found a higher N-efficiency on organic mixed farms compared with conventional ones (Halberg, Kristensen and Kristensen, 1995; Dalgaard et al., 1998).

While in conventional livestock production the emphasis lies on strategies to increase feed conversion ratio and to decrease nutrient excretion in relation to the quantity of products by using among others bought-in feedstuffs of high quality such as soybean meal and synthetic amino acids, the system-orientated approach in organic agriculture is striving for the avoidance of nutrient inputs and nutrient losses on the farm level (Sundrum, 2002). If the excess nitrogen can be caught and retained in the agricultural nutrient cycle, the environmental effects are relatively low. If the nutrients are discharged from the cycle and emitted into the environment, this can mean correspondingly high environmental damage. This includes the release of greenhouse gases, particularly of N_2O from cultivated soils, due to increased inputs by mineral fertilizer, animal wastes and biological N-fixation (IPCC, 1996). On average, 0.025 of total N input by synthetic N fertilizer, organic fertilizer and crop residues are emitted as N_2O-N (Flessa, Ruser, Dörsch, Kamp, Jimenez, Munch and Beese, 2002). In this respect it is of central importance to know how nutrients imported on to the farm are used in a targeted and efficient way, and how excess nitrogen given off from the feed is dealt with.

In the future the demands concerning a reduction in nutrient losses from livestock farms will further increase. In Germany, the implementation of the Council Directive 91/676/EEC (referred to as Nitrates Directive) prescribes that the nutrient surplus of nitrogen calculated by nitrogen balance sheets should not exceed 60 kg of nitrogen per ha per year in the average of the years 2009, 2010 and 2011. While this goal is already achieved by most organic farms (Haas et al., 2001; Scheringer, 2002), many conventional farms are currently far from reaching this threshold in a comparable farm situation. With respect to the future demands of livestock production, to achieve an environmentally-compatible production it can be argued that organic agriculture anticipates what will also be a challenge in the next years for conventional production.

Strategies to the disposal of feed millers

Currently, organic feed millers (particularly for protein feeds) rely on approved conventional feeds in their compound diets. Appendix II (of Regulation (EEC) 2092/91) provides a list of conventional feed ingredients that millers can use in compounds feed within the specified non-organic proportions. There have been requests to extend this list, due both to the shortage of many organic proteins and some conventionally-produced protein feeds (e.g. potato protein) but this could only provide a short-term solution as the derogation for the use of conventional feed will be phased out and organic systems have to move towards the complete use of organic feedstuffs by December 2011.

Apart from a general shortage in the availability of organic feed across the EU in 2007, some countries (e.g. the UK) are also experiencing long-term logistical problems with the supply of organic feeds. Continuity of supply and crop quality are very variable, and this can add to problems of undersupply and create problems for both the feed milling industry and for farmers trying to source feed. There appears to be a certain level of market failure, whereby even if demand and prices paid for organic livestock feed are high, the arable sector still does not respond adequately.

The best crop-based sources of essential amino acids are soya, or from industrial co-products such as potato protein or maize gluten. However, the co-products are available only from conventional sources and will be phased out by the end of 2011, while soya is quite difficult to grow in many parts of the EU or sourced in sufficient quantity and quality. Feed millers may therefore need to consider other grain legume crops or source soya from countries where the cultivation of organic soya is possible.

Feed mills have identified starter feeds as being the most difficult to produce to meet specifications under organic feeding regulations. This is due to a combination of the fast-growing breeds that are used in many organic systems and the lack of organically-grown protein feeds of suitable quality. Most millers make full use of the derogation for conventional feeds in their diets, particularly in starter diets and many feel that there is absolutely no flexibility left in the starter feed specification. Unless structural changes can be made in the organic livestock sector it will be very difficult to feed organic young stock when the conventional feed derogation is removed. One such change in the organic industry could be to reduce the use of organic soya to balance the diet of organic dairy cows and encourage ruminant farmers to rely more strongly on protein forages and home-grown grain legumes. This could result in increased availability of high quality organic protein for non-ruminant animal production.

Home-grown corn legumes (faba beans, peas and lupins) are the main home-grown protein source in organic livestock production. Although home-grown legumes are characterised by high crude protein content, the content of essential amino acids and their digestibility are low compared to soya beans (Jeroch, Flachowsky and Weißbach, 1993). The crude protein contents increase in the sequence peas, faba beans and lupins. However, the mean crude protein content of lupins can vary markedly between 258 and 440 g/kg DM (Van Barneveld, 1999; Sundrum et al., 2005). Due to the large variation in the protein content of lupins there is a need for a separate storage of the different batches.

Because of the occurrence of anti-nutritional factors (ANFs), legume protein sources can only be fed to a limited extent. Plant breeding research has developed methods to select for lower levels of ANFs in legumes, but relevant legume crops still contain significant amounts of ANFs, which reduces the use of the legumes as a protein source. Substances in grain legumes that have a performance-reducing effect on the animal are tannins, lectins, protease-inhibitors and glycosides. An overview of ANF in legume seeds is provided by Huismann, van der Poel and Liener (1989) and Gordon (1999). There are several processes to minimize the content of anti-nutritional factors in grain legumes: For instance, the husks that contain the highest concentration of trypsin inhibitors can be removed. De-hulled seeds are also lower in crude fibre and thus more easily digestible by poultry. ANFs can be deactivated by autoclaving, expanding, extruding, toasting or steam-pelleting. A practical process is the pelleting of feed using steam. The alkaloid content is reduced substantially by swelling the grains and washing them. Water-saving extraction processes have already been developed. However, due to the limited scale of organic livestock production, the large scale feed processors are still hesitant in developing separate organic production lines for the different types of processing grain legumes.

Available organic grain is often supplied to millers in small batches, requiring grain to be stored until there is sufficient quantity to process. Storage difficulties are further increased if the mill processes both conventional and organic feed and essential storage is tied up by small batches of organic grain. Millers prefer to buy their organic grains and legumes on the spot market and are not prepared to commit to forward supply contracts with farmers. This is one of the key problems highlighted by cereal farmers when asked for the reasons for their reluctance to convert to organic production (Nicholas, Sundrum and Padel, 2007). Some organic farmers are known to hold on to organic feed cereals in the expectation that feed prices will rise further as demand continues to increase. Organic farmers also prefer to grow a range of cereals (including barley, oats and triticale) in their crop rotations to maintain soil fertility and reduce disease pressure. Millers, however, prefer to buy mainly feed wheat as this can be used in a wide range of rations for all types of farm animals. Finally, the premiums available to farmers for growing crops for bio-fuels are also dissuading farmers from converting to organic production. Conversion to organic is also seen as the much riskier diversification option.

A number of steps could be taken to improve the continuity and quality of supply of organic livestock feeds. Millers and farmers need to be prepared to enter forward supply contracts so that there is some degree of security for both parties. The farmer will know what price they will receive for the grain and the miller will be assured of both the quantity and quality of the grain supplied. Farmers need to work together to ensure that sufficient quantities of a suitable quality feed grain can be delivered to fulfil supply contracts with millers. Retailers also need to be prepared to enter supply contracts with organic farmers so that there is some degree of security for both parties in relation to the quantity and quality of organic products of animal origin.

Conclusions

The EU-Regulation on organic livestock production limits the availability of feedstuffs with high quality protein and thereby reduces the potential for increasing productivity and decreasing production costs. Due to a restricted availability of high quality protein feed, it is clearly more difficult to formulate diets that accurately meet the requirements of the animals than in conventional production. On the other hand, it appears a consensus within all sectors of the organic industry that organic livestock should be fed complete organic diets, as this is one of the key principles of organic farming and contributes to the integrity of organic livestock products. Phasing out of the derogations to use non-organic feed as set out in the Regulation (EEC) 2092/91 is necessary to maintain consumer trust for the future development of organic farming and the organic market. Removal of the derogations means that the supply of organic livestock feed, especially high quality protein feed, needs to grow to meet increasing demand from an expanding organic livestock sector. There are still significant advances to be made by both farmers and feed millers before the derogation allowing conventional feed expires at the end of 2011.

Due to the limited availability of high quality feed, organic farms in general cannot compete with conventional farms with respect to production costs. In order to compensate for the higher production costs, organic farmers have to focus primarily on a quality-oriented production, including a high eating quality of animal products and a high level of animal health and environmentally friendly production, to meet the expectations of consumers and correspond to their willingness to pay premium prices for organic products.

The farmers are required to think through the complexity of the production processes and therefore need accurate information about the nutrient flow within the farm system. Farm-gate feed balance, feed analysis of all feedstuffs available, calculation of feed rations as well as assessing feed intake, considering the different stages of development of the animals, are appropriate tools to deal with the complexity with regard to the nutrient flow, to improve the efficiency in the use of nutrients and to prevent imbalances that may cause harm to the animals. Due to a large variation in relation to the availability of high quality feedstuffs and utilization of nutrients between farms there is need for the development of feeding strategies that are closely related to the farm specific situation.

To adapt livestock production to the availability of nutrients from home-grown and external feed within the specific farm system and to increase the efficiency in the use of nutrients on the farm level is the real challenge in organic farming. It covers the different demands of the organic principles and the different interests of the farmers as well as the consumers. Hence, organic livestock production could play a pioneering role for other livestock systems which have to face limitations in the availability of nutrients or which are challenged by the Council Directive (91/676/EEC) not to exceed the nutrient losses from the farm beyond the gradually decreasing thresholds.

There are different environmental loads at the subsystem and total system levels. Farmers, feed millers and animal nutritionists should be aware of these differences and ought to take responsibility for the total system by striving for a high efficiency in the use of nutrients within the total system rather than focussing only on the level of the farm animals. To increase the efficiency and to compensate for the limitations in the availability of feedstuffs, expertise and knowledge about the internal processes has to be increased, requiring skilled farm management. In this context the question arises to what degree the farmer can be supported by the feed millers, not only with respect to the shortage in feed of high quality but also with respect to the knowledge about the nutrient flow within the farm system. Feed millers should not only provide a high variety of different components that are suited to supplement home-grown feedstuffs but should also provide tools to support for a better advisory service for the farmer.

Acknowledgement

The authors gratefully acknowledge financial support for the project "Research to support revision of the EU-Regulation on organic agriculture " (Contract No FP6-502397) from the Commission of the European Communities under the Sixth Framework Programme for Research.

References

Alroe, H.F., Noel, E. (2007) What makes organic agriculture move - protest, meaning or market? A polyocular approach to the dynamics and governance of organic agriculture. Forthcoming in IJARGE special issue on "Continuity and change in organic farming - philosophy, practice and policy" (in press).

Auckland, J.N., Morris, T.R. (1971) Compensatory growth in turkeys: effect of under nutrition on subsequent protein requirements. *British Poultry Science*, **12**, 41-48.

Bellof, E., Schmidt, E. (2005) Broiler production with 100 % organic feed is possible. In *Proceedings of the 8th Conference on Organic Farming - 2005*, pp 321-324. Edited by J. Hess and G. Rahmann. Kassel University Press GmbH.

Bessei, W. (1993) Der Einfluss der Besatzdichte auf Leistung, Verhalten und Gesundheit von Broilern - Literaturbersicht. *Archiv Geflügelkunde*, **57**, 97-102.

D'Mello, J.P.F. (2003) Amino acid in animal nutrition. 2nd ed. CAB International, Wallingford (UK).

Black, J.L., Mullan, B.P., Lorschy, M.L., Giles, L.R. (1993) Lactation in the sow during heat stress. *Livestock Production Science*, **35**, 153-170.

CEC (2007) Council Regulation (EEC 2092/91) on Organic Agricultural Products and indications referring thereto on agricultural products and foodstuff. Committee of the European Communities, Brussels.

Chamruspollert, M., Pesti, G.M., Bakalli, R.I. (2002) Determination of the methionine requirement of male and female broiler chickens using an indirect amino acid oxidation method. *Poultry Science*, **81**, 1004-1013.

Cherry, J.A., Siegel, P.B. (1981) Compensatory increases in feed consumption in response to marginal level of the sulphur containing amino acids. *Archiv Geflügelkunde*, **6**, 269-273.

Chiba, L.I., Ivey, H.W., Cummins, K.A., Gamble, B.E. (1999) Growth performance and carcass traits of pigs subjected to marginal dietary restrictions during the grower phase. *Journal of Animal Science*, 77, 1769-1776.

Dalgaard, T., Halberg, N, Kristensen, E.S. (1998) Can organic farming help reduce N-losses? Experiences from Denmark. *Nutrient Cycling in Agroecosystems*, 52, 277-287.

Dalgaard, T., Heidmann, T., Mogensen, L. (2002) Potential N-losses in three scenarios for conversion to organic farming in a local area of Denmark. *European Journal of Agronomy*, 16, 207-217.

Damme, K. (2000) Bedarfsgerechte Nährstoffversorgung des Geflügels bei unterschiedlichem genetischen Leistungspotential: Möglichkeiten und Grenzen der Ökobetriebe. Tierärztl. Praxis 28, 289-293.

De Boer, I.J. (2003) Environmental impact assessment of conventional and organic milk production. *Livestock Production Science*, 80, 69-77.

Dietze, K., Werner, C., Sundrum, A. (2007) Status quo of animal health of sows and piglets in organic farms. In *Proceedings of the 3rd QLIF Congress - 2007*, pp 366-369. Edited by U. Niggli, C. Leiffert, T. Alföldi, L. Lück, and H. Willer. Hohenheim, Germany.

Elbers, A.R., Den Hartog, L.A., Verstegen, M.W., Zandstra, T. (1989) Between- and within-herd variation in the digestibility of feed for growing-finishing pigs. *Livestock Production Science*, 23, 183-193.

Erisman, J.W., Monteny, G.J. (1998) Consequences of new scientific findings for future abatement of ammonia emissions. *Environmental Pollution*, 102, 275-282.

European Commission (2000) Report of the Scientific Committee on Animal Health and Animal Welfare. The welfare of chickens kept for meat production (broilers). Adopted 21.03.2000.

European Environment Agency (2003). Water. Europe's Environment: the Third Assessment. *Environmental Assessment Report* 10, 165-197.

Fabian, J., Chiba, L.I., Kuhlers, D.L., Frobish, L.T., Nadarajah, K., Kerth, C.R., McElhenney, W.H., Lewis, A.J. (2002) Degree of amino acid restrictions during the grower phase and compensatory growth in pigs selected for lean growth efficiency. *Journal of Animal Science*, 80, 2610-2618.

Ferguson, N.S. (1999) Nutrition x environmental interactions: Predicting performance of young pigs. In *Recent advances in animal nutrition - 1999*, pp 169-188. Edited by P.C. Garnsworthy, W. Haresign and D.J.A. Cole. Butterworth Heinemann, Oxford.

Flachowsky, G. (2002) Efficiency of energy and nutrient use in the production of edible protein of animal origin. *Journal of Applied Animal Research*, 22, 1-24.

Flachowsky, G. (2007) Humans need, nutrient economy and ecological challenges for animal production. In *Proceedings of the 13th International Conference on Production Diseases in Farm Animals - 2007*, pp 43-54. Edited by M. Fürll. Leipzig.

Flessa, H., Ruser, R., Dörsch, P., Kamp, T., Jimenez, M.A., Munch, J.C., Beese, F. (2002) Integrated evaluation of greenhouse gas emissions (CO_2, CH_4, N_2O) from two farming systems in southern Germany. *Agriculture, Ecosystems and Environment*, **91**, 175-189.

Franckenpohl, U. (2002) Deutsche Putenmast – Wohin geht die Reise? DGS Magazin **34**, 15-17.

Fuller, M.F., Franklin, M.F., McWilliam, R., Pennie, K. (1995) The responses of growing pigs, of a different sex and genotype, to dietary energy and protein. *Journal of Animal Science*, **60**, 291-298.

Gordon, S.H. (1999) The use of home-grown protein sources in organic poultry rations. ADAS-report. ADAS Gleadthorpe, Meden Vale, Mansfield, Nottinghamshire NG20 9PF.

Günther, R. (2001) Putenhaltung - Wie Licht Verhalten, Wachstum und Gesundheit beeinflusst. DGS Magazin 35, 39-41.

Haas, G., Wetterich F., Köpke, U. (2001) Comparing intensive, extensified and organic grassland farming in southern Germany by process life cycle assessment. *Agriculture, Ecosystems and Environment,* 83, 43-53.

Halberg, N., Kristensen, E.S., Kristensen, I.S. (1995) Nitrogen turnover on organic and conventional mixed farms. *Journal of Agriculture and Environmental Ethics*, 8, 30-51.

Hansen, B., Kristensen, E.S., Grant, R., Hogh-Jensen, H., Simmelsgaard, S.E., Olesen, J.E. (2000) Nitrogen leaching from conventional versus organic farming systems – a system modelling approach. *European Journal of Agronomy*, 13, 65-82.

Hermansen, J.E. (2003) Organic livestock productions systems and appropriate development in relation to public expectations. *Livestock Production Science*, 80, 3-15.

Huismann, J., van der Poel, T.F., Liener, I.E. (1989) Recent advances of research in antinutritional factors in legume seeds. Proceeding 1st International Workshop on Antinutritional Factors (ANF) in Legume seeds. Wageningen, Pudoc press, Wageningen.

Hyun, Y., Ellis, M., Johnson, R.W. (1998) Effects of feeder type, space allowance, and mixing on the growth performance and feed intake pattern of growing pigs. *Journal of Animal Science*, 76, 2771-2778.

IPCC (Intergovernmental Panel on Climate Change) (1996) Climate Change 2005. Contribution of the Working Group I to the Second Assessment Report of the IPCC. Cambridge, University Press, Cambridge, UK.

Jeroch, H., Flachowsky, G., Weißbach, F. (1993) Futtermittelkunde. Gustav-Fischer-Verlag, Jena, Stuttgart.

Knudsen, M.T., Kristensen, I.S., Berntsen, J., Petersen, B.M., Kristensen, E.S. (2006) Estimated N leaching losses for organic and conventional farming in Denmark. *Journal of Agricultural Science*, 144, 135-149.

Köpke, U. (1995) Nutrient management in Organic Farming Systems: The case of nitrogen. *Biological Agriculture and Horticulture*, **11**, 15-29.

Köpke, U. (1998) Optimized rotation and nutrient management in Organic Agriculture: The example experimental farm Wiesengut Hennef, Germany. In *Proceedings on Workshop on Mixed Farming Systems in Europe- 1998*, pp 159-164. Edited by H. van Keulen, E.A. Lantinga and H.H. van Laar. Dronten, The Netherlands.

Krutzinna, C., Boehncke, E., Herrmann, H.-J. (1996) Die Milchviehhaltung im ökologischen Landbau. *Berichte über Landwirtschaft,* **74**, 461-480.

Martens, H. (2007) The dairy cow: physiological facts and concerns. In *Proceedings of the 13th International Conference on Production Diseases in Farm Animals - 2007*, pp 26-42. Edited by M. Fürll. Leipzig.

Meunier-Salaun, M.-C. (1999) Fibre in the diets of sows. In *Recent advances in animal nutrition - 1999*, pp 257-273. Edited by P.C. Garnsworthy, W. Haresign and D.J.A. Cole. Butterworth Heinemann, Oxford.

Nicholas, P.K., Sundrum, A., Padel, S. (2007) Guidance notes to operators including recommendations in relation to nutrient supply. EEC 2092/91 (Organic) Revision: Project report D 4.3. Institute of Rural Sciences, University of Wales (UWA) and University of Kassel (UNKA). Aberystwyth and Kassel.

NRC - National Research Council (1994) Nutrient requirements of poultry. Nutrient requirements of domestic animals. National academy press, Washington D.C. (USA).

NRC - National Research Council (1998) Nutrient requirements of swine. Nutrient requirements of domestic animals. National academy press, Washington D.C. (USA).

NRC - National Research Council (2001) Nutrient requirements of dairy cattle. Nutrient requirements of domestic animals. National academy press, Washington D.C. (USA).

Padel, S. (2005) Overview of supply and demand for concentrated organic feed in the EU in 2002 and 2003 with a particular focus on protein sources for mono-gastric animals D4.1 (2) EEC 2092/91 (Organic) Revision SSPE-CT-2004-502397. Institute of Rural Sciences, University of Wales, Aberystwyth.

Padel, S., Lowman, S. (2005) 2004 update of supply and demand for concentrated organic feed in the EU (WP42). Aberystwyth, University of Wales, Aberystwyth. http://orgprints.org/10980/.

Padel, S., Sundrum, A. (2006) How can we achieve 100% organic diets for pigs and poultry. In *Aspects of Applied Biology 79, What will organic farming deliver? COR 2006.* Edited by C. Atkinson, B. Ball, D.H.K. Davies, R. Rees, G. Russell, E.A. Stockdale, C.A. Watson, R. Walker and D. Younie. *Association of Applied Biologists*, Wellesborne, pp 237-241.

Parr, J.F., Summers, J.D. (1991) The effect of minimizing amino acid excesses in broiler diets, *Poultry Science*, **70**, 1540-1549.

Rauw, W.M., Kanis, E., Noordhuizen-Stassen, E.N., Grommers, F.J. (1998) Undesirable side effects of selection for high production efficiency in farm animals: a review. *Livestock Production Science*, **56**, 15-33.

Peter, W., Dänicke, S., Jeroch, H., Wicke, M., von Lengerken, G. (1997a): Einfluss der Ernährungsintensität auf den Wachstumsverlauf und die Mastleistung französischer „Label"-Broiler. *Archiv Tierzucht*, 40, 69-84.

Peter, W., Dänicke, S., Jeroch, H., Wicke, M., von Lengerken, G. (1997b) Einfluss der Ernährungsintensität auf ausgewählte Parameter der Schlachtkörper- und Fleischqualität französischer „Label"-Broiler. *Archiv Geflügelkunde*, 61, 110-116.

Pluske, J.R., Pethick, D.W., Durmic, Z., Hampson, D.J., Mullan, B.P. (1999) Non-starch polysaccharides in pig diets and their influence on intestinal microflora, digestive physiology and enteric disease. In *Recent advances in animal nutrition - 1999*, pp 189-226. Edited by P.C. Garnsworthy, W. Haresign and D.J.A. Cole. Butterworth Heinemann, Oxford.

Scheringer, J. (2002) Nitrogen on dairy farms: balances and efficiency. In *Göttinger Agrarwissenschaftliche Beiträge – 2002*. Edited by J. Isselstein and R. Marggraf. publisher excelsior p.s..

Schinkel, A.P., Smith, J.W., Tokach, M.D., Dritz, S.S., Einstein, M., Nelssen, J.L., Goodband, R.D. (2002) Two on-farm data collection method to determine dynamics of swine compositional growth and estimates of dietary lysine requirements. *Journal of Animal Science*, 80, 1419-1432.

Schutte, J.B., Pack, M. (1995) Sulphur amino acid requirement of broiler chickens for fourteen to thirty-eight days of age 1. Performance and carcass yield. *Poultry Science*, 74, 480-487.

Sundrum, A. (1998) Grundzüge der Ökologischen Tierhaltung. Deutsche Tierärztliche Wochenschrift, 105, 293-298.

Sundrum, A. (2001): Organic livestock farming - A critical review. *Livestock Production Science*, **67**, 207-215.

Sundrum, A. (2002) Verfahrenstechnische und systemorientierte Strategien zur Emissionsminderung in der Nutztierhaltung im Vergleich. *Berichte über Landwirtschaft*, **80**, 556-570.

Sundrum, A. and Ebke, M. (2004) Problems and challenges with the certification of organic pigs. In *Proceedings of the 2nd SAFO-Workshop* . 2004, pp 193-198. Edited by M. Hovi, A. Sundrum and S. Padel. University of Kassel, Germany.

Sundrum, A. and Padel, S. (2006) Evaluation criteria for including feed materials in Annex II C and dietary supplements in Annex II D of the Regulation (EEC) 2092/91. D 4.2 EEC 2092/91 (Organic) Revision. SSPE-CT-2004-502397. University of Kassel.

Sundrum, A., Schneider, K. and Richter, U. (2005) Possibilities and limitations of protein supply in organic poultry and pig production. Report D4.1 EEC 2092/91 (Organic) Revision – Project, SSPE-CT-2004-502397. University of Kassel.

Van Barneveld, R.J. (1999) Understanding the nutritional chemistry of lupin (Lupinus spp.) seed to improve livestock production efficiency. *Nutrition Research Reviews*, 12, 203-230.

Willer, H., Yussefi, M. (2007) The world of organic agriculture 2007: Statistics and emerging trends. *International Federation of Organic Agriculture Movements Publication (IFOAM)*, 7th ed. Online at http://www.soel.de/oekolandbau/weltweit.html.

13

HOW DOES VARIABILITY IN FEEDSTUFF COMPOSITION AFFECT THE DECISIONS WE MAKE IN FORMULATING RATIONS?

MARTIN GREEN[1], JAMES HUSBAND[2], RICHARD VECQUERAY[2], LAURA GREEN[3]

[1]School of Mathematics and School of Veterinary Medicine and Science, University of Nottingham; [2]Evidence Based Veterinary Consultancy, 68 Arthur Street, Penrith; [3]Ecology and Epidemiology Group, Department of Biological Sciences, University of Warwick

Introduction

The fact that feedstuffs used in animal diets have variable composition is well recognised and it is also accepted that this variability will lead to uncertainty in final diet composition (Kertz, 1998; Zhang, 1999; St-Pierre, 2001; Roush, 2004; Gizzi and Givens, 2007; Weiss, 2007). The current chapter will discuss sources of variation that lead to uncertainty in diet specification, examine the effects of variability in feed components in diet formulation and propose that a Bayesian, decision-theoretic framework may be useful in working with the variability that inevitably occurs, to improve on-farm decision-making. The objective is to stimulate thought and discussion on how to deal practically with uncertainty in the nutritional value of feed components.

What do we mean by variability in feedstuff nutrient composition?

The nutritional value of any particular raw material or forage is not the same for all batches used in animal feed. For example, the ruminant energy concentration for rolled wheat used in a particular mill over a six month period may have a mean value of 13.5 MJ ME/kg DM but, for any given diet formulation during that six month period, there will be some variation around this mean value. For example 0.70 of batches may have an energy density between 13.4 and 13.6 MJ/kg DM and if it is assumed that the probability of energy concentrations is distributed normally, a probability distribution that approximates to that in Figure 1 emerges.

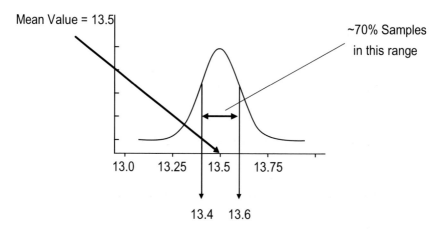

Figure 1. Example of a probability distribution for the metabolisable energy of rolled wheat.

Another way to look at variability is that there is uncertainty associated with the compositional value of a particular sample. The degree of uncertainty may be expressed as a credibility interval (an interval within which there is a specified probability that the true value lies) or assuming a normal distribution, as a standard deviation (SD) or variance (SD^2), as presented in Figure 2.

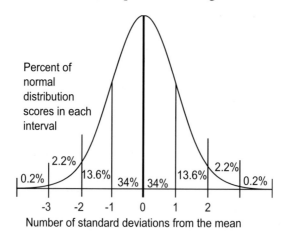

Figure 2. Properties of a normal distribution.

Similarly, a forage sample can be considered. Suppose a grass silage analysis is returned as 10.8 MJ/Kg DM, it is not CERTAIN that is the true value. It may be reasonably assumed (possibly 95% certain) that the true value lies between 10.2 and 11.4, or 70% sure that it lies between 10.5 and 11.1. If many samples of this grass silage were obtained and analysed, the mean and variation in composition could be estimated directly but this is too expensive and time consuming to be carried out each time components are measured.

A crucial aspect of understanding the relevance of variability in feedstuffs is the question "How does variability in feedstuff affect the decisions we make in formulating rations?" is considered subsequently.

Where does variability in feed components arise?

Variability in feedstuff composition can arise from two general sources; random variation (often termed 'error'), or systematic variation ('bias'):

Random variation may arise from:-

- Natural variation in a product (e.g. silage through a clamp, sequential loads of raw materials delivered to a mill, products harvested in different conditions, genetic variation)
- Measurement error in laboratory methods (e.g. 50 results for the 'same' sample will not be precisely the same)

Systematic variation may arise from:-

- An analytic machine that always reads 'low' or 'high' for a particular nutrient
- Decomposition of feeds in certain storage conditions
- Poor sampling technique.

So is variability in feed components of any importance?

When formulating animal diets there is always uncertainty arising from variation in the nutrient composition of feeds. This results in uncertainty in final cake, meal, mix or whole diet formulations and is therefore potentially of great importance. There are many choices available in handling this uncertainty. Solutions include:-

1) Ignore variation and hope that 'things even out'.
2) Minimise sources of variability where possible (and then ignore residual uncertainty).
3) Minimise sources of variability where possible and make allowances for residual uncertainty in farm level decision-making.

If uncertainty is ignored and diets formulated based on a mean figure, then a ration will be under-specified on 0.50 of occasions. Intuitively it would appear that the third choice is best, though most difficult, and a framework for achieving this ideal is proposed. First, ways to reduce the uncertainty in final diet specifications are examined and second how knowledge of the residual uncertainty can be used to enlighten decision-making at farm level is illustrated.

Reducing uncertainty in diet specification

Random variation in feed component nutritional values is usually more difficult to identify and remove from diet formulation than systematic variation. In general, random variation is better estimated by increasing the number of samples analysed and can be reduced by increasing the accuracy of the testing procedures. Realistically, for economic reasons, there is a limit to the number of tests that can be undertaken on any raw material or forage component although increasing the number taken will help. In terms of sample testing, there are technical limitations to methods of nutrient analysis and thus some error will be inevitable. Estimating the size of this random variation may be difficult but sources of information are available, such as literature reports, test data from individual laboratories and information on test characteristics from equipment manufacturers. Use of a reputable accredited laboratory may reduce random error.

In a Bayesian setting, information on random error can be incorporated as prior (or 'currently believed') information and can be used to model diet components in a way that includes this uncertainty (stochasticity). This will be considered subsequently.

Systematic variation can and should be minimised wherever possible, by identifying the source of the bias. This may mean improving sampling techniques, storage methods, machine maintenance or calibration, etc. Systematic variation also occurs from farm management procedures and this is considered later.

Having minimised random and systematic variation, there are some pragmatic principles, as outlined by Weiss (2007), to reduce the impact of uncertainty in feed components in a final diet specification:-

- Do not use highly variable feedstuffs.
- Reduce the proportion of variable products used in a diet.
- Increase the number of dietary components (this has the effect of 'averaging' feeds that may be higher or lower than their expected mean value – see example below)
- Consider adjusting a feedstuff by a proportion of the SD to allow for the probability of the feed being above a specified nutrient level.

A potential problem with the principle of reducing the use of variable feedstuffs is that there may be occasions when it is unavoidable (feeds in short supply) or cost effective (variable feeds being advantageously priced). A problem with using individual feed adjustments is that it can be difficult to assess the final output probabilities for the overall diet (combinations of distributions are needed for this). Rations that use individual component 'safety margins' have been shown to be less cost effective than full probability based models (Roush, 2004).

Additions can be made to the list above; careful and regular monitoring of farm performance. If monitoring reveals that predicted outputs are not achieved, one reason could simply be unexpected variation in nutritional components. Reformulation can then be considered promptly to avoid long term financial implications.

To illustrate the importance of mixing dietary components the example below is provided.

EXAMPLE 1 - MIXING FOUR FEEDS TO MAKE A CONCENTRATE BLEND

Consider a mix of 0.25 kg of each of four raw materials, a, b, c, and d. It is assumed all products have an energy concentration of 11 MJ ME/kg DM.

The mean ME value of the mix is therefore 11 MJ/kg DM
{ie = (0.25 x 11) + (0.25 x 11) + (0.25 x 11) + (0.25 x 11) }

It may now (more realistically) be assumed that each constituent has an ME value with some uncertainty attached to it, such that the value fits a probability distribution with a mean of 11 and standard deviation of 0.2 (variance = 0.04), as shown below in Figure 3.

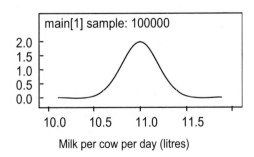

Figure 3. The probability distribution for the energy concentration of raw materials a,b,c and d.

The probability distribution for the energy concentration of the final mix has a mean of 11.0 MJ/kg DM and SD of 0.10. Thus the variation is now reduced for the mix compared to the individual components and this can be thought of as averaging out across all feeds the likelihood of taking a sample either above or below their mean value. As indicated above (Weiss, 2007) this principle is of importance when formulating diets because it means that, in general, mixing of dietary components reduces uncertainty in the final specification.

A decision-theoretic framework can now be considered with the question, "what is the probability that the mix has an energy concentration > 10.9 or > 10.8 MJ/kg DM?" This can be calculated from a closed formula or (in this case) using simulation methods. The resulting probabilities are:-

Probability > 10.9 MJ/kg DM = 0.84 (84%)
Probability > 10.8 MJ/kg DM = 0.98 (98%)

Informative decisions on the probability that the mix reaches certain levels of ME can now be made. Some rationale for decision making is required, such as what is an acceptable probability of exceeding different thresholds in formulation. Put another way, the acceptable 'risk' that the current least cost formulation does not meet requirements needs to be considered.

Calculating diets to incorporate feedstuff probability distributions (uncertainty in feed components)

Feed programs that incorporate variability of feed components have been developed (Zhang, 1999, St Pierre, 2001). Researchers at Ohio State have made economic assessments of feed levels using stochasticity with the software "Optimu7m". Interestingly Roush (2004) reports that, by using probability distributions rather than simple safety margins for feedstuffs, a reduced cost per tonne of a final feed is achieved, for a given strategy of accepted risk. This is expanded subsequently.

MOVING TOWARDS A DECISION-BASED BAYESIAN APPROACH

The essence of a Bayesian approach is to combine reasonable known evidence/ information of a parameter (prior knowledge) with new data on the parameter, to determine a final probability for the parameter (posterior distribution). The combination is carried out using Bayes Theorem and effectively weights the new data by the prior information. The method is flexible, is able to include diverse sources of evidence and is particularly useful at allowing predictions to be made.

The results give the probability of future events, given prior knowledge and current data.

It is possible to incorporate information on the variability of feedstuffs alongside recent sample analyses in a Bayesian context to provide outputs in a decision-theoretic framework. Thus, results can take the form of a meaningful decision parameter such as the probability distribution of the diet cost, the cost per unit of meat/milk/eggs produced, the herd/flock daily or annual margin and so on. Specific thresholds can be evaluated, according to attitudes on the associated risks, to improve decision-making. For example, on a particular dairy farm in a particular quota situation, it may be decided that an 80% probability is required for a specified minimum bulk tank output and a least cost formulation can be based on this. Aspects of farm management can also be included in this decision, such as variability in feed preparation and variability in animal intakes. An extended example is provided below.

EXAMPLE 2: EFFECTS OF VARIABILITY IN FEED COMPONENTS AND FARM MANAGEMENT ON OUTPUT, COSTS AND PRODUCTION DECISIONS

Consider a dairy farm with 100 high yielding cows for which a partial TMR diet is being formulated. Using a particular feed software, a traditional best cost formulation for a medium-high yield group was estimated as:-

Dry matter intakes;
Maize silage = 6 kg DM per head per day
Grass silage = 6 kg DM per head per day
Wheat = 2 kg DM per head per day
Soya = 2 kg DM per head per day
Compound = 5 kg DM per head per day

For simplicity in the illustration, only energy (in terms of metabolisable energy, ME) will be considered in the formulation and output. The estimates of ME in the feed components were;

Maize silage = 11.5 MJ/kg DM
Grass silage = 10.8 MJ/kg DM
Wheat = 13.5 MJ/kg DM
Soya = 13.5 MJ/kg DM
Compound = 12.7 MJ/kg DM

This provided a total daily ME intake per cow of 251.3 MJ and we assume that there is no other nutrient limiting milk production. Thus if we take rounded figures of 70MJ/day for maintenance and 5 MJ required per litre of milk produced, the expected output from this diet was (251.3-70)/5 =36.26 litres per cow per day.

Including probability distributions for feed components

In reality the ME values cannot be known for certain and it is known from data and experience that there is some uncertainty associated with estimates of the feed component ME values above. Normal probability distributions are now included in the example;

In MJ/kg DM:-

> Maize silage - mean = 11.5, SD = 0. 2
> Grass silage - mean = 10.8, SD = 0. 2
> (i.e. 68% probability that the results are +/- 0.2 MJ/kg DM and 95% probability +/- 0.4 MJ/kg DM)

> Wheat – mean = 13.5, SD = 0.1
> Soya – mean = 13.5, SD = 0.1
> Concentrate - mean = 12.7, SD = 0.1
> (i.e. 68% probability that the results are +/- 0.1 MJ/kg DM and 95% probability +/- 0.2 MJ/kg DM)

By combining these probabilities a mean ration ME of 251.3 and a mean expected production of 36.2 litres / day is maintained, but the uncertainty around these estimates can now be calculated.

The expected litres produced per cow has a probability distribution such that there is a 68% probability the actual production will be +/- 0.36 litres /cow/day and 95% probability it will between 35.56 and 36.96 litres /day. Another way to look at this is that, if this ration were set up 20 times, due to the uncertainty in feed component values, on one occasion the yield per cow would be at least 0.7 litres above or below the expected mean value.

In this case, if the milk price was 19 pence per litre (ppl), and feed costs of maize silage = £80 per tonne DM, grass silage = £70 / tonne DM, wheat = £100 tonne DM, soya = £160 / tonne DM and cake = £120 / tonne DM, then further calculations to assess the impact of this variability on the farm can be made. The expected production from these 100 cows is 3620 litres /day (mean) with a SD ~

35.7. Therefore there is a 16% probability that this output would be more than the 35.7 litres below expected At 19ppl the value of this 35.7 is approximately £6.80 per day which over a three month period is around £625.

This variation in milk volume is relatively modest. If there was less certainty of the actual value of the grass silage ME such that the SD is increased by a factor of two to 0.4 MJ /kg DM, this would result in an increased uncertainty in the bulk tank milk (SD = 54.7) and now a 16% probability that the actual daily production for 100 cows would be more than 54.7 litres below expected. Such a milk loss would be worth approximately £10.40 per day which over a three month period is around £950, a more significant loss. This illustrates the potential importance of variability and uncertainty in feed components. However, in rations in which a variety of feeds are mixed and none tend to have extreme variation, the variability in the final ration will often be of limited importance.

Using this method, a probabilistic and decision-based approach to feeding can be taken. Depending on risk, quota, current farm finances and client relationships, final diets can be formulated transparently with specified objectives. The best cost formulation to provide (say) an 80% certainty of a specified milk output or margin per litre (or per cow) may be required. Having specified a ration, there also needs to be clarity about the uncertainty of the final diet. The final probability distributions of key features of the diet, such as the predicted milk per cow per day or milk value per day may be illustrated. Such graphical representations allows a visualisation of the uncertainty associated with a suggested ration as illustrated in Figure 4.

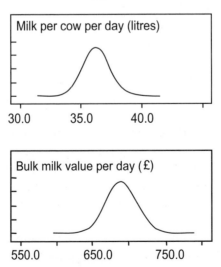

Figure 4. Probability distributions illustrating the output of milk per cow per day and bulk milk value per day for an example dairy cow diet.

Why variability in feed component nutrients affects the cost of a diet

The variability of different raw materials means that a best cost formulation will change depending on feed variability as well as the expected mean value. Feeds with more variability (greater uncertainty of the true value) represent a greater risk and this itself effectively has a cost when probabilities are used to formulate diets in this manner. This can be illustrated by including some more variable feeds in our current example ration and comparing the expected milk yield per cow (Figure 5).

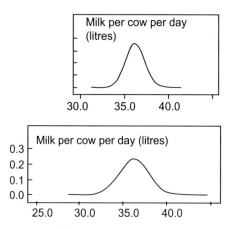

Figure 5. An illustration of the probability of milk output per cow per day (litres) for two diets that provide the same mean metabolisable energy content but with different variability in feed constituents.

Thus, although the mean expected output remains the same, there is a higher probability that the ration with more variable ingredients will not exceed specific yields below this. For example, there is an 86% probability that cows consuming the less variable ration would exceed 35.7 litres whereas this probability is reduced to 62% for the more variable diet. Therefore, more nutrients (at greater cost) would need to be added for the more variable diet to reach the same probability of producing this minimum milk production. Using this approach, least cost formulation can be used such that a cost is attributed to feed variability in the context of farm risk acceptance. Approximate variabilities in feedstuffs are included in the NRC feeding recommendations (2001).

The impact of variation in farm management

The example to include variability in farm feed management and examine how this affects final performance can now be extended. Farm variability can be split into two general areas; i. variation that occurs because the storage, mixing, preparation and feeding practices may be variable (the extent of our uncertainty that the specified ration is actually fed), and ii. variation that occurs because there is uncertainty in the cows or herds dry matter intakes arising from factors such as feed access, quality of presentation and standard of equipment (extent of uncertainty that the specified feeds are actually eaten). These farm factors may vary within a farm over time or between farms.

The initial ration that includes uncertainty in forages (SD = 0.2MJ/kg DM) and concentrate feeds (SD = 0.1 MJ/kg DM) can now be reconsidered. In this extension, it is assumed that storage/mixing/preparation causes the DMI to vary with a normal probability distribution with mean = 1 (ration is fed 100% as specified) and SD = 0.03 (68% probability that the ration is +/- 3% of the mean). It is assumed that there is added uncertainty due to feed access/presentation with the same probability distribution.

The expected production from these 100 cows remains at 3620 litres/day (mean) but now the uncertainty around this has increased such that the SD = 163 (1.63 litres per cow per day). Therefore there is now a 16% probability that this output would be more than 163 kg (1.63 x 100 cows) below expected, and this may be an 'unacceptable' risk for a relatively large reduction in daily yield. At 19ppl the value of the 163 litres of milk is approximately £31 per day which over a three month period is over £2,800, a sizeable sum. This illustrates the principle that since farm factors generally affect the whole diet, they will often have a larger impact on farm outputs than variability that arises from individual feed components in a diverse diet. If, as some experts believe, farm management varies more than this, such that the SD in storage/mixing/preparation and also feed access/presentation is 7%, the variability in milk production is such that there is now a 16% probability of a loss in milk production per day worth approximately £71.00 or over a 3 month period, around £6,400.

The situation in which a specific farm management problem is thought to occur can also be modelled. It may be believed that on a certain farm, food access is restricted and the possibility (for example) that DMI is reduced by 3% (with a SD of 1%) can be examined. These beliefs can be incorporated as probability distributions into the model along with our other feed probability distributions. Again, this will influence the probability of achieving specified outputs and hence the approach taken to formulating a new diet. In our example, this DMI reduction would result in a 50% probability of a reduced yield per cow per day of 2.15 litres (worth ~£3,700 for 100 cows in three months) and a 16% probability that a reduction of 3.2 litres per cow per day would occur (worth over £5000 in three months). The importance of small changes in dry matter intakes is clear and can be included in probability-based models.

The examples and discussion to date have, for the sake of simplicity, considered only metabolisable energy in the diet. Including other dietary components is a matter of incorporating the relevant probability distributions and interrelationships. Whilst these are rather complex (particularly for ruminants) and depend upon the animal feed models used, final diet and production predictions can still be made in the form of probability distributions and interpreted in the way described.

Incorporating "prior" probabilities and a full Bayesian approach

Modelling of sources of variability can be further extended by combining some prior beliefs alongside new data from a particular farm. For example, we may have laboratory data for the ME of rolled wheat from a particular source. From this (assuming normality) a mean and standard deviation can be estimated and used as prior knowledge of the probability distribution for the ME of wheat. If recent samples of wheat for a farm are analysed, the new data can be used to modify previous information to estimate a new (posterior) probability distribution for the ME of wheat. In this way the strength of previous knowledge is used alongside new information to (hopefully) make a better estimate.

If the probability distribution for the ME of wheat is taken as our 'prior' (wheat; mean = 13.5 MJ/kg DM, SD = 0.1), but now add a further four current wheat ME measurements; 13.6, 13.4, 13.3, 13.1.Combining these develops a posterior estimate;

mean = 13.45, SD = 0.08 and 95% credibility interval = 13.29 to 13.63.

The distributions are illustrated in figure 6.

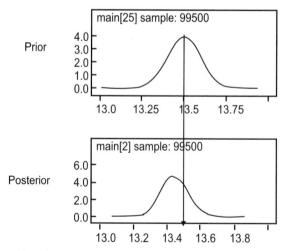

Figure 6. Prior and posterior probability distributions in the example of incorporating previous and new knowledge into a feed model.

The posterior distribution can be used for subsequent ration prediction and may be thought of as a weighted mean of the prior knowledge and the data from current samples. This may work well for forage analysis, when a prior distribution for a specific silage cut (e.g. mid May, new grass variety, good making conditions) could be combined with a relatively small number of analyses from the silage clamp in question. This has the effect of averaging, between the current (few) sample results and the 'expected' probability distribution for such silages. This limits the influence of one or two very unusual sample results.

This concept can be extended to all feed components for which there is reasonable prior knowledge from literature, laboratory data or expert advice, and used to formulate diets with outputs in the form of probability distributions. Different prior information can be used, such as solely the variability of each feed component (using the mean from current samples), the variability of a subset of feeds (e.g. forages and wet feeds), or full prior information for as many components as are available. It is also possible to make different assumptions about prior information, such as being more optimistic or pessimistic about the figures, to examine how this affects final probabilities and hence decisions on feed components.

Conclusions

In summary, variation in feed components used to produce animal diets is unavoidable and leads to uncertainty in the final diet specified. Approaches to handling this uncertainty are:-

- Minimise variation by:
  - Reducing random and systematic variation wherever possible.
  - Using a variety of different feeds to make a diet.
  - Limiting the use of highly variable feeds in general and particularly if they are the dedicated protein or energy component of the diet.
- Allow for uncertainty in feed components:-
  - A decision-based approach can be used to model uncertainty – feeds with more variability have a greater risk of under-performing and are therefore worth less than the mean value may represent. Decisions need to be set in the context of each farm situation.
  - Probability based models can easily be extended from diet specifications, to probability distributions of expected output of production and expected farm returns, and can also incorporate variability in farm feeding practices.
  - A Bayesian approach that incorporates prior knowledge of feed component characteristics as well as results of recent farm samples may provide improved estimates for decision-making.

• Expect formulation to be an iterative process. Monitor animal performance and farm outputs regularly and carefully as a guide for possible errors in dietary assumptions. It should not be assumed that a diet is correct just because it is 'right' on paper and vice versa.

Acknowledgements

Martin Green is currently funded by a Wellcome Trust Intermediate Clinical Fellowship.

References

Berry, D. A. and Stangl, D. K. (1996). *Bayesian Biostatistics*. Marcel Dekker Inc. New York, USA.

Gizzi, G. and Givens, D. I. (2007). Variability in feed composition and its impact on animal production. www.fao.org/agrippa/publications/ToC4.htm

Kertz, A.F. (1998). Variability in delivery of nutrients to lactating dairy cows. *Journal of Dairy Science*. **81**, 3075-3084.

Roush, W.B. (2004). Stochastic programming: Addressing risk due to variability. *Aqua Feeds: Formulation & Beyond*, **1** (3)

Spiegelhalter, D. J., Abrams, K. R. and Myles, J. P. (2004). *Bayesian Approaches to Clinical Trials and Health-Care Evaluation* (Statistics in Practice). John Wiley and sons, Chichester, UK

St-Pierre, N. (2001). Managing variability in feed programs. Pennsylvania State Dairy Cattle Nutrition Workshop, Grantville, PA. November 6-7.

Weiss, B. (2007). Understanding and managing variation in nutrient composition. Western Dairy Management Conference, Reno, Nevada. March 7-9.

Zhang, F. (1999). Stochastic models and software design for feed formulation. Ph.D. Thesis, Penn State University.

14

WATER MEASUREMENT IN PIG AND POULTRY PRODUCTION

NICK BIRD

Farm Energy & Control Services Ltd, Pingewood Business Estate, Pingewood, Reading, RG30 3UR

Introduction

Water makes up the greater part of body tissues, and the greater part of dietary intake of farmed animals. Without water, animals quickly become ill and die. Water is more important than feed, temperature and genetics. It makes up a far greater proportion of dietary intake than any of the complex assortment of carbohydrates, vitamins, amino acids in feed that are the very substance of the role of nutritionists.

When considering feed it is in the context of "optimisation". When considering water, this usually means "adequate". As long as animals have "adequate" access to an "adequate" supply of "adequate" water, then water is not an issue.

This is partly because animals seem to "get what they need" - or it is assumed they do - but rather more because there is just no money in it as it is not "economically interesting". Farms pay hundreds of millions of pounds a year on feed, and though feed companies may well complain there is no profit in it, they could divert a little of that to research and development, study. Water is just pumped out of the ground and, if not entirely free, is not costed. No value is attached to it and the general view is that it does not matter that much. There is somewhat more concern over what comes out the other end.

This is an unfortunate situation because there is a lot of useful information in water intake, if examined correctly. The problem is that it is not examined properly and it has not been measured it in a way that reveals the relevant information.

The data shown in the current chapter are mostly from pig production. This is partly because pigs - as the most highly evolved of the farmed species - offer a range of issues that may not be present, or present in a different way, in other species.

Much of what appears is somewhat speculative and opinion-based. It is not claimed that all - or indeed any - of the interpretations placed on the data

275

presented are fact, or true in any absolute sense. It is, perhaps, a tribute to the lack of significant extensive academic - or even commercial - research that this is necessarily the case.

The hardware

WATER METERS

Measuring water - sufficient for purpose in commercial-scale production - is very easy, and there is little point in going into the whys, wherefores and details of different types of meter here.

In typical buildings, a 15 mm (1/2") or 20mm (3/4") or sometimes 25mm (1") standard "utility" meter - as installed in homes and offices - is perfectly adequate. They are cheap and widely available from many plumbing supply companies, priced from £50 to £150.

To be of any use for the specific purposes intended, they must have a "pulse" output - a pair of contacts operated by a magnet attached to part of the meter, that allows an electronic connection to a "pulse counter" for remote display or data logging.

Water meters are "integrating" or "quantising" meters in nature. That is, giving a pulse per "unit" of volume delivered - usually 1 pulse per 0.5 or 1.0 litre. Meters with 1 pulse per m^3 are commonly used for charging purposes by some utility companies but are not useful for intake monitoring.

For more specialist applications - such as for lower volumes - other types are available such as "Titan" turbines and ultrasonic flow meters.

WATER METER ISSUES

Water meters have a limited dynamic range because they are mechanical - the water drives the mechanism. Within their intended flow range, they are typically sufficiently accurate for purpose (normally specified +/- 2%).

At low flow rates, they become inaccurate, but at lower flow rates they register no flow at all, though there may be some flow.

For example a typical 15mm meter has a nominal flow of 1500 lph (litres per hour) and down to 23 lph @ +/- 2%. However, below 6 lph, they register no flow. Accordingly there might be as much as 150 litres per day with none registering at all. If flow is always very slow, as much as 500 litres may register only half that or less. This is often a significant problem in UK systems with header tanks and worn float (ball) valves.

Pressure drop - a loss of water pressure between the inlet and outlet of the meter - increases with flow rate. This can be an issue, particularly where supplies are poor in the first place. It is impractical in most cases to measure flow rate in low pressure systems, i.e. from a header tank to drinkers.

Scaling and particulate matter (silt and sediment) are a common problem on farms, since supplies are usually from a borehole. Farms are often reluctant to use filters because they silt up. To put it another way, they would rather have sediment clogging up pipes and drinkers, which is why water provision may well be a problem. High levels of scale and sediment do not affect meter accuracy so much, rather the meters stop working, and impede water flow completely.

DATA LOGGING

Data can only provide useful information if they are accessible and in a usable form. For reasons explained subsequently, manual daily readings of water use in poultry may yield useful and usable data although not very accessible, and labour intensive. For any other purpose, data logging is essential.

Water is recorded by connecting pulse contacts to a data logger, which counts the pulses as an accumulating count. The recommended logging (storing the value) - along with other related factors – is at 15 minute intervals. This gives sufficient data rate to assess most of the signals in the data without excessive redundancy.

For very short term use by students and hobbyists, a host of data logging units is available. With modern microprocessors, making something that can log readings at some set interval is not that difficult, and most microprocessor engineers could install something suitable using standard components in a couple of days.

However, for serious long term use amid the rigours of agricultural installations, a fixed installation is necessary, recording more than just water. For example, if a specific change is considered to be attributable to temperature, then temperature information as well is needed. In practice, more benefits accrue from long-term fixed monitoring than short-term "investigations" for a week or two.

Most farms are spread out, and yet it is necessary to get data all to one place, so cost is actually dominated by installation cost due to the long wiring runs. Despite numerous press releases representing wireless data networks as a firmly established, wireless data gathering - which may significantly reduce the cost - has yet to make any significant inroads into data logging in industrial-type situations. This is partly because of the distances. Using available licence-free radio bands and signal strengths, distances of a few metres are no problem, but flexible, robust systems over hundreds of metres definitely are. Practical commercial systems are expected within the next 3 years, but for time being hard-wired systems are still standard. Whilst installation cost is a distinct disincentive, a well-engineered - and even more importantly well-installed - logging system should last at least 10 to 15 years.

The most economical way to install logging on livestock farms is using integrated controller networks. That is, using ventilation and other regulators that are networked (such as for alarm purposes) and can also gather data. This reduces the effective cost of data logging on farm considerably - the only additional cost is for "additional data connection" rather than the whole thing. However, the data logging capabilities vary considerably from brand to brand, and in some cases control unit to control unit.

In practice, on-site use of primary data is - and always will be - extremely limited. Whilst the idea that a stockperson or unit manager labouring over their computer will see readings and instantly make changes to correct any and all issues is an attractive idea, it has little practical application. Of greater value would be computer programs that automatically analyse the readings, calculate corrective action and instruct site managers accordingly. This may well be somewhat futuristic and is unlikely to be realised in the short term.

Most use of real-time data is "off site" - whether at farm office, production company headquarters or in the hands of advisers and consultants. Hence, remote retrieval and management of data is crucial. Landline modems are useful, although competing for use on shared lines is often difficult. In the UK, with good cellular coverage, cellular modems and GPRS are an effective alternative. The future, however, is broadband - a shared, always-on high-speed connection, largely because of its low and falling cost. Any system that may be modem connected can be converted to broadband, using adapters.

On-unit display of current readings (or via a modem or PC link) is useful for installation and maintenance purposes, but is of little use otherwise. Typical cost for a data logger suitable for long term use in agricultural surroundings is from around £1000 for 8 input channels, plus £200 per additional 8 inputs.

Data Logging Software

Recording the data is straightforward, but to be of any use they must accessed, displayed, summarised and analysed.

Whilst the current chapter is about water measurement, no particular distinction can be drawn between logging of water intake, and data logging for other purposes. Thus, in order to include the underlying information sufficiently well (depending on the purpose), data must be sampled sufficiently frequently and accurately. For example, to know how fast cars go, recording mileage once a week would not only be inadequate, but very deceptive indeed.

There is some trade-off between volume and cost of data (especially of recording and storage). For typical purposes in livestock, recording readings every 15 minutes appears adequate.

One of the biggest - and most common - errors is to mistake or misunderstand the nature and volume of the data. Real time data logging on farms generates large data sets. For example, a modest scale producer with just 50 buildings, each with only 10 data factors recorded, generates 17.5 million readings a year.

Large data sets are not such an issue for modern computers - gone are the days when databases needed to operate within 640k of RAM. One current database is around 70Gb and runs well on an ordinary PC. However, readily accessing such large data sets remains an important factor in the design of software for real time data. A popular - and often repeated - mistake, for example, is to use a web-based charting tool with an on-line database query engine. It works perfectly well only until real volumes of data are entered.

Although spreadsheets are useful for small volumes of data (up to a few tens of thousands of data points), they need a lot of skill, experience and practice. Beyond that, there are no easy-to-use "general purpose" presentation and analysis tools for this type of data. Hence, presentation tools are almost all "bespoke" - designed by the manufacturers of the equipment. The style and facilities vary considerably.

The illustrations used in the currrent paper are all derived (directly from screen captures, or with further analysis) from Barn Report, the market leader in real-time monitoring systems in pig production the UK and US.

DATA SIGNALS

Whilst water is interesting in itself, it is rather more useful to think of it as an indicator of underlying processes. By analogy, the sound of a car engine can tell us things including rpm, the state of the bearings, or how much force it is exerting.

Water data is a complex waveform containing signals of varying intensity and frequency. To make sense of it, it is important to attempt to understand these data signals.

Data signals are information or factors within the data that affect the measured value - that is, a change in the measured value indicates a changed parameter or circumstance.

The main signals are -

- Growth
- Body clock and lighting
- Temperature
- Feed type and taste
- Health
- Feed availability

- Socialisation, behaviour and habit
- Water quality
- Water availability
  Leakage and dribbling

Signals have varying frequencies. For example, larger pigs drink more, so increased consumption is an indication of growth. However, this takes place over a long period of time (low frequency data).

The body clock means that water intake varies considerably over each day. This higher frequency is superimposed on the lower frequency growth data. The measured data is therefore a waveform of greater or lesser complexity.

Characteristic trace

When lights are switched on (see figure 1), there is an initial peak, but otherwise the intake is relatively flat until lights are dimmed. At night, there is almost no consumption.

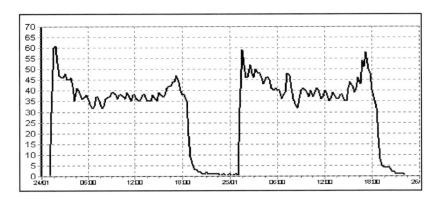

Figure 1. Characteristic trace of water consumption in a typical poultry building. (turkeys) with timer controlled lighting.

The responses of pigs are quite different (Figure 2). Water intake rises gradually from around zero (at 6 am) to a peak at sunset, when it falls sharply. During the night there are cycles of intake which fall gradually to zero at 6am.

A key difference in the housing of pigs and poultry is that poultry houses are usually artificially lit, with timers. It is well known that the activity of poultry is regulated by lighting, and even when given access to outside, are closed in at night.

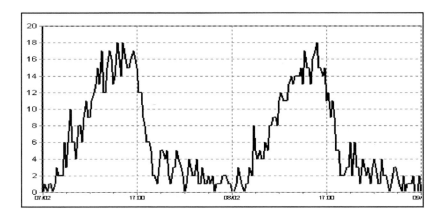

Figure 2. Characteristic trace of pigs (in natural lighting).

By contrast, pigs tend to have natural light - either partly or wholly - and artificial lighting (if used) is usually manually switched. Many producers leave some lighting switched on all the time (not in this building in Figure 2) in the belief that this helps pigs find feed. Whilst pigs may synchronise to daylight, it is clear that they have significant activity even in the dark.

Since poultry have little or no water intake in the dark, measuring daily intake simply means counting from one dark period to the next. For manual readings it does not matter when the reading is taken, as long as it is during the dark period - from zero intake to the next zero intake - it is one "day".

The pig "day" is also, clearly, from one zero to the next zero but this is a narrow time frame. Unless readings are taken at a precise time, readings will be part of one day, and part of another - giving significant indeterminacy or "noise".

Feed intake

Ad lib, dry fed pigs - at least - drink when they eat, and eat when they drink. The two are the same activity. This is hardly surprising - the "cream cracker test" shows how difficult it is to eat dry food without drinking. This is not necessarily obvious from logged data (Figure 3) since feed systems only run periodically - refilling hoppers that may be depleted to a greater or lesser extent.

However, where there are feed systems that run semi-continuously or "on demand" - the pattern is clear (Figure 4).

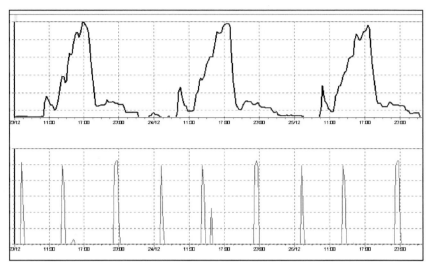

Figure 3. The auger run time (lower trace) shows refilling operations at arbitrary times, whilst the water tank refills semi-continuously

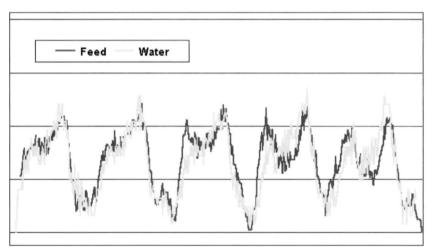

Figure 4. Feed delivery (by auger run time in each 15 minutes) against water delivery in the same period over 4 days in a finishing building.

An interesting aspect is that feed intake appears not to be the main driver, but the only driver of water intake. Water taken with feed is the only water intake. This has important implications for the design and layout of feed and water systems.

Usefully, it suggests that when and how much they eat can be estimated reasonably well by measuring when and how much they drink. Water use is easier to measure than feed use (Figure 5).

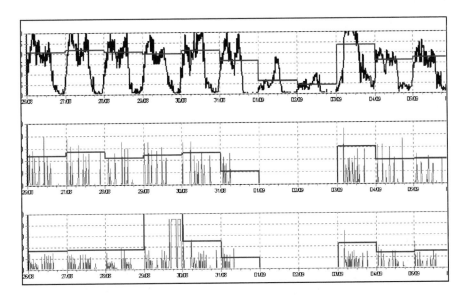

Figure 5. A building with one water reading and two auger run time readings - we can see where the augers stopped working - they ran out of feed for two days. Although the pigs still drank some water (daily total red line), it fell to only 25% of the normal value.

Typically - though there is limited data - the ratio of water to dry feed is 2.7 to 1 in grow/finishing, but a lower ratio for younger pigs.

Growth

Clearly, the normal trend for water intake is upward (figure 7), indicating growth. It is a constant ssource of amazement that producers and feed companies alike see fit to summarise this as a single figure of "ADFI" or "ADG" when, clearly, it is a slope. It is like defining a hill in terms of average height.

If these data are further clarified, it is clear that there is not even one single slope but three. Apart from the initial fall in water intake in the first few days (not uncommon) there are two other reductions - intake falls and then rises again. The second and third slopes are lower than the previous - suggesting that rate of growth is declining. The reductions are where the feed ration is changed.

Since water intake is reduced for several days, there is a strong implication of loss of growth rate. It is not entirely clear whether - or to what extent - nutritionists "factor in" a loss of growth to their feed optimisation calculations or are even aware of it.

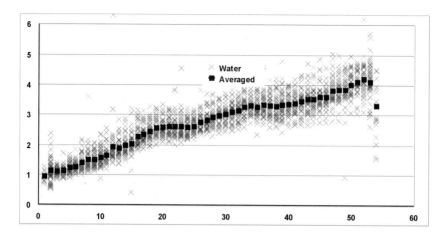

Figure 6. Daily intake - litres per pig - of pigs in nursery buildings on a particular farm. Individual data points are average water intake per pig in a room, for each day in the production batch. (Bottom axis is relative day number - the pigs are housed from weaning at 28 days old, for 54 days.) The averaged line is the average of all pigs. This covers 42 batches of pigs across 7 buildings - roughly 25,000 in all.

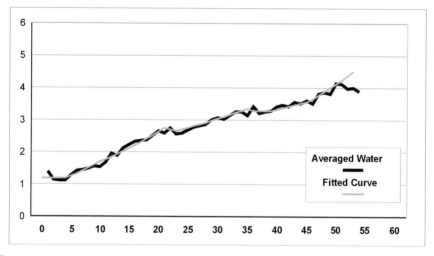

F
igure 7. Pattern of increasing water intake with age (days)

Temperature

It is well known and sufficiently obvious that higher temperatures mean greater water intake. In hot weather, it is very important to keep the water system functional efficiently, as the animals have greater need of water.

Except that higher water intake on rising temperatures seems not to be particularly the case (Figure 8).

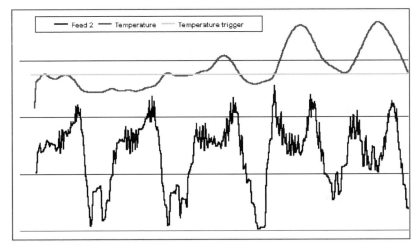

Figure 8. Feed intake in finishing pigs as influenced by temperature

In this example (Figure 9) a sudden "blip" in temperature (caused by rising outside temperature) causes a reduction in intake in the middle of the day. Pigs drink less not more. The reason being that they are "put off their feed" in the middle of the day by rising temperature.

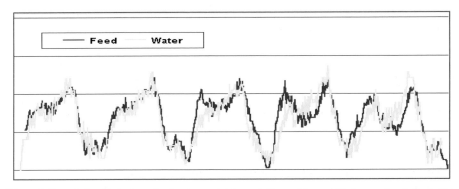

Figure 9. The relationship between feed and water intake, as influenced by variable temperature indicated in Figure 8.

Interestingly the "trigger temperature" (which is estimated, not measured) is actually only 22°C - just a few degrees higher than the normal operating temperature, and nowhere near the "UCT" (upper critical temperature).

After a few days of high peak temperatures, pigs develop the habit of reduced intake in the middle of the day, with more consumed in the early morning and late evening. It should be emphasised that this is not normal in the sense of what pigs would do if temperatures were not an issue - it is a pattern of behaviour induced by high temperatures. It takes pigs several days to "lose the habit" - depressed middle of day drinking remains for several days after temperatures return to normal.

Under extreme conditions, behavioural modification - eating and drinking early and later - is more extreme Overall, indications are that pigs drink marginally more - per unit of feed - in hot conditions than cold conditions, but the impact is marginal, and probably due to marginally greater evaporative loss from the lungs. Water intake remains related to feed intake (Figure 10).

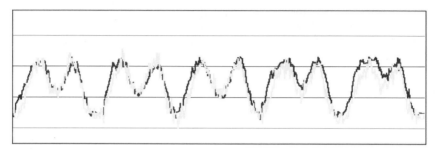

Figure 10. Further evidence for the relationship between water and feed intake

Body clock

The body clock is a system of regulation that determines that animals respond to - and are prepared for - the conditions they experience. Light is an important factor in the body clock. In the case of poultry, it appears to dominate entirely - if light is above a certain level it is day, and below that it is night with birds eating and drinking in the day, sleeping at night. Poultry are so evidently affected by light that most producers have lighting timers, or are very careful to switch lighting consistently.

Pigs have an endogenous body clock, their bodies "know" roughly what time it is, whether the lights are on or off.

The two snapshots (Figure 12) show water intake pattern in the same naturally lit (ACNV ventilated) continuously stocked pig finishing building in North of Scotland. Drinking pattern is slightly longer and perhaps starts slightly earlier in June but - given that night is very short indeed in the North of Scotland in June, the differences are not so great as one might expect.

This seems to be because the pig body clock synchronises with the "real" day, but is not - as with poultry - controlled by it. The total daily water intake (Figure 12) is not very different, and the difference may be simply due to slight difference in average pig weight at the different times.

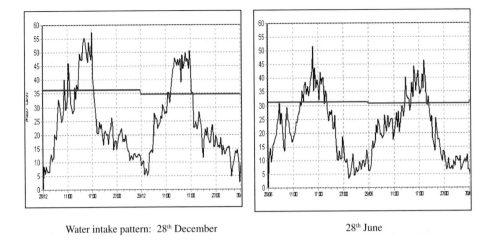

Water intake pattern: 28th December   28th June

Figure 11. Water intake at different times of the year

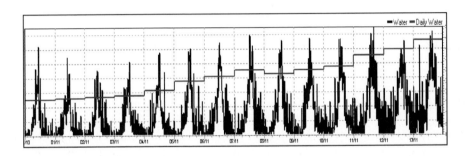

Figure 12. Water and fed intake under 24 hour light.

The endogenous body clock tends to run slightly longer than 24 hours. In this artificially-lit pig nursery, lights are kept on at high level all the time - shown for 2 weeks.

At the beginning of the response in Figure 11, the peak of consumption is at about 4 pm. By the end, it is at 11 pm. A key issue here is that, since the pig day and real day fall out of step, there must - at some point - be a reckoning. When the pigs are eventually moved to follow on accommodation this may be "in the middle of their night" - that is, jetlag.

Whether pigs grow better with an endogenous or "real" body clock is an important question. In this case, the unit manager believes that pigs need continuous lighting to "find the feed". Whilst this is not appreciated, this means an endogenous rather than body clock. This is, incidentally, illegal in the EU (continuous artificial lighting is banned), although it is not expressed in terms of body clock.

Health

There is increasing evidence that water intake may decline some time before clinical signs of illness are apparent - up to 10 days before. This is probably due to a decline in feed intake. Whether this is all or most animals dropping a little intake, or a small but increasing number dropping intake a lot is not clear.

The potential for this to be used as a *predictive* tool on which to base *preventative* treatment is unclear. However, one small US producer (100,000 pigs finished per year) has developed a protocol to prevent Swine Flu, based on analysis of previous data. They give a low cost water based treatment of aspirin and antibiotics if there are three clear days of water decline (that are not due to other causes). This has eliminated clinical incidence of swine flu in their herd (previously around 5 - 7 incidents a year) with a net value of $20,000 per year.

Water may be useful indicator of the success - or otherwise - of treatment (Figure 13). These data - covering 3 weeks - are from two groups of weaners dosed with E Coli and treated (Pen 1)   or not (Pen 2. Whilst both decline initially, treatment success - or otherwise - is self evident.

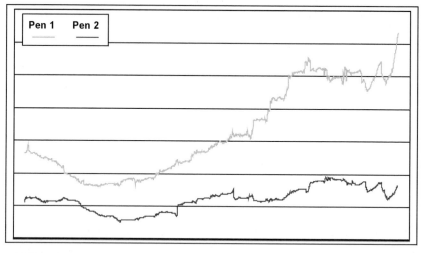

Figure 13. Water intake as an indicator of the success of treatment for E. coli infection (Pen 1) compared with untreated control (Pen 2)

Feed availability

Feed availability - or lack of it - is a significant factor in pig production. A rough estimate based on typical feed outages alone suggest that "feed outage" is a far greater cost to pig production than major diseases such as PMWS. However, since animals do not die, and it is assumed they "make up the difference", it is largely unregarded.

The causes are principally feed system issues as such - trip outs, bridging, etc. - and failing to order feed. The earlier example shown was due to forgetting to order it before a public holiday weekend. On that farm, it was part of a general pattern of poor availability and conversion rates were regularly 4 or even 5 on a batch to batch basis (compared to 3.1 for the producer in general.)

Water monitoring helps to distinguish between mere "interruptions" - temporary issues with the feed system that have no impact on actual feed intake - and actual feed loss.

In Figure 14, temporary feed interruptions (as shown by the lower trace of feed system operation) are relatively commonplace. The water trace makes it rather more obvious when they actually run out of feed.

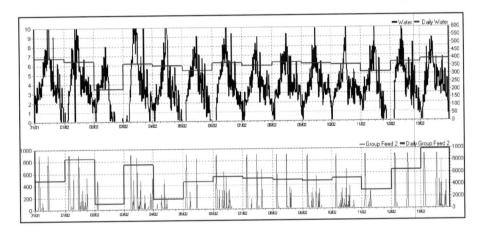

Figure 14. Effect of feed limitation on water intake.

However, feed may be "relatively unavailable". That is, it may be harder to get at. In the example (Figure 14), water intake in a pig finishing building (which is taken to be closely related to feed intake) is expressed in terms of "Min-Max Ratio (MMR)". That is, the lowest water intake recorded in any 15 minute period as a percentage of the highest in any 15 minute period, on a daily basis, for a batch of grow-finish pigs. This is, in a sense, an extreme simplification of a complex waveform. Since total daily volumes increase with time, minimum and maximum are expressed as a percentage of total daily volume.

MMR is typically a very low value - there is some point in the day when intake is zero. In the following case, the minimum and maximum daily lines are surprisingly close together. Minimum intake is as much as 1/3rd of maximum. Over time, this ratio falls. At the end of the chart MMR falls to zero.

The probable cause in this case is the type, style and number of feeders - which are a common type of wet/dry feeder. Younger pigs took longer to eat - and this is probably far worse with wet/dry feeders. The result is that they must eat around the clock to get their fill. This may well imply a reduction in feed intake as such - and loss of growth potential. Over time, they get faster, so they can - to a greater extent - fulfil their desires to eat during the day. However, it is only at the end of the batch - when some pigs are removed (there is a sudden fall in intake) that the restriction disappears altogether.

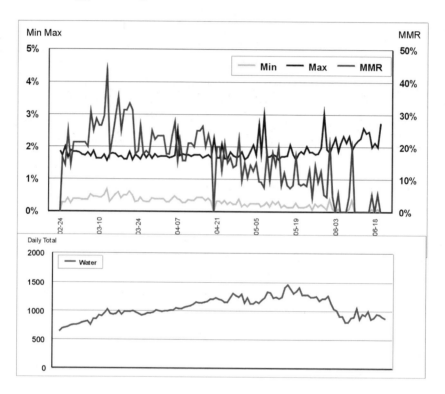

Figure 15. Ratio of minimum to maximum water intake (MMR)

Leakage

One drop a second is 6.3 tonnes of water a year. If that were feed at £140 a tonne it might be of some small concern, but as it is only water, it may not seem to matter that much. However multiply that by the number of drinkers on a typical livestock farm - and bear in mind that it is not just a drop a second and then consider that farm staff have no particular plumbing training, nor any way to readily detect leaks, and the scale of the problem is apparent. Incoming water is cheap but slurry is expensive - typically around £1 to £1.50 a tonne. Wet litter causes big problems.

As well as a problem in production itself, it is a real headache in water monitoring as it is a signal of unknown magnitude imposed up on the data (Figure 16). It presents itself in a number of ways.

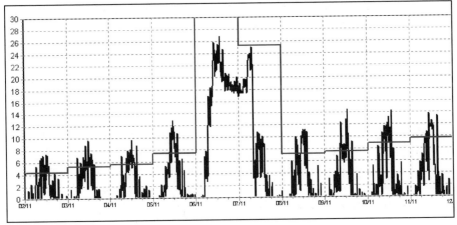

Figure 16. Changes in water intake attributable to a leak (6/11 to 8/11).

This is by far the easiest to recognise – a dramatic change from the normal pattern, and an exceptional daily value. This was relatively quickly detected by the operator, but for all that resulted in almost 2 tonnes of extra slurry. The obvious exceptional nature of the problem makes it relatively easy to filter out.

However, the following data - which are all too common - makes it far more difficulty to distinguish the noise from the data. The giveaway is the lack of a "zero point" in consumption where there is leakage (Figure 17).

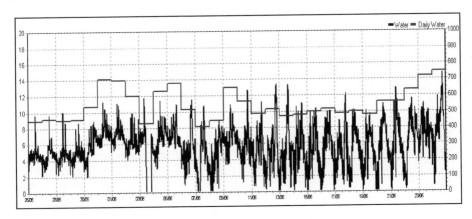

Figure 17. Patterns of water intake that may indicate leak(s)

A less obvious form of leakage is presented in Figure 18.The problem here is a faulty header tank ball valve. It does not shut off properly - dribbling at a rate too low to register on the meter. This over fills the tank, and the first drinking is of the over fill. For young animals, this may be the entire consumption. "Proper" flow is not registered until pigs are older.

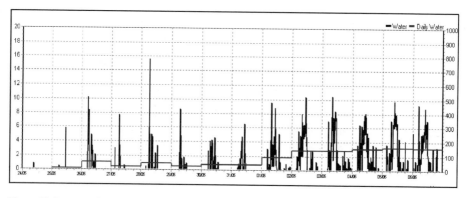

Figure 18. Patterns of water intake that may indicate leak(s) or another problem

For reference, the standard specification for a header tank float valve is 200,000 operations. In a home or office, that is probably quite adequate for a long term life. In a livestock building, with 8,760 hours in a year, and operating many times an hour, the design life may be exceeded within a year or less.

Uses of water intake data

- detecting acute issues such as water and feed system failures
- detecting maintenance issues such as leaking drinkers
- monitoring growth and batch to batch comparison
- detecting illness
- assessing performance and suitability of feed and water delivery systems
- impact of housing including lighting
- monitoring labour

At its simplest, measuring water is a way of checking that things are working and that the feed system and water supply are operating. By far the easiest way to do that, incidentally, is to just "look at the pictures". Humans have a highly developed sense of pattern recognition - even in fuzzy data. Simply seeing it "looks like yesterday" is a useful technique, even if there is no clear idea what it should be in an absolute sense.

In "normal" growth, water intake simply goes up a little each day as the animals grow, because water is related to feed intake – that is almost all that regular producers need to know. Exactly how much it should go up each day is really down to nutritionists. Water intake does not go down, if things are going to plan. It may go down because of illness.

Feed and water systems - and limitations thereof - can readily have a negative impact on growth and feed conversion ratio, but this can easily be put down to feed itself. Similarly, lack of space and the impact of erratic lighting, ventilation,etc. can have similar effects. Abnormal intake pattern is one way of detecting such issues.

Farm staff probably have more impact on production than any other factor, although what they do is often hidden, and there may be no clear evidence of impact on the livestock. Water monitoring (along with other factors) can offer a great deal of insight. For example, going into a building usually causes a rise in water consumption.

Closing remarks

Water is crucial to livestock production, but has been relatively little studied - in pigs at least, and only to a limited extent in other species.

Some poultry producers record daily water use as a matter of routine - although it is not clear how much use is made of the information. Few, if any, pig producers record water use. Although this could be because it genuinely does not matter to livestock - and that this fact was clearly established may years ago - a more likely explanation is that no one has really noticed, and water is too cheap to be bothered too much about.

However, it may be concluded that water monitoring not only offers a great deal of insight into what is going on, but is cheap, non-invasive, and very easy to achieve - even if the information it offers is not as "simple" as some might like it to be.

The current chapter has only provided some basic guidance on some the issues, but it is to be hoped that it will stimulate the desire for both more research, and greater uptake in livestock production as a matter of routine.

15

NUTRITIONAL APPROACHES TO REDUCING THE ENVIRONMENTAL IMPACT OF OUTDOOR PIGS

S A EDWARDS
Newcastle University, School of Agriculture, Food and Rural Development Agriculture Building, Newcastle upon Tyne NE1 7RU

The challenges of outdoor pigs

The growth of outdoor pig production in the UK has been driven by a combination of economic, marketing and agronomic advantages. Outdoor pigs offer the producer a cost effective production system, with favourable consumer perception of animal welfare that has resulted in niche marketing opportunities (Edwards, 2005). They also offer the landowner a good "break crop" in an arable rotation, giving effective land clearance of volunteers and a significant manurial residue for the subsequent crop which allows savings in inorganic fertiliser (Thornton, 1988). This has resulted in an expansion of outdoor production systems for breeding sows in the UK, with approximately 0.14 of English herds and 0.27 of sows now in such systems (Sheppard, 2002). Outdoor systems are less common for weaned pigs (0.07 of herds and 0.13 of pigs) and finishing pigs (0.03 of herds and 0.013 of pigs), because of their greater difficulty of management and climatic effects on performance. The current chapter will therefore focus on the breeding sow herd, although most of the principles discussed are equally applicable to the growing pig.

Management of the environmental impact of outdoor pig systems poses challenges under conditions of year-round land occupation and high nutrient deposition. Based on a simple calculation of nitrogen (N) in feed inputs and weaners produced, Worthington and Danks (1992) estimated the nitrogen residue from an outdoor pig breeding herd to be 541 kg N/ha/year, of which 419 kg was available for leaching after allowance for gaseous losses. Looking more specifically at nutrient deposition rates on paddocks within the pig area under current management practices, even higher values can be calculated (Table 1). Whilst such calculations are simplistic, and details will vary significantly between units depending on stocking rate, feed formulation and performance level, they indicate the magnitude of risk.

Table 1. Calculated nutrient excretion from outdoor sows

	Gestation paddocks	Lactation paddocks	
Stocking density (sows/ha)	27	19	Abbot *et al.* (1994)
Feed intake per pig (kg/day)	3.2	6.5	
N content of feed (g/kg)	20	28	130 g CP/kg gestation diet 175g CP/kg lactation diet
N excreted in faeces (g/pig/day)	11.5	32.8	Coefficient of total tract apparent digestibility of N = 0.82
N excreted in urine (g/pig/day)	36.5	74.2	16g N retained in gestation 80g N retained in lactation
Total N deposition (kg/ha/year)	473	593	Gestation paddocks occupied 365 days Lactation paddocks occupied 292 days
P content of feed (g/kg)	7	7	
P excreted in faeces (g/pig/day)	14.6	29.6	Coefficient of P retention = 0.35
Total P deposition (kg/ha/year)	144	164	

The consequences of such high levels of deposition for soil nutrient content have been assessed in several studies. On a light loam soil in Scotland, paddocks with dry sows stocked at 18 sows/ha reached an autumn soil nitrate-N level of 170 kg/ha in the top 45 cm after 8 months of occupation. As autumn rainfall commenced, this level fell to 50 kg/ha as a result of substantial leaching and denitrification (Edwards and Watson, 1997). In a parallel study, paddocks stocked with lactating sows at 10 sows/ha reached a soil nitrate-N level of 100 kg/ha in the top 45 cm after 7 months of occupation, and then fell to 40 kg/ha by the late autumn. The values for dry sow paddocks are in line with those from a study in Southern England, which indicated an autumn soil mineral N level of 200-300 kg/ha in the top 90 cm (130-270 in the top 60 cm) after 1 and 2 years of pig occupation at stocking rates ranging from 12-25 sows/ha (Williams, Chambers, Hartley, Ellis and Guise, 2000). A subsequent detailed Danish study on lactation paddocks stocked at 32 sows/ha for a 6 month period showed inorganic N levels of 34 mg/kg in the top 20 cm of soil, and of 17 mg/kg in the 20-40 cm layer. These levels were reduced by more than 80% by the following spring, as a result of leaching and emission losses equivalent to 150 kg/ha (Eriksen and Kristensen, 2000). More detailed studies of the fate of deposited

N indicated a leaching loss of 126-276 kg N/ha over a 2 year period as a result of 6 months of sow occupation (Eriksen, 2001). Denitrification losses averaged 0.5 kg N/ha/day during the pig occupation period, falling to 0.1 kg/ha/day by the following spring (Petersen, Kristensen and Eriksen, 2001), and totaled 69 kg N/ha/annum or 0.11 of net N input. In the same study, measured ammonia volatilisation ranged between 0.1 and 2.1 kg N/ha/day and in total accounted for 4.8 kg N/sow/annum (Sommer, Sogaard, Moller, and Morsing, 2001).

Whilst nitrogen has received the greatest attention, further environmental risk is posed by other excreted nutrients, in particular phosphorus which has the potential to cause eutrophication of watercourses. A Scottish study reported that 15 months of occupation by dry sows at typical stocking densities resulted in saturation of the soil profile with respect to P in some areas of the field, which represented a significant environmental risk (Watson, Atkins, Bento, Edwards and Edwards, 2003). In Danish studies, levels of extractable P in lactation paddocks stocked at 32 sows/ha for a 6 month were increased by 12% (Eriksen and Kristensen, 2000).

The fate of excreted nutrients within the environment depends on their chemical form, the soil type, climate and paddock management system. Because the free-draining soils best suited to pig production are also those giving greatest risk of nutrient leaching to groundwater, plant capture and utilisation of these deposited nutrients is highly desirable. However, the nature of rotation management and land rental arrangements often results in pigs moving onto autumn stubbles, where vegetation cover has little opportunity to establish. A survey of practice in 2001 indicated that the majority of sows were not managed on grass (Table 2). In an unreplicated study of 3 management systems (Williams *et al.*, 2000), nitrate leaching in the first winter varied from 28 mg/l in the worst system (25 dry sows/ha, no grass cover) to 8 mg/l in the best system (12 sows/ha on established grass). By the second winter however, when grass cover had been destroyed in all systems, N leaching had increased to similar levels of 111 and 105 mg/l respectively. Ammonia volatilisation measurements failed to distinguish between systems, with an average loss of ~11 g/sow/day.

Table 2. Rotation practice of outdoor pig herds (Newcastle University survey, 2001)

	Gestation paddocks	*Lactation paddocks*
Proportion of herds moving pigs onto:		
Established grass sward	0.30	0.34
Undersown cereal stubble	0.15	0.17
Cereal stubble	0.53	0.46

Meeting the challenges

There is no single, or simple, solution to preventing environmental impact of outdoor pigs. Producers must therefore combine nutritional, management and agronomic approaches to target key risk factors. Strategies include increasing efficiency of feed utilisation, by better matching of diets to nutrient requirements and reduction in feed wastage, and reducing environmental losses from excreta, by dietary modifications designed to reduce nutrient mobility and increased vegetation capture of nutrients.

REDUCING LEVELS OF EXCRETED NUTRIENTS

The simplest approach to reducing environmental impact is to match dietary inputs more closely to animal requirements, and hence reduce excess nutrients excreted onto land. Historically, diet formulation for outdoor pigs has focused more on simplicity of management and physical quality of feed than on minimising nutrient excretion, and these objectives may sometimes be in conflict. The principles of reducing dietary nutrient excess are common to both indoor and outdoor systems, and have been extensively studied in the indoor context (Lenis and Jongbloed, 1999; Aarnink and Verstegen, 2007). Significant reductions in excreted nutrients can be made by raw material selection for higher digestibility, optimisation of amino acid balance toward "ideal protein", and use of enzymes such as phytase to increase nutrient availability. The environmental benefits of such diet modifications in an outdoor pig system were illustrated in the study of Edwards, Jamieson, Riddoch and Watson (1998). Applying these principles to sow gestation diets, the level of crude protein was reduced from 156 to 119 g/kg, and that of phosphorus from 7.6 to 4.6 g/kg, whilst still meeting animal requirements for ileal digestible ideal protein and digestible phosphorus. Monitoring of soil nutrient content over a 17 month period showed significant reductions in both inorganic and soluble organic N, and in resin extractable P (Watson *et al.*, 2000).

The levels of digestible lysine adequate to meet the requirements of gestating and lactating sows under experimental conditions have been determined as 3.8-5.0 g/day at the beginning of pregnancy, 13.2-13.8 g/day at the end of pregnancy and 38-47g/day during lactation, for gilts and older sows respectively (Everts, 1994). However, much higher levels than this are generally provided in current outdoor practice. Limitations to the extent of reduction in dietary inputs are imposed by raw material costs, lack of a wider range of commercially available synthetic amino acids to permit further idealisation of dietary protein, and uncertainties about the safety margins needed to avoid detrimental effects on performance. These safety margins arise from a necessary allowance for inherent raw material variability, and uncertainties about required levels of the less commonly limiting amino acids as dietary crude protein is reduced. The suggested ideal protein composition for pregnant and lactating sows shows significant differences between British (Whittemore, Hazzledine and Close, 2003), American (NRC, 1998) and Danish (Danske Slagterier, 2002) recommendations. Some of these differences arise from assumptions about the level of production, the extent of body tissue mobilisation or accretion at different stages of the reproductive cycle, and therefore the balance between maintenance and production requirements. For example, theoretical modelling of specific production scenarios indicates that the limiting order of essential amino acids (lysine, valine and threonine) in a maize-soya diet changes depending on feed intake and tissue mobilisation in the lactating sow (Kim, Baker and Easter, 2001). Since the climatic influences on outdoor sows show large seasonal differences, often resulting in reduced lactation feed intake and greater body tissue mobilisation in summer, this might suggest a need for different seasonal amino acid composition if low protein diets are adopted. Uncertainties about raw material variability may be increased if greater reliance is placed on enzyme technology to increase digestibility. For example, different studies measuring digestible phosphorus contents in sow diets from phytase enzyme addition have shown not only markedly different levels of response between experiments, but also consistent differences in efficacy of the same enzyme at different stages of the reproductive cycle (Kemme, Radcliffe, Jongbloed, and Mroz, 1997; Kemme, Jongbloed, Mroz and Benyon, 1997; Jongbloed, van Diepen, Kemme and Broz, 2004).

Once these initial formulation strategies have been adopted, further reductions in dietary excess are only possible if a more detailed "precision feeding" approach is utilised. This involves the use of a greater number of diets, geared specifically to the changing requirements of parity, reproductive stage and season. Such a detailed strategy is often limited by the practicalities of handling many different diets in a situation where infrastructure for feed storage and distribution is limited. However, this approach is particularly worthy of consideration under outdoor conditions, where seasonal effects are more extreme and where many herds have adopted a policy of all-in-all-out batch stocking by site, giving single parity groups of animals at any particular point in time. By using pig models to estimate requirements over any specific period, diets can be more precisely formulated and efficiency increased. The extent of possible nutrient savings offered by these approaches can be indicated by simple calculations. When considering parity-specific diets, it is well known that the lysine: energy requirement reduces as the sow ages because of the greater body size, maintenance requirement and milk yield of the older sow, in contrast with the greater requirement for maternal tissue growth of the young animal (Table 3).

Table 3. The changing nutrient requirements with parity (after Whittemore *et al.*, 1993).

	Net energy (MJ/day)	Digestible lysine (g/day)	Dig lysine: NE ratio
Gestation:			
Gilt	20.9	11.7	0.56
Young sow	25.0	9.6	0.38
Old sow	26.0	8.9	0.34
Lactation:			
Gilt	51.5	43.2	0.84
Young sow	72.3	59.4	0.82
Old sow	81.7	64.4	0.78

Feeding a diet with the optimal lysine: energy balance for a gilt, at a level necessary to supply the daily energy needs of an old sow, results in oversupply of N by approximately 18g/day in gestation and 13g/day in lactation, equivalent on a whole herd basis to deposition on land of an extra 174 and 74 kg N/ha/year respectively at current stocking rates. In herds with a continuous replacement policy, such savings would apply only to a proportion of the animals present at any given time, and the logistics of managing single parity groups are complex.

Similarly, when looking at the seasonal requirements, the required lysine: energy ratio for the gestating sow is lower in winter because additional energy is required for thermoregulation below the lower critical temperature of 13-15 °C (Close and Cole, 2000; Table 4). Feeding a diet with the optimal lysine: energy ratio for thermoneutral conditions at the level necessary to supply the daily energy needs during colder winter weather results in an oversupply of N by approximately 18-19 g/day for half the year, equivalent to deposition on land of an extra 89 kg N/ha/year at current stocking rates.

Table 4. The changing gestation nutrient requirements with season (after Whittemore *et al.*, 1993; Close and Cole, 2000)

	Gilt (150 kg)		Old sow (300 kg)	
	Summer	Winter	Summer	Winter
Requirement for:				
Energy (MJ NE/day)	21.5	27.4	26.8	34.9
Digestible lysine (g/day)	11.7	11.7	8.9	8.9
Dig lysine: NE ration	0.54	0.32	0.43	0.26

Whilst it is now common practice to feed different diets in gestation and lactation, the further refinement of feeding for stage of gestation has received less attention. It is well known that the requirements for growth of foetal and reproductive tissues increase exponentially at the end of gestation, with N accretion in the conceptus increasing from 2g/day in the first trimester to 14 g/day in the final trimester (Noblet, Close, Heavens and Brown, 1985). Comparison of a phased three-diet gestation regime in comparison with a single gestation diet indicated a 7% reduction in N excretion, with no adverse effects on performance over three parities (Clowes, Kirkwood, Cegielski and Aherne, 2003). However, caution must still be exercised in the use of very low protein diets in early pregnancy, since a subsequent experiment examining use of a comparable low protein diet (3.4 g digestible lysine/kg) in early pregnancy reported a substantial reduction in conception rate in parity one and two sows (van der Peet-Schwering and Smolders, 2004). A similar detrimental effect of a low protein gestation diet on gilt litter size was also found in a large UK study (Edge, Edwards, Taylor and Gill, 2003), and the precise amino acid requirements for optimal early embryo establishment require further investigation in different genotypes. These uncertainties, together with the practical difficulties of handling a number of different gestation diets concurrently, make phase feeding in gestation currently unattractive.

In the recent UK "Ecopig" project (data not yet published), commercial application of the diet modification and precision feeding approaches showed that it was possible to maintain satisfactory performance whilst reducing N input by 10% and P input by 20% on a whole herd basis. This was against a background where the current conventional best cost diets already contained relatively low crude protein content.

MODIFYING THE FORM OF EXCRETED NUTRIENTS

An alternative nutritional approach to reducing environmental impact of pig production is to manipulate the diet to give alterations in the composition of excreta that reduce subsequent environmental losses. One method of achieving this is to shift nitrogen excretion from urea in urine, which can be rapidly broken down to release ammonia-N, to protein in faeces where it is incorporated in more stable chemical compounds. Bacterial fermentation in the colon incorporates nitrogen in digesta into bacterial protein. It has further been shown that urea excreted from the blood into the colon can similarly be incorporated, thus reducing nitrogen excretion in urine (Bakker, Bakker, Dekker, Jongbloed, Everts, van der Meulen, Ying, and Lenis, 1996). Jongbloed (2001) analysed data from a number of studies to show a significant relationship between increasing NSP content of the diet and a reduction in urinary: faecal N ratio. However, since raw materials high in

NSP frequently have lower protein digestibility, total dietary N excretion may be increased by this strategy.

A further way to reduce loses from excreta as a result of ammonia volatilisation is to acidify the excreta. The pH of faeces is reduced by inclusion of higher levels of NSP in the diet, as a result of volatile fatty acid production during hind gut fermentation (Canh, Sutton, Aarnink, Verstegen, Schrama and Bakker, 1998). The pH of urine can be reduced by changing the dietary electrolyte balance, for example by replacing calcium carbonate by calcium sulphate or calcium benzoate (Canh, Aarnink, Mroz, Jongbloed, Schrama and Verstegen, 1998). This approach has been studied in the context of reducing ammonia emissions from slurry in housed pigs and shown to offer significant benefit. However, its applicability to outdoor production, where faeces and urine are deposited separately directly onto soil, rather than mixed for a period of storage, is uncertain. Velthof, Nelemans, Oenema and Kuikman (2005) carried out laboratory studies to investigate the gaseous nitrogen and carbon losses from slurry of different compositions, generated by dietary manipulations including reduced protein, increased NSP and addition of acidifying calcium sulphate. It was shown that the consequences for emission of nitrous oxide after soil application depended on soil type, indicating interactions with soil properties such as the organic matter content. Larger scale studies of efficacy of approaches involving modification of excreta composition under outdoor conditions are therefore required.

REDUCING NUTRIENT LOSS FROM FEED WASTAGE

It is not only the efficiency of nutrient utilisation by the animal which will determine the level of nutrient loss to the environment, but also the extent of feed wastage which necessitates higher total nutrient inputs to the system. Outdoor systems require significantly higher feed inputs than indoor systems (typically by 10-15%; MLC, 1990-2007), arising from climatic penalties and wastage through ground feeding losses and wildlife scavenging. The relative contribution of these sources of poorer feed utilisation is still uncertain. In order to target nutrient inputs more accurately, it is important to know and maximise actual intake, and minimise wastage of feed provided. Evidence from the spatial distribution of soil nutrients in paddocks after pig occupation suggests significant wastage might be occurring around feeding areas (Eriksen and Kristensen, 2000; Eriksen, 2001). In indoor sows, it has been suggested that floor feeding in yards, compared to trough feeding, requires 5-10% more food as a result of wastage and the need to feed higher average levels to safeguard low ranking sows in mixed-size groups competing for the daily ration (Edwards, 2000). Given these considerations, it is possible that improved efficiency of feed use, and hence reduction in pollution, could be achieved under outdoor conditions by trough feeding rather then the current commercial practice of scattering feed on the ground. Unpublished results from the "Ecopig" study have shown that liveweight loss during lactation was significantly reduced (by 27%) in trough-fed compared to ground-fed sows. In gestation paddocks, trough feeding significantly improved liveweight gain (by 13%) and efficiency of feed use (by 17%), but also increased within group variation in gain, indicating that the restricted feeding area penalized lower ranking sows in the group. This highlights the need for great care in implementation of such a strategy. A further finding from the study was a significant reduction in bird numbers on trough-fed paddocks, offering potential benefits for feed loss and biosecurity.

MANAGING PIG EXCRETORY BEHAVIOUR

Even when nutrient excretion is minimised by good diet formulation, the excretory behaviour of pigs can still result in localised areas of high soil nutrient loading and hence pollution risk. Nutrient budgeting models generally assume even uptake or deposition within each individual cropping area. However, this is not the case with outdoor pigs, and a particular pollution risk and problem for nutrient utilisation by the following crop is posed by the spatial heterogeneity of soil nutrients seen in pig paddocks. A detailed study in Denmark on spatial distribution of excreted nutrients in lactation paddocks showed that this accounted for 0.17 of the spatial variation in dry matter yield of the subsequent potato crop (Eriksen and Kristensen, 2000). More detailed studies of the fate of deposited N demonstrated a higher level of leaching, denitrification and ammonia volatilisation from 'hotspots' with high soil N where sows tended to urinate (Eriksen, 2001, Petersen *et al.*, 2001; Sommer *et al.*, 2001).

A series of behavioural studies have shown that both pregnant and lactating sows have clearly preferred excretory areas within the paddock (Watson, Anssems, Kuhne, Scholzel and Edwards, 1998; Marcellis, Kelly, Browning, Day and Edwards, 2002). These observations, supported by subsequent commercial scale studies in the "Ecopig" project, showed that the incidence of both urination and defaecation was lower than expected in the feeding area and in the region immediately adjacent to the hut, with excretion being highly focussed at the paddock fencelines lateral to the hut in small paddocks. This behaviour is consistent with the recorded excretory patterns of sows under semi-natural conditions, which defaecate in a region 5-15 m from the nest site. The preference for the fenceline areas appears to result from both their position relative to the hut, and to a territorial motivation. These observed behaviour patterns gave rise to substantial differences in soil chemistry, with soil inorganic N levels being 4-fold higher at these preferred excretory sites. By changing the location of the feeding site across time, as well as the location of huts and fencelines, more even distribution of excreta can be encouraged and nutrient losses reduced.

PROMOTING AND UTILISING VEGETATION COVER

A number of studies highlight the importance of vegetation cover in pig paddocks for reducing N losses by uptake and immobilisation of inorganic N, an important mechanism for reducing leaching and gaseous emissions (Williams *et al.*, 2000; Jarvis, 1997). Capture of excreted inorganic nutrients by vegetation and their fixation in slow release organic forms therefore offers the greatest potential for minimising short term nutrient losses and maximising long term nutrient utilisation in rotations incorporating pigs. However, the maintenance of vegetation cover poses a major challenge in outdoor pig systems because of the rapid destruction of vegetation through foraging and rooting activities of the sows. Studies have shown that, at typical commercial stocking rates, a well-established full grass cover can be reduced to less than 0.10 cover within 4 weeks by dry sows (Edwards *et al.*, 1998), although cover of >0.50 can persist in lactating sow paddocks with lower stocking densities and higher feed inputs (Edwards and Watson, 1997). Nose-ringing of sows is a very effective way to maintain vegetation cover and hence reduce pollution risk. In a replicated experiment on dry sow paddocks, autumn soil inorganic N levels in the top 45cm were reduced by more than 50% in paddocks with rung compared to unrung sows, thus reducing winter leaching risk (Edwards *et al.*, 1998). However, nose-ringing of sows to protect pasture raises concerns about animal welfare (Horrell, A'Ness, Edwards and Eddison, 2001), and a UK survey carried out by Newcastle University in 2001 indicated that 0.62 of outdoor herds did not ring sows. Attempts to maintain acceptable vegetation cover by dietary modification in the absence of nose-ringing have met with limited success. It has been demonstrated that foraging and rooting activity is motivated by hunger, resulting from the low level of concentrate diet provided as adequate to meet requirements for health and production. Increasing the level of feed, or the bulk of the diet, can reduce rooting activity (Braund, Edwards, Riddoch and Buckner, 1998), as can providing supplementary roughage in the form of silage or root crops (Edge, Bornett, Newton and Edwards, 2004; Edge, Bulman and Edwards, 2005). However, rooting is not completely abolished by these strategies, and vegetation destruction may be slowed but not prevented. An alternative strategy of seeking to establish a favored "sacrifice" rooting area has met with some success in small-scale experiments, where sows have been encouraged to forage in this area by the presence of a root crop (Swedes: Edge *et al.*, 2005; sugar beet: "Ecopig" project), providing both occupation and dietary bulk. However, this approach still requires commercial scale evaluation.

If vegetation cover is maintained, or additional bulky feeds are provided as a strategy to reduce pasture damage, predicting and adjusting for nutrient intake from pasture and forages will then become important in refining dietary inputs. Data on this subject are currently limited, but indicate that significant contributions to overall nutrition could be achieved. The intake of grazed ryegrass by pregnant sows showed seasonal variation, with increasing intake compensating for reduced nutrient quality as summer progressed (Rivera Ferre, Edwards, Mayes, Riddoch and Hovell, 2001). Based on the data obtained in this study, it was estimated that grazing can contribute approximately 0.50 of daily maintenance requirements for energy and ideal protein over the spring and summer periods (Edwards, 2003). Reports on intake of foraged root crops are scarce, but fresh weight intakes of 30 kg/day for strip-grazed fodder beet (Chambers, Hardy and Pugh, 1986) and 2 kg/ day for sugar beet ("Ecopig" project) have been estimated. Such large differences may relate to the nature of the crop, the length of experience of the sows involved or other nutritional and environmental factors, and require further investigation.

A major challenge in integrating pigs within rotations is synchronising nutrient supply with crop demand. An important factor in crop choice will be the timing of placement and removal of pigs from the land. High nutrient-demanding crops such as winter cereals are obvious candidates to follow summer pig production. It may also be economic to sow good N scavenging cover crops like mustard prior to summer cash crops such as potatoes. Where pigs are removed in spring, following potatoes would be expected to yield well. Due to the long-term nature of rotations, there are few data available on the impact of outdoor pig production on subsequent crops and the consequences for environmental impact. Calculated nutrient budgets for two organic rotations with pigs found that stocking rate had a major influence on rotational nutrient budget (Berry, Stockdale, Sylvester-Bradley, Phillips, Smith, Lord, Watson and Fortune, 2003). The balance between subsequent utilisation and losses of nutrients for different rotation scenarios can be estimated using nutrient budgeting models. These highlight the importance of whole rotation assessments, since short term effects brought about by changes in the pig phase of the rotation may also have converse longer term effects through modifications of subsequent cropping (Topp and Watson, 2007).

Conclusions

Managing the nutrition of outdoor pigs for reduced environmental impact, in addition to maximal reproductive performance, requires more closely targeted nutrient inputs than in the past, in combination with skilled system management and careful rotation planning. By achieving this, outdoor pigs can continue to be regarded as a valuable rotation option rather than an environmental hazard.

Acknowledgements

Work described in this paper has been funded by SEERAD and by the Defra "Ecopig" project (IS0215). I gratefully acknowledge the input of many collaborators and students at Newcastle University, SAC, CEH and BQP, and the co-operation of commercial producers in carrying out trial work.

References

Aarnink, A.J.A. and Verstegen, M.W.A. (2007) Nutrition, key factor to reduce environmental load from pig production. *Livestock Science*, **109**, 194-203.

Abbott, T.A., Hunter, E.J., Guise, H.J., Penny, R.H.C. (1994) Outdoor breeding herds: preliminary results of a survey. *Pig Veterinary Journal*, **33,** 79-83.

Bakker, C.G.M., Bakker, J.G.M., Dekker, R.A., Jongbloed, R., Everts H., van der Meulen, J., Ying, S.C. and Lenis, N.P. (1996) The quantitative relationship between absorption of nitrogen and starch from the hindgut of pigs. *Journal of Animal Science*, **74**, 188.

Berry, P.M., Stockdale, E.A., Sylvester-Bradley, R., Phillips, L., Smith, K.A., Lord, E.I., Watson, C.A. and Fortune, S. (2003) N, P and K budgets for crop rotations on nine organic farms in the UK. *Soil Use & Management*, **19**, 112-118.

Braund, J.P., Edwards, S.A., Riddoch, I. and Buckner, L.J. (1998) Modification of foraging behaviour and pasture damage by dietary manipulation in outdoor sows. *Applied Animal Behaviour Science*, **56**, 173-186.

Canh, T.T., Aarnink, A.J.A., Mroz, Z., Jongbloed, A.W., Schrama, J.W. and Verstegen, M.W.A. (1998) Influence of electrolyte balance and acidifying calcium salts in the diet of growing finishing pigs on urinary pH, slurry pH and ammonia volatilization from slurry. *Livestock Production Science*, **56**, 1-13.

Canh, T.T., Sutton, A.L., Aarnink, A.J.A., Verstegen, M.W.A., Schrama, J.W. and Bakker, G.C.M. (1998) Dietary carbohydrates alter the faecal composition and pH and ammonia emission from slurry of growing pigs. *Journal of Animal Science*, **76**, 1887-1895.

Chambers, J., Hardy, B. and Pugh, O. (1986) The use of an electronically controlled sow feeder to supply a compound feed as a balancer to sows grazing fodder beet. *Proceedings of the British Society of Animal Science*, p121.

Close, W.H. and Cole, D.J.A. (2000) *Nutrition of sows and boars*. Nottingham University Press, Nottingham.

Clowes, E.J., Kirkwood, R., Cegielski, A. and Aherne, F.X. (2003) Phase-feeding protein to gestating sows over three parities reduced nitrogen excretion without affecting sow performance. *Livestock Production Science*, **81**, 235-246.

Edge, H.L., Bornett, H.L.I., Newton, E. and Edwards, S.A. (2004). Alternatives to nose ringing in outdoor sows: 2. The provision of edible or inedible overground enrichment. *Animal Welfare*, **13**, 233-237.

Edge, H.L., Bulman, C.A. and Edwards, S.A. (2005) Alternatives to nose ringing in outdoor sows: 3. The provision of root crops. *Applied Animal Behaviour Science*, **92**, 15-26.

Edge, H., Edwards, S., Taylor, L. and Gill, B.P. (2003) Feeding for sow lifetime productivity. *Proceedings of the Society of Feed Technologists*, Coventry, 6 November 2003.

Edwards, S.A. (2000) Alternative housing for dry sows: system studies or component analysis? In *Improving health and welfare in animal production*, pp 99-107. Edited by H.J. Blokhuis, E.D. Ekkel and B. Wechsler. EAAP Publication 102. Wageningen Pers, Wageningen.

Edwards, S.A. (2003) Intake of nutrients from pasture by pigs. *Proceedings of the Nutrition Society*, **62**, 257-265.

Edwards, S.A. (2005) Product quality attributes associated with outdoor pig production. *Livestock Production Science*, **94**, 5-14.

Edwards, S.A., Jamieson, W., Riddoch, I. and Watson, C.A. (1998) Effect of nose ringing and dietary modification in outdoor pig production on temporal changes in soil nitrogen status. *Proceedings of the British Society of Animal Science*, p42.

Edwards, S. A. and Watson, C. (1997) An approach to investigating the environmental impact of an outdoor pig production system. In *Livestock Farming Systems - more than food production*, pp 335-340. Edited by J.T. Sorensen. EAAP Publication 89, Wageningen Pers, Wageningen.

Eriksen, J. (2001) Implications of grazing by sows for nitrate leaching from grassland and the succeeding crop. *Grass and Forage Science*, **56**, 317-322.

Eriksen, J. and Kristensen, K. (2000) Nutrient excretion by outdoor pigs: a case study of distribution, utilisation and potential for environmental impact. *Soil Use and Management*, **16**, 1-10.

Everts, H. (1994) *Nitrogen and energy metabolism of sows during several reproductive cycles in relation to nitrogen intake*. Doctoral thesis. Wageningen Agricultural University, Wageningen.

Horrell, R.I., A'Ness, P.J.A., Edwards, S.A. and Eddison, J. (2001). The use of nose rings in pigs: consequences for rooting, other functional activities and welfare. *Animal Welfare*, **10,** 3-22.

Jarvis, S.C. (1997) Emission processes and their interactions in grassland soils. In *Gaseous nitrogen emissions from grasslands*, pp 1-17. Edited by S.C. Jarvis and B.F. Pain. CAB International, Slough.

Jongbloed, A.W. (2001) Hebben voermaatregelen ter verlaging van de ammoniakemissie een negatief effect op de vertering en benutting van nutrienten? In *Veevoeding en Ammoniakemissie uit Varkensstallen,* pp 11-23. Editors A.W. Jongbloed and M.C.Blok. Samenvattingen van de themamiddag, volume 2174. Productschap Diervoeder, The Hague.

Jongbloed, A.W., van Diepen, J.Th.M., Kemme, P.A. and Broz, J. (2004) Efficacy of microbial phytase on mineral digestibility in diets for gestating and lactating sows. *Journal of Animal Science,* **91**, 143-155.

Kemme, P.A., Radcliffe, J.S., Jongbloed, A.W. and Mroz, Z. (1997) The effect of sow parity on digestibility of proximate components and minerals during lactation is influenced by diet and microbial phytase supplementation. *Journal of Animal Science,* **75**, 2147-2153.

Kemme, P.A., Jongbloed, A.W., Mroz, Z. and Benyon, A.C. (1997) The efficacy of *Aspergillus niger* phytase in rendering phytate phosphorus available for absorption in pigs is influenced by pig physiological status. *Journal of Animal Science,* **75**, 2129-2138.

Kim, S.W., Baker, D.H. and Easter, R.A. (2001). Dynamic ideal protein and limiting amino acids for lactating sows: the impact of amino acid mobilization. *Journal of Animal Science,* **79**, 2356-2366.

Lenis, N.P. and Jongbloed, A.W. (1999) New technologies in low pollution swine diets: diet manipulation and use of synthetic amino acids, phytase and phase feeding for reduction of nitrogen and phosphorus excretion and ammonia emission. – review. *Asian-Australasian Journal of Animal Science,* **12**, 305-327.

Marcellis, J., Kelly, H., Browning, H., Day, J. and Edwards S. (2002) Excretory behaviour of lactating sows in an outdoor organic production system. *Proceedings of the British Society of Animal Science,* p 225.

MLC (1990-2007) *Pig Yearbooks.* Meat and Livestock Commission, Milton Keynes.

Noblet, J., Close, W.H., Heavens, R.P. and Brown, D. (1985) Studies on the energy metabolism of the pregnant sow. 1. Uterus and mammary tissue development. *British Journal of Nutrition,* **53**, 251-265.

NRC (1998) *Nutrient requirements of swine. Tenth revised edition.* National Academy Press, Washington.

Petersen, S.O., Kristensen, K. and Eriksen, J. (2001) Denitrification losses from outdoor piglet production: spatial and temporal availability. *Journal of Environmental Quality,* **30**, 1051-1058.

Rivera Ferre, M.G., Edwards, S.A., Mayes. R.W., Riddoch. I. and Hovell, F de B. (2001) The effects of season and level of concentrate on the voluntary intake and digestibility of herbage by outdoor sows. *Animal Science,* **72**,

501-510.

Sheppard, A. (2002) *The structure of pig production in England.* Special Studies in Agricultural Economics No 55, University of Exeter, Exeter. 35pp.

Sommer, S.G., Sogaard, H.T., Moller, H.B. and Morsing, S. (2001). Ammonia volatilisation from sows on grassland. *Atmospheric Environment*, **35**, 2023-2032.

Thornton, K. (1988) *Outdoor pig production.* Farming Press, Ipswich.

Topp, C.F.E. and Watson, C.A. (2007) Outdoor pigs: their impact on the environment. In *Farming Systems Design "007*: an International Symposium in Methodologies for Integrated Analysis of Farming Systems. Field -farm scale design and improvement, p171-172. September 10-12, 2007, Catania, Italy.

Williams, J.R., Chambers, B.J., Hartley, A.R., Ellis, S. and Guise, H.J. (2000) Nitrogen losses from outdoor pig farming systems. *Soil Use and Management*, **16**, 237-243.

Van der Peet-Schwering, C. and Smolders, M. (2004) Phase feeding for sows. *Pig Progress*, **20** (8), 15.

Velthof, G.L., Nelemans, J.A., Oenema, O. and Kuikman, P.J. (2005) Gaseous nitrogen and carbon losses from pig manure derived from different diets. *Journal of Environmental Quality*, **34**, 698-706.

Watson, C.A., Anssems, E., Kuhne, B., Scholzel, Y. and Edwards S.A. (1998) Assessing the nitrogen pollution risk from outdoor pig systems. In *Diffuse Pollution and Agriculture II*, pp 230-235. Edited by A. Petchey, B. d'Arcy and A. Frost. SAC, Aberdeen.

Watson, C.A., Atkins, T., Bento, S., Edwards, A.C, and Edwards, S.A. (2003) Appropriateness of nutrient budgets for environmental risk assessment: a case study of outdoor pig production. *European Journal of Agronomy*, **20**, 117-126

Whittemore, C.T., Hazzledine, M.J. and Close, W.H. (2003) *Nutrient requirement standards for pigs.* British Society of Animal Science, Penicuik.

Worthington, T.R. and Danks, P.W. (1992) Nitrate leaching and intensive outdoor pig production. *Soil Use and Management*, **8**, 56-60.

16

SALMONELLA: A PIG PRODUCER'S PERSPECTIVE

MERYL WARD
Ermine Farms Ltd, Waddingham Grange, Waddingham, Gainsborough
Lincolnshire, DN21 4TB

Introduction

Ermine Farms operates in North Lincolnshire with three breeding units and several third party grow-out units, and has recently expanded into a farmshop with butchery and restaurant. A respectable start to the Zoonosis Action Plan (ZAP) scoring system in 2002 for all units deteriorated rapidly in 2005 with a misjudged change to feed specifications (Figure 1). The situation has proved difficult to reverse, but has given invaluable experience in the ZAP scheme and different aspects of salmonella control.

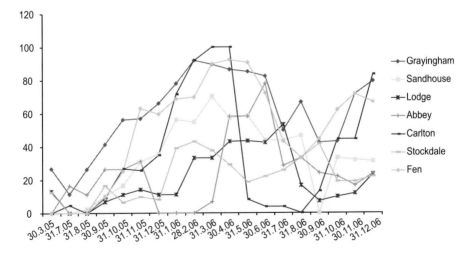

Figure 1. Deterioration in the Zoonosis Action Plan (ZAP) scoring system in seven pig units.

311

Previous experiences of salmonella-based food safety scares in the poultry sector has led to a greater understanding of the consequences of a similar problem hitting the pig industry. The industry knows that it needs a positive improvement in the national ZAP scores. All producers have a duty of care to supply safe food but, for a variety of reasons, the ZAP programme, measured against its original objectives, has failed to date. A recent attitude survey by the British Pig Executive (BPEX) reported that producers supported the principle of the programme but had many concerns over its effectiveness as a tool to support salmonella reduction, not least because of the several £millions spent since 2002 – including producer levy money – with no discernible outcome. This should be compared with the Danish scheme, that started in 1995, where the annual spend has been about £2.5 million **per year** and where, for herds producing over 200 pigs, 97% are virtually free of salmonella. The EC regulation requiring a National Control Plan and the industry's own desire to position its product at a premium are key drivers to motivate the industry to do better. Key elements of the scheme are Regulation (EC) No 1260/2003 which stipulates:

-       Survey of 600 meat samples (80% throughput covered)
-       EC to set target 11/2007
-       National Control Plan 04/2008

EU Hygiene legislation is a HACCP- based approach to safe food across all food business operators.

The objectives of ZAP were to monitor trends in levels of salmonella on individual units and achieve a 25% reduction in prevalence in the first 3 years of the programme. It should be no surprise that what in effect has been a simple 'monitoring tool' has not achieved solutions at an individual level to improve a complex and multifactorial problem, where different solutions are needed for different producers (Figure 2). A paradox within the current scheme is that it has given a statistically reliable level of information at a national level but a poor indication of performance at the individual unit level. From a producer point of view, it does not measure the level of actual salmonella at the critical control point of delivery to slaughter house, and is therefore also ineffective in providing an enforceable penalty scheme within the industry.

The objectives of the current chapter are to:

a)   Address some of the concerns of the ZAP programme and why it apparently has not motivated the industry to improve.
b)   Examine local experiences.
c)   Provide some practical suggestions for improvements to the current scheme.

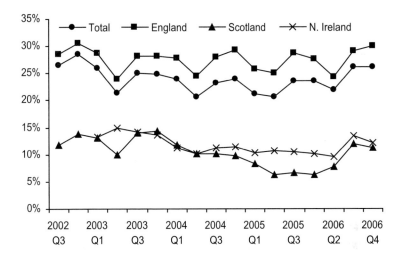

Figure 2. Trends in ZAP salmonella meat-juice sample positive percentage.

Recent revisions to the ZAP scheme

Over the last six months, the scheme has been substantially revised as follows:

1. Early problems in the scheme relating to sample errors and statistical accuracy of results have improved with recent updates to the database. There is improved information flow with test results available on-line within 2 weeks of the pigs being slaughtered.
2. More cost-effective targeted testing has been introduced with sites below 25% positives reduced to one sample per month until a positive is found. Other sites remain at 5 samples per month. A review of sampling frequency options informed these decisions.
3. The system of three levels has been retained with the level cut-off points reduced from 85% at Level 3 and 65% at level 2 reduced to 75% and 50%. The scheme is still under review to a potential two levels. The issue with three levels is that it gives the appearance that ZAP level 1 is acceptable. That is fatal to the scheme. If the national average is 23% and only producers over 50% are engaged, then any improvement is likely to be negated by changes in the levels of producers in ZAP level 1. Are producers who are being asked to sort the problems statistically any more of a risk (Research has shown that any producer who is over a 20% level is at risk of delivering active salmonella to the factory)?
4. On-farm salmonella investigations and microbiological testing is available to farms in level 2 and 3 but is not compulsory.

5.   A knowledge review of has been undertaken relating to the control of salmonella on-farm, that has been used to identify the main interventions suitable for on-farm use and to evaluate the feasibility of implementation as large scale field trials.

Local experiences

Our own experience has shown that, once established, it is difficult to reduce scores to acceptable levels. Salmonella is well adapted to living in the gut, survives well in the environment and has a wide host range.

One finishing herd that had a very high score and is a straw-based scrape-through system was completely depopulated and cleaned down in the summer of 2006 and the scores have already risen again to 65%. The breeding supply unit was tested and found to be negative pre the restocking but on a retest found to be positive. The aim must be to clean up the supply farms with restraints on breeding herd supply and a new focus on testing herd supplying weaners to level 2 and 3 farms. The Danish system requires all breeding herds to be blood sampled for antibodies. If the scores exceed a certain index level, pen faecal sampling is undertaken. When the index exceeds 15, a sales ban on breeding pigs is imposed until the index falls. Vaccination of breeding stock or weaners needs investigation but is currently not an option due to practical difficulties, but until control is achieved within breeding herds progress will be hampered.

Once established on farm, a heavy burden of salmonella is difficult to reduce. Any programme to reduce levels will fail without good basic management practices including good hygiene, rodent control, all-in all out systems, management of sick pigs and improvement of the overall health of the pig. Over-use of anti-microbials will destabilise the gut flora and leave a niche that may be filled by salmonella which readily develop antimicrobial resistance. Recent BPEX trial work highlighted the ineffectiveness of many disinfectants – none were effective against salmonella typhimurium in the presence of organic matter and only two were effective in its absence. On 80% of ZAP2 and 3 farms, salmonella was isolated from empty pens after cleansing and disinfection, demonstrating the difficulties of providing effective cleansing systems. We have found that old-fashioned lime-wash is more effective especially where floors are cracked and worn.

The main culprit for transmission of the problem remains the pig. Our problem started from changes to feed specifications and we have concentrated on feed changes to find solutions. Meal-feeding and wet-feeding are not options through our bin and feeding systems. Initial changes were made to the barley levels to around 400g/kg which had some effect. The difficulty is selecting the feed or water additives that provide the most cost-effective solution. An individual's best options depend on the farm's own feed and water equipment, health status of the herd and feed raw material costs. More information is required on the cost-effectiveness of different products in a UK situation.

In our situation, use of an acid product through the water to the weaned pig has proved cost-effective for us and aims to provide a clean pig at point of supply to the grow-outs. Salmonella inhabit mainly the end of the small intestine and the large intestine. However most acids are absorbed in the stomach and upper digestive tract and thus they are better as a barrier to re-infection used early in the pig's life rather than a treatment for existing salmonellosis. Protected acids (about 10 available) are effective in theory but data are limited – are they supplying enough acid to the hind gut to do the job? The net cost of acidification is often negligible through improvements in FCE and DLWG.

Probiotics work through competitive exclusion and some are also lactic acid-secreting so deliver acid to the hind gut. Some compounds show promise at a cost of around £3.50/t. Enzymes increase feed digestibility and therefore supply of nutrients to the hindgut. Generally their use leads to reduced coliforms in the hindgut but there are few specific data on salmonella. The cost is 60-150p/t feed and there are around 10 products available. Again, cost may be negated by improvements in FCE and DLWG.

General strategies are based on: shower when entering units, forget disinfectant dips, limewash wherever possible, concerted efforts on eliminating rodents, no hospital pens, check water quality and general unit tidiness and cleanliness.

Solutions at industry level

The revised ZAP scheme has the potential to make a difference by reducing ZAP levels to 2, with the cut-off point the national average. Implementation of breeding herd testing would be valuable. Co-ordination of independent British research into clear guide-lines with costings by using case-studies where appropriate and joint industry initiatives with comparisons with other countries is essential. It is important to create an HACCP based system of control to include identifying the problem farms at slaughter-house delivery and segregate. Better communication through the chain to develop cost-effective solutions that are whole chain is recommended. Finally it is important to motivate producers with cost benefits.

Conclusions

The conclusion is that there are solutions to reducing farm infection levels which can be guided and encouraged by the industry bodies. However, to be cost effective, the solution for the industry needs to be whole-chain. The Danes have found that their Salmonella programme made progress in reduding salmonella at farm level in the first five years of the programme but has made little progress since. It has become more cost-effective to take action post-farmgate e.g hot washes in the abattoir. Given the structure of the UK industry with 30% of herds outdoors and a significant proportion in straw based accommodation, the cost effectiveness of post-slaughter controls needs evaluating against the cost of farm measures.

17

SUPPLEMENTS TO FACILITATE PARTURITION AND REDUCE PERINATAL MORTALITY IN PIGS

THEO VAN KEMPEN

Provimi RIC, Brussels, Belgium, and North Carolina State University, Raleigh, NC, USA

Summary

Perinatal mortality, which includes stillbirths and neonatal mortality in the first days after parturition, is a serious challenge for the pig industry. It is common that 1 in 5 piglets do not survive this period. Approximately half of this loss is due to stillbirths and the other half due to neonatal mortality. Besides being a considerable economic loss, this also represents a serious welfare problem.

Perinatal mortality has been extensively studied, with environmental and metabolic challenges for the piglets as the major focus. The practical impact of these studies, however, has been rather limited. Perinatal mortality has not decreased proportionally in the last 50 years. Clearly, this is not an objective evaluation as litter size has increased significantly during this same period which complicates the management of perinatal mortality. Nevertheless, the fact remains that much can be gained from a better understanding and management of perinatal mortality.

Evaluation of the problem underlying perinatal mortality suggests that it is mainly driven by the dam, not by the piglets. Based on published literature and internal observations, a hypothesis has emerged that dystocia (abnormally long and difficult birth) is at the basis of a large proportion of perinatal mortality.

Sows in modern housing systems are not accustomed to strenuous exercise as they are typically in stalls with limited freedom to move. Parturition, or *labour*, however, is a serious physical challenge for the sow, both in intensity and duration. Typically parturition lasts 6 hours but in extreme cases it can last well over a day. The animals are not prepared for such an extended period of intensive labour and become exhausted. At the point of exhaustion, the sow will interrupt the process of labour, independent of where foetuses are in the birth process.

During the birth process, the frail umbilical cord has a high chance of being squeezed or, worse, ruptured. Either case leads to an interruption in blood flow to the foetus and the consequence is a lack of oxygen supply. and accumulation of CO_2 and lactic acid with a concomitant decrease in blood pH. Most piglets are born quick enough and this interruption in blood flow does not jeopardize health. However, if the birth process of a foetus has been initiated and the mother interrupts labour due to fatigue, the foetus may experience a prolonged period of respiratory failure. Interruptions of respiration of less than 2 minutes typically are well tolerated. Interruptions of more than 5 minutes result in stillbirths. Intermediate interruptions result in piglets that are born with metabolic damage (acidosis). These piglets will require additional time to recover from the birth process, making them very vulnerable to hypothermia and over-laying by the sow. These piglets will also have more difficulty finding the teats or competing at the udder. These piglets are thus much more likely to die during the first days after birth.

Periparturient fatigue is also common in humans. Dystocia during human labour is well recognized as a problem but is equally not treated in practice (although women are advised to exercise prior to parturition). Similarly, during intense exercise, athletes suffer from fatigue. To combat this problem, a large industry has developed that supplies 'sports drinks'. These products typically contain easily-digestible energy sources, minerals and vitamins, all critical during intense exercise. Scientific studies have shown that these supplements can delay the onset of fatigue and speed up the recovery from fatigue. To date, there has been no scientific evaluation of such supplements for helping mammals in labour.

The objective of the current programme was to develop a sports supplement specifically to help during the process of labour. For this purpose, the metabolic demands of labour were studied and a tailored energy, mineral, vitamin and antioxidant blend was developed named ParturAid®. For pigs, this blend is delivered to the animal rally.

Concept testing of this product showed that indeed as the birth process proceeded, more piglets were born with low blood pH, in line with our working hypothesis. Providing ParturAid to the sows at the start of parturition improved blood pH of the piglets at birth and reduced the time interval between the birth of piglets for those born towards the end of parturition. When tested in sows with minimum intervention, ParturAid prevented delays in labour and also numerically reduced both stillbirths and neonatal piglet mortality.

Subsequent field trials with over 800 sows across 8 locations showed that, on average, ParturAid reduced stillbirths by 0.44 pigs and neonatal mortality by 0.26 pigs per litter giving a total increase in litter size of 0.70 pigs. This effect was greater in farms with problems (>2 stillbirths and neonatal mortality combined) where ParturAid reduced this mortality by nearly 50%. Sows that received ParturAid also consumed more feed post-partum and farmers observed that piglets were more vital and that sows had less health complications. It is expected that these benefits of ParturAid will increase with time, as farmers will become better at predicting the onset of labour and thus able to better implement the product at the appropriate time.

In conclusion, fatigue during parturition is a major contributor to perinatal mortality. By providing sports supplements such as ParturAid to sows pre-partum, fatigue problems can be lessened. This results in speedier recovery and better feed intake post-partum and in up to 50% lower stillbirths and lower neonatal mortality.

Introduction

Perinatal mortality (stillbirths and neonatal mortality) is a serious problem for the pig industry. Estimates suggest that roughly 1 in 4 to 5 piglets do not survive this period (SIVA, 1999). The etiology underlying this has been described by several researchers (e.g., English and Morisson, 1984; Randall et al., 1971). It appears that sows tire easily causing them to interrupt the parturition process (*labour*). If the expulsion of a foetus was in progress at this time then this foetus may well suffer from a lack of blood exchange with the placenta because its umbilical cord may be pinched or ruptured or because the pig itself was pinched inside the birth canal reducing blood flow. These interruptions in blood flow impede or prevent the supply of oxygen and the removal of carbon dioxide, resulting in metabolic damage and a reduction in blood pH. Short periods of interruption lead to weak piglets that have an increased risk of crushing and failing to thrive. Long periods of interruption lead to stillbirths.

In sports and athletics, supplements like Gatorade® and Powerade® are common tools to fight fatigue. These supplements typically contain readily-available sources of energy, minerals that are critical during intense activity (for example magnesium), and vitamins (for example the B vitamins, C, and E) to support intense metabolism and prevent oxidative damage. Scientific studies have shown that such supplements indeed can extend the performance of athletes. The use of such supplements during parturition is not recognized as a means to reduce complications in mother, foetuses, and newborns. The objective of this research was to test a sport-type supplement specifically formulated for sows in labour for effects on sow health, stillbirths, and neonatal survival.

Materials and methods

PARTURAID

The sport supplement for parturient mammals (ParturAid) was formulated based on a literature review of metabolic needs during parturition and a study on the utilization of key nutrients during parturition. One complicating factor was the mode of administration. Many pig production facilities do not allow for the delivery of liquids other than water to the sow in the farrowing crates. Instead, administration as an oral paste was chosen as the preferred route as this was deemed as much more practical.

The test product was a paste that was administered orally immediately preceding parturition (up to 8 hours before the birth of the first piglet). The paste contains glycerine, dicalcium phosphate, invert sugar syrup, sorbitol, taurine, magnesium sulphate, natural antioxidants, zinc sulphate, flavour, sodium chloride, potassium chloride, citric acid, silicon dioxide, potassium sorbate, alpha tocopherol acetate, ascorbic acid, menadione sodium bisulphite, and sodium selenite. The final dose volume per sow was 30 ml (based on 140g moisture, 5g sodium, 7g potassium, 35g calcium, 35g phosphorus, 7g fiber, 250g ash, 2g oil, 6 mg tocopherol acetate, and 0.11 mg selenium).

ANIMAL TESTS

All animal protocols were in compliance with local ethical regulations.

Experiment 1. The objective of the experiment was to determine if respiratory problems occurred in piglets during the birth process, and if treatment reduced the incidence of this problem.

Sows (Dutch Landrace x Yorkshire, n=13) were assigned to either control or treatment based on parity. Immediately after the birth of the first piglet, 30 ml of the test product was dosed on the tongue of sows assigned to the treatment group. Control animals did not receive a sham treatment. Parameters recorded were the time of the birth of each piglet, skin radiation temperature as a measure of metabolic activity (D501 microscanner, Exergen corp, Watertown, MA, USA) and umbilical venous blood pH using an MI-413 pH micro-probe (Microelectrodes Inc., Bedford, NH, USA) attached to a Cyberscan pH 11 reader (Eutech Instruments, Nijkerk, NL). Piglets served as the experimental unit for statistical purposes. This blood pH was used as a measure of respiration; a low pH is indicative of CO_2 and lactic acid accumulation in blood caused by interruptions in respiration (Randall et al., 1971).

Experiment 2. The objective of the experiment was to test the product for effects on ease of labour and effects on piglet survival under controlled conditions. Sows (Dutch Landrace x Yorkshire, n=56) were assigned to either control or treatment based on parity. Immediately after the birth of the first piglet, 30 ml of the test product was dosed on the tongue of the sows assigned to the treatment group. Control animals did not receive a sham treatment. Interventions in the birth process were minimized to those sows that required assistance in order to prevent health complications for the sow. Parameters recorded were time of birth of each piglet, stillbirths, weak piglets at birth, and piglet mortality in the first 24h post farrowing.

Field trials. Commercial farms in Brazil (Br), Denmark (DK), the Netherlands (NL), Spain (SP), and the United Kingdom (UK) volunteered to participate in the trials (Table 1).

Table 1. Field trial location, trial size, and farm information.

Code	Trial sows	Herd size (sows)	Induction	Genetics
BR	189	2000	Not routine	PIC
DK	95	1000	Not routine	Not identified
NL	85	600	Not routine	Topics: GY x DL
SP A	87	500	Routine	Pietrain x LR x LW
SP B	91	650	Not routine	Duroc x LR x LW
SP C	80	700	Not routine	Dalland
UK A	168	1200	Not routine	JSR: LW x LR
UK B	54	5500	Not routine	ACMC: LW x LR x Meishan

Farms were instructed to assign sows, based on parity, either to the control or test group. Sows were identified with a red tag for controls and a green tag for sows to be treated. The protocol stipulated that the person in charge of the study was to inspect the sows three times a day (morning, early afternoon, and evening), and if a sow assigned to the treatment group was expected to start farrowing in the next 8 hours or had just started to farrow then 30 ml of the test product was administered on the tongue. The person in charge of the study was also instructed to record the timing of the dose, milk-letdown, start and end of parturition, stillbirths, weak piglets at birth, and mortality in the first 5 days post birth. Compliance to these requests varied by farm. The recording of mortality was especially variable as farms often cross-fostered immediately after birth.

Data from one farm (DK B) were excluded prior to the final analysis as protocol adherence was grossly inadequate (e.g., according to the records, all piglets were born at 07:00). A second farm (DK C) did not record any parity information and as parity was an important parameter in the statistical analysis, data from this farm were excluded as well. For the remaining, actual data recorded were analyzed as-is (no outliers were removed, even if dosing did not occur according to protocol).

STATISTICAL ANALYSIS

Data were analyzed using SPSS 11.0 using unconditional ANOVA. In each analysis, litter size (foetuses carried to term) was included as a covariate, and treatment, location, and parity, as well as interactions (full factorial) were included in the model. Parameters, other than treatment, not significant were removed prior to the final statistical analysis.

Results

EXPERIMENT 1: METABOLIC EFFECTS

The sows produced 13.7 pigs on average, of which 0.54 were stillborn and 0.69 were crushed by the sow within 24 h. The birth weight of the piglets was 1.26 kg and piglets gained 0.07 kg over the first 24 h. The average umbilical blood pH at birth was 7.2, and the interval between births of subsequent piglets was 20 min. The low pH of the piglet blood at birth showed that virtually all piglets suffer from some interruption in respiration during the birth process. This pH, on average, dropped when parturition proceeded, indicating that piglets were suffocated for longer periods of time likely as a consequence of fatigue in the sow.

Both pH and birth interval were affected by treatment. Umbilical blood pH decreased quadratically with time interval, being significantly higher (0.044±0.020, P=0.03) for piglets from treated sows. The time interval between individual births increased with 0.15±0.04 min/min (P=0.00) from the start of parturition for controls sows. For treated sows, this increase was 0.06±0.04 min and not significantly different from 0 (P=0.11) but it was significantly lower than the value for the control sows (P<0.05). Radiation temperature was 0.60±0.29°C higher in piglets from sows that received the test compound (P=0.04).

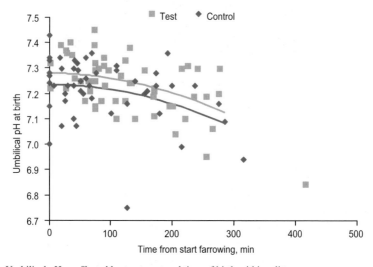

Figure 1. Umbilical pH as affected by treatment and time of birth within a litter.

EXPERIMENT 2: PERFORMANCE SCREEN

The sows produced 13.6 pigs on average. In the controls, there were 0.96±0.18 stillbirths/litter, and in the treated sows 0.63±0.27. In the controls, 0.22±0.09 pigs/litter were scored as weak, which was only 0.01±0.14 in the treated group. Mortality averaged 1.14±0.18 in the controls, and 0.68±0.25 in the treated sows. Although these trends were encouraging, none of the differences were significant (P>0.10).

The interval between the birth of the first and 10th pig was also analyzed as a means to compare objectively the ease of labour between groups (Fig. 2). For control sows this averaged 159±21 minutes, and for the treated sows it was significantly less at 110±12 minutes. For control sows, the distribution of these time intervals showed significant kurtosis (3.2±0.5, flattening compared to a normal distribution) and skewness (1.4±0.5, a tail in the distribution to one side, in this case towards an extended time interval). Neither was observed in the treated animals (skewness = 0.5±0.5, kurtosis = -0.7±1.0). These observations indicate fewer fatigue problems during labour due to the administration of this sports supplement.

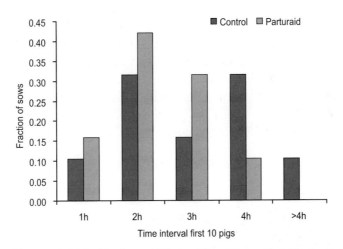

Figure 2. Interval between the birth of the first and 10th pig within a litter as affected by treatment.

FIELD TRIALS

The general feedback from those in charge of the studies was that the administration of the product was a lot easier than anticipated. Problems with aggression towards the person administering were not noted. In some cases, a small quantity of product would fall from the sow's mouth but typically the sow would lick this off the ground again suggesting good palatability. Farmers were also generally positive about the results they observed on their farm, which included speedier recovery of the sows, reductions in stillbirths and weak piglets at birth and also improvements in piglet vigour. No quantitative data on the latter were obtained.

Data from parity 9 and higher were excluded prior to analysis as the number of sows in these categories were deemed too small to properly estimate treatment effects. In addition, only one location (NL) had such sows. Otherwise, no data points were excluded.

Stillbirth data were obtained for 440 control sows and 409 treated sows. Average litter size was 13.4 (which includes stillbirths) and parity 3.48. The stillbirth figure was 1.33 ± 0.08 for the controls, and 0.89 ± 0.08 for the treated sows (P=0.001), a difference of 0.44 pigs/litter. Data per farm are provided in Fig. 3. This graph suggests that the treatment effect is larger for farms with a larger stillbirth problem which is in line with expectations.

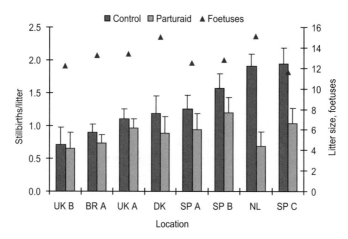

Figure 3. Litter size and stillbirths per litter (LSMeans + SEM) for each farm as affected by treatment.

Farm and parity both had a strong effect on the expression of stillbirths. In control sows, the lowest rate of stillbirths was observed in gilts and young sows, increasing nearly linearly with parity (Fig. 4). In the treated animals there was no significant increase in stillbirths with increasing parity when treating parity as a covariate.

Litter size expressed as the number of foetuses carried to term, is a strong determinant of stillbirths. The larger the litter, the higher the stillbirth rate. In the controls, there was effectively a linear relationship between stillbirths and litter size (Fig. 5). In the treated group, this relationship is somewhat more variable. Overall it is clear that stillbirths are less of a problem, especially in larger litters. Using linear regression for predicting stillbirths, the regression coefficient assigned to litter size for the controls is 0.17 ± 0.02, and that for the treated group 0.11 ± 0.02 (different at P<0.05). The parity and litter size data combined indicate that the treatment is most interesting in higher parity sows with larger litters.

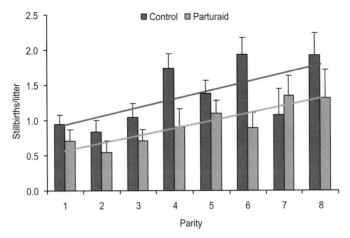

Figure 4. Stillbirths as affected by treatment and parity.

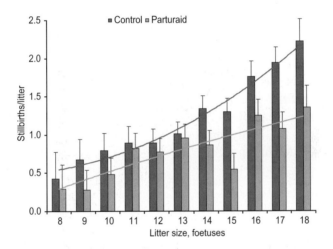

Figure 5. Stillbirths as affected by litter size (number of foetuses) and treatment. Litter sizes with less than 25 data points were excluded from this graph. For this graph, litter size was treated as a discrete variable.

The interval between dosing and stillbirths showed that there were large differences between farms. Brazil had the shortest interval, averaging 3.5 h, while Denmark had the largest interval (22.9 h). Dividing the dose interval into discrete groups (Fig. 6) showed that the dosing interval did affect the efficacy of the product, with dosing within 8 hours of the start of parturition (per the recommendation) having the best effect. Dosing between 8 and 10 hours only numerically improved stillbirths compared to the control group. Especially since a larger dose interval again showed improvements compared to the control stillbirth rates, it is not clear if this represents a true dose-interval effect or simply a data anomaly.

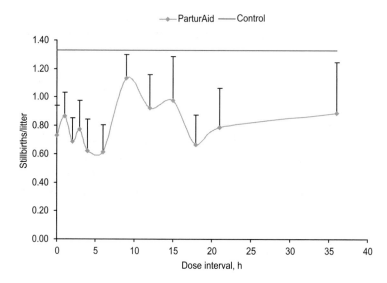

Figure 6. Stillbirth count as affected by the interval between dosing the treatment and the start of parturition. The average stillbirth level in the controls is shown for comparison.

The weak pig count was 0.84±0.08 for the controls, and 0.58±0.08 for the treated sows (P=0.01), a difference of 0.26 pigs/litter. Litter size again was an important determinant for the weak piglet count, increasing with 0.14±0.01 for every extra foetus carried to term. Parity, however, was not significant in this respect. Data per farm are included in Fig. 7.

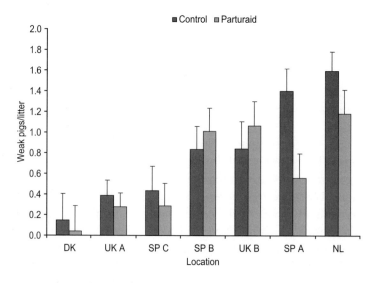

Figure 7. Weak piglet count as affected by treatment and location.

Parturition length was not recorded for Spain C and there were several missing observations in the other datasets. The total number of observations was 268 for the controls and 250 for the treatment. The average parturition length was 6 hours. It was not affected by litter size, but it was strongly affected by trial location (P<0.01) and parity (P=0.03, Fig. 8). Overall, the treatment reduced the length of labour from 6.2 to 5.6 h (P=0.09).

Piglet mortality in the first 5 days post-farrowing was only recorded in the Spanish and Dutch farms. On average, 0.90 pigs/litter died during this period. For the control sows, this number was 1.01±0.10, and in the ParturAid treated sows 0.76±0.11, a difference of 0.26 pigs/sow (P=0.07, numerically identical to the reduction in weak piglets at birth observed on all farms). Litter size

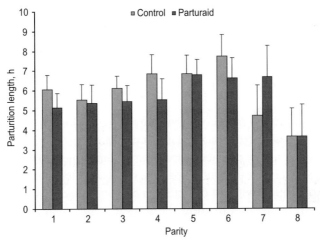

Figure 8. Parturition length as affected by parity and treatment. For parity 7 and 8, only 17 and 16 data points were recorded, respectively.

had a significant effect on this mortality, increasing with 0.1±0.02 for each extra foetus. Like for weak piglets, parity had no significant effect on piglet mortality (P=0.23).

For the UK trial A, sow feed intake data were recorded as they were fed by a computerized sensor-operated liquid feeding system. For the control sows, feed intake averaged 82.3±1.9 MJ/d, and for the treated sows 88.2±1.9 MJ/d, an increase of 7% (P=0.03). UK trial B also recorded feed intake during the first five days of lactation and recorded a 5% (NS) increase in feed intake during this period. Several farmers indicated that treated sows required less oxytocin shots during parturition and health support post parturition. Also, piglets from treated sows appeared heavier and healthier, and the observation on feed intake is in line with this.

One farm (NL) was particularly good at recording data and administering the product within the time-frame specified (75% of sows were dosed within the 8 h window). At this farm, stillbirths dropped from 1.64 to 0.84 (P=0.01), and weak piglets dropped from 1.97 to 1.08 (P=0.04). Mortality decreased from 1.81 to 1.18 (P=0.21), in line with the differences in weak pigs seen at the same farm. The bottom line for this farm was an extra 1.4 pigs per litter. This farmer actually cut the experiment short, as in his words, he couldn't afford to not treat the control sows.

Discussion

In large mammals like humans, pigs, and cattle, parturition is often a physically-demanding process. The duration of this intense activity is typically hours, but in extreme cases it can exceed a day (33 h was the longest recorded parturition in these field trials). For swine, the typical interval between the birth of the first piglet to expulsion of afterbirth is around 6 hours (current experiments). However, the process of parturition starts well before the expulsion of the first piglet, and thus the total period of intense activity is substantially longer than this.

Breeding females in modern housing systems typically live a very sedentary life style. Their activities consist of eating with some exploratory behaviour and on rare occasions they walk from one housing unit to another. None of these activities prepare the sow for intense physical activity around the time of parturition. It should thus not come as a surprise that during parturition, sows often don't have the stamina to complete parturition without difficulty. The consequence is interruptions and delays in parturition in order to allow the sows to 'catch their breath'.

The umbilical cord of a pig foetus is approximately 25 cm long (Leenhouwers, Knol, de Groot, Vos, and van der Lende, 2002). During expulsion of the foetus this cord has a high chance of being ruptured as the distance travelled is typically more than 25 cm. This cord can also get wrapped around the foetus which reduces its effective length and in itself reduces blood flow to the foetus. In either case, respiration of the piglets is impeded. Interruptions in blood flow are tolerated up to approximately 2 minutes. Longer interruptions, caused by the sow interrupting parturition due to, for example fatigue, result in a shortage of oxygen and accumulation of carbon dioxide and lactic acid resulting in a drop in blood pH. Both these processes result in metabolic damage in the foetus. When the interruption in blood flow exceeds approximately 5 minutes, the foetus is delivered stillborn. Piglets born with intermediate interruptions in blood flow are born alive but with such metabolic damage that their ability to survive is compromised (English and Morisson, 1984). Besides the metabolic complications which may be fatal, these piglets have a lower heat production predisposing them to hypothermia, and they are also likely to suffer from lack of orientation hindering their ability to compete and suckle.

In order to reduce perinatal mortality it is thus of key importance to fight fatigue during parturition. The physiology of fatigue is complex. It involves depletion of readily available energy sources, accumulation of lactic acid, and depletion of minerals such as calcium, magnesium, sodium, and phosphorus. Sports nutritionists have long recognized this problem and have developed supplements for athletes to fight fatigue. The best of these products are supported by sound scientific data showing that they do improve endurance. Key ingredients in these products are readily available energy (typically simple carbohydrates) and minerals (e.g., Von Duvillard et al., 2004).

The test product, ParturAid, is based on the same principle. However, because of the limitations imposed when working with farm animals the decision was made to use a small volume of paste rather than a large volume liquid product as the means for delivery. This imposed limitations on the ingredients, especially energy, that could be included in the product.

The first trial with ParturAid confirmed that most piglets are born with some interruption in respiration, as blood pH was below 7.4 for nearly all piglets. As parturition proceeded, blood pH in newly born piglets dropped even further, in line with what English and Morisson (1984) and Randall et al. (1971) described. This indicates that as parturition progresses, the birth of piglets has a higher chance of being interrupted resulting in failure of respiration. More importantly, it showed that in sows treated with the sports supplement, piglet blood pH was raised suggesting that fatigue-induced interruptions in labour were less common.

In the subsequent trial, effects on stillbirths, weak piglets, and piglet mortality were investigated. Numerically, improvements in these parameters were seen in this trial, but because of large variation relative to the number of sows used these improvements failed to reach statistical significance. A significant shift in the time required to birth 10 piglets was observed, being shorter and normally distributed in the treated sows instead of a seriously skewed distribution towards drawn-out labour in the controls.

The field trials with much larger numbers of sows did confirm that treatment reduced stillbirths by 0.44 and weak piglets and neonatal mortality both by 0.26 ($P<0.01$) for a total of 0.70 piglets extra per litter. The smaller response seen in the field trial as compared to the research farm is likely linked to poorer protocol adherence in the field trials. Estimating if sows were to farrow in the next 8 hours proved difficult at several farms, although feedback suggests that farmers got better at this over time (which isn't captured in these trials). Another factor is that in the field trials farmers were probably more aggressive in intervening in difficult births, possibly obscuring some of the negative effects of nutritionally unsupported births.

These trials also showed that the product is practical to use. Farmers reported back that the administration was much easier than expected and generally were positive about continuing to use the product after the trial period. Estimating the time of birth of the piglets remained the biggest challenge, and several farmers considered combining the test product with induction with prostaglandins so that the time of parturition would be easier to predict.

Conclusions

Parturition is a physically challenging process for which many sows are ill prepared. By providing a sports supplement such as ParturAid, fatigue during parturition can be delayed. Delaying fatigue reduces birth complications resulting in quicker farrowing and improved feed intake for the sow during lactation. Delaying fatigue also reduces stillbirths and neonatal piglet mortality. This effect depends on the severity of the problem, litter size, and parity. The average reduction observed was 0.70 pigs/litter, and reductions as high as 1.4 pigs per litter in highly productive farms were observed. ParturAid thus presents an attractive and cost-effective nutritional means to facilitate parturition resulting in healthier sows and substantially improved piglet survival, and thus annual sow productivity.

References

English, P.R., and Morrison, V. (1984) A review of survival problems of the neonatal pig. *Proceedings of the Pig Veterinary Society,* **11**, 39-55.

Leenhouwers, J. I., Knol, E. F., de Groot, P. N., Vos, H., and van der Lende, T. (2002) Fetal development in the pig in relation to genetic merit for piglet survival. *Journal of Animal Science,* **80**, 1759-1770.

Randall, G. C. (1971) The relationship of arterial blood pH and pCO2 to the viability of the newborn piglet. *Canadian Journal of Comparative Medicine Medicine*, **35**, 141-146.

SIVA (1999) Bedrijfsvergelijking Siva-produkten.

Von Duvillard, S. P., Braun, W. A., Markofski, M., Beneke, R., and Leithauser, R. (2004) Fluids and Hydration in Prolonged Endurance Performance. *Nutrition* **20**, 651– 656.

18

COMPENSATORY GROWTH IN PIGS

H.R. MARTÍNEZ-RAMÍREZ AND C.F.M. DE LANGE
Centre for Nutrition Modelling, Department of Animal and Poultry Science, University of Guelph, Guelph, Ontario, Canada. N1G 2W1

Introduction

Growth can be defined as an increased in the size (volume, length, height or girth) or weight of an animal over time as it develops towards maturity (Reeds *et al.*, 1993). Growth is accomplished by cellular hyperplasia early in life and cellular hypertrophy thereafter (Lawrence and Flower, 2002). The animal's potential for growth is ultimately determined by its genotype (Schinckel, 1999). Maximum growth can be achieved by maintaining animals in a stress-free environment and by supplying diets with sufficient and balanced energy nutrient contents (Reeds *et al.*, 1993; Lawrence and Flower, 2002).

Periods of food abundance and deficiency have a direct influence on the animal's growth patters (Lawrence and Flower, 2002). Already at the beginning of last century, Waters (1908) and Osborne and Mendel (1916) reported that animals with retarded growth due to undernutrition can achieve a growth rate higher than normal for chronological age, after removal of feed restrictions. This phenomenon was called compensatory growth (CG) by Bohman (1955). According to Hornick *et al.* (2000) CG may be defined as a physiological process whereby an animal accelerates its growth following a period of growth restriction compared to control animals.

In the pork industry CG may be explored as a means to improve carcass and meat quality (Kristensen *et al.*, 2002; Therkildsen *et al.*, 2002; Oksbjerg *et al.*, 2002) and nutrient utilization (Tullis *et al.*, 1986), to reduce gut health problems due to excess protein intake in growing pigs, to simplify feeding strategies such as phase feeding (O'Connell *et al.*, 2006), and thus to improve pork production efficiencies (Gill, 1998; MLC, 2004). Indeed, well-controlled studies such as these on phase feeding at the MLC in the UK using pigs with high lean tissue growth potentials and between 35 and 102 kg body weight (BW), show that pigs fed a single diet achieve the same or better growth performance than pigs that were exposed to phase feeding to meet closely changing amino acid requirements at the various stages of growth, when cumulative amino acid intakes are kept similar for both feeding strategies (MLC, 2004).

Many investigators have attempted to demonstrate that CG takes place in pigs following a period of either feed intake restriction (e.g. Bikker *et al.,* 1996a,b; Skiba and Fandrejewski, 1998) or amino acid intake restriction (e.g. Wyllie *et al.,* 1969; Whittemore *et al.,* 1978; Campbell and Dukin 1983; Fabian *et al.,* 2004). Studies have shown complete (Wyllie *et al.,* 1969; Donker *et al.,* 1983; Fabian *et al.,* 2004; Martínez and de Lange, 2005; Collins *et al.,* 2006; Skiba *et al.,* 2006a,b), incomplete (Campbell and Dunkin, 1983a; Kyriazakis *et al.,* 1991; Stramataris *et al.,* 1991; de Greef *et al.,* 1992; Critser *et al.,* 1995; Bikker *et al.,* 1996b; Skiba and Fandrejewski, 1998) or no CG in pigs (Hogberg and Zimmerman, 1978; Pond *et al.,* 1980; Pond and Mersmann, 1990; Chiba *et al.,* 1999, 2002; Ferguson and Theeruth, 2002). Extensive literature reviews have been written on the phenomenon of CG in farm animals (Wilson and Osbourn, 1960; Allden, 1970; O'Donovan, 1984; Doyle and Leeson, 1998; Lovatto *et al.,* 2000; Lawrence and Flower, 2002). These studies indicate that the extent and rate of CG vary with the type, degree, timing and duration of energy and nutrient intake restriction, as well as the pig's genotype, and energy and nutrient availability following the period of energy and nutrient intake restriction. However, the underlying mechanisms and control of CG remain to be elucidated, limiting the ability to predict the extent and rate of CG. Indeed, many investigations on CG are merely descriptive and empirical in nature and do not explore the potential underlying mechanisms that control CG (Chiba, 1994, 1995; Crister *et al.,* 1995; Chiba *et al.,* 1999, 2002; Whang *et al.,* 2000a,b, 2003; Fabian *et al.,* 2002, 2004; Collins *et al.,* 2006; O'Connell *et al.,* 2006; Reynolds and O'Doherty; 2006). Tanner (1963), Pits (1986), Mosier (1990), Baron *et al.* (1994), Zubair (1994) and Hornick *et al.* (2000) have proposed potential mechanisms that are involved in the control of CG. However, these theories have largely appeared inadequate to represent the dynamics of CG (i.e. Tanner, 1963; Mosier, 1990; Kyriazakis and Emmans, 1992b; Baron *et al.,* 1994).

The main objective of the current Chapter is to explore a framework that may be used to predict the rate and extent of CG following periods of qualitative (i.e. amino acid) and quantitative (i.e. feed intake) intake restriction in growing pigs. The complex issue of potential CG following growth retardation induced by other environmental stresses, such as disease, will not be addressed.

Basic principles

To understand better the potential mechanism underlying CG, key concepts regarding the partitioning of available energy and amino acid intake as well as chemical and physical body composition must be understood. For extensive reviews on these concepts the reader is referred to Black *et al.* (1986), Ferguson and Gous (1993), Schinckel and de Lange (1996), Emmans and Kyriazakis (1997), Moughan (1999), and de Lange *et al.* (2003). Two key aspects are the upper limit to body protein deposition (PdMax) and constraints on the whole body lipid to whole body protein ratio (TargetL/P) in growing pigs. These two aspects will be described briefly. Moreover, some evidence is provided, based on the animal's physiology, to consider TargetL/P in the utilization of available energy and nutrient intake for body protein deposition (Pd) and body lipid deposition (Ld) in growing pigs.

UPPER LIMIT TO BODY PROTEIN DEPOSITION (PDMAX)

The PdMax can be defined as the intrinsic impetus for maximum protein growth and dominates the partitioning of available energy and nutrients (Moughan and Verstegen, 1988; Schinckel and de Lange, 1996). PdMax represents the maximum difference between whole body protein synthesis and degradation and is ultimately defined by genotype. Under practical conditions, the expression of PdMax is limited by environmental factors such as energy and nutrient allowance, social and physical and thermal environments, and exposure to pathogens. PdMax varies with the stage of maturity and decreases to zero when the pig approaches to maturity (Figure 1).

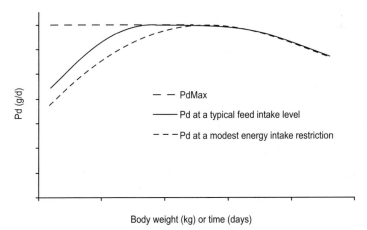

Body weight (kg) or time (days)

Figure 1. Schematic representation of the dynamics of body protein deposition (Pd) in pigs fed non-limiting diets, either at a typical feed intake level or a modest energy intake restriction. At the lower body weight, the period in which Pd increases with body weight denotes the energy dependent phase of Pd.

The relationship between BW and PdMax in young growing pigs before they start to mature is still a matter of debate. One view is that PdMax is best represented by a sigmoidal relationship between body protein mass (P) and time (Black *et al.*, 1986; Ferguson and Gous, 1993; Emmans and Kyriazakis, 1997), implying that PdMax increases with P until the inflexion point in the P growth curve is reached. This approach is not supported strongly by experimental observations. Indeed, in many pig growth experiments sigmoidal relationships between P and time have been observed. However, only in very few studies has it been confirmed that a slight change in nutrient intake at the various stages of growth does not alter Pd, which is a pragmatic means to assess whether PdMax has been achieved (Moughan and Verstegen, 1988; Schinckel and de Lange, 1996). Another view is that PdMax is constant and independent of BW or P until pigs start to mature (Whittemore and Faucett, 1976; Moughan and Verstegen, 1988; Moughan, 1999; de Lange *et al.*, 2001) (Figure 1). This is supported by experimental observations where pigs were exposed to varying intake levels of non-limiting diets at different BW ranges (Quiniou *et al.*, 1995, 1996; Möhn and de Lange, 1998; Moughan *et al.*, 2006). According to these studies, PdMax remains constant between 45 and 100 kg BW (Quiniou *et al.*, 1995, 1996), 25 and more than 70 kg BW (Möhn and de Lange, 1998), and 25 and 85 kg BW (Moughan *et al.*, 2006). Similarly, Martínez-Ramírez (2005) observed in recent CG experiments at the University of Guelph that Pd in castrates (156 g/d) and entire male pigs (215 g/d) remained constant between 35 and 83 kg BW when pigs were fed at high levels of energy and nutrient intake.

Procedures to estimate PdMax for specific populations of pigs have been suggested previously (e.g. Moughan and Verstegen, 1988; Schinckel and de Lange, 1996; de Lange *et al.*, 2001). It may be suggested that the assumption that PdMax is independent of BW up to about 85 kg BW is acceptable for the routine characterization of pig genotypes and allows accurate representation of the dynamics of CG following a period of amino acid intake restriction.

A refinement of the PdMax concept is to apply it to the carcass component only (PdMaxCarc; de Lange *et al.*, 2003). Such a refinement allows for a quantitative representation of substantial feeding level and diet composition effects on the size and chemical composition of visceral organs and thus the development of feeding strategies to optimize the proportion of whole body protein that is present in the carcass fraction (de Lange *et al.*, 2001, 2003). The latter is also relevant when quantifying CG in pigs following a period of feed intake restriction (Stamataris *et al.*, 1991; Bikker *et al.*, 1996a,b). Based on the review by Skiba (2005), protein intake restriction and subsequent re-alimentation has little or no influence on visceral protein mass.

CONSTRAINTS ON THE WHOLE BODY PROTEIN TO WHOLE BODY LIPID RATIO (TARGETL/P)

There is an implicit association between feed intake (energy intake) and Pd in growing pigs. Several researchers have focused on this relationship and its consequences for lean tissue growth (e.g. Campbell *et al.,* 1983a; de Greef, 1992; Bikker, 1994). To describe this relationship, a linear-plateau model has been proposed (Whittemore and Fawcett, 1976). This model is supported by empirical observations in which different groups of pigs of similar genotype are exposed to five or more levels of energy intake pigs (e.g. Campbell and Taverner, 1988; Bikker, 1994; Möhn *et al.,* 2000). This model describes Pd and Ld in response to different energy levels over a specific BW range. According to this model, and when intake of essential nutrients is not limiting, Pd and Ld increase linearly with increasing energy intake until PdMax is reached. Once energy intake exceeds requirement for PdMax, additional energy intake is used for Ld only. During the energy intake dependent phase of Pd, when energy intake limits the expression of Pd, the relationship between energy intake and Pd is closely associated with a minimum Ld to Pd ratio (Ld/Pd), which is the minimal amount of Ld that accompanies Pd. This ratio varies with pig genotype, gender, BW and even energy intake (Cambell and Taverner, 1998; de Greef, 1992; Quiniou *et al.,* 1995, 1996; Möhn and de Lange, 1998).

During the energy dependent phase of Pd, there is a close association between Ld/Pd and the ratio between body lipid mass (L) and P (L/P)(de Greef, 1992). This implies that constraints on either Ld/Pd or L/P can be used to characterize the partitioning of retained energy in the pig. However, unlike constraints on Ld/Pd, constraints on L/P can be used to represent impacts of nutritional history on the composition of growth (Verstegen and Moughan, 1998; Schinckel and de Lange, 1996; Kyriazakis and Emmans, 1992a,b; Martínez-Ramírez, 2005). Within a population of pigs, minimum L/P, or more appropriately TargetL/P, is known to increase with both level of energy intake and BW (de Greef, 1992; Weis *et al.,* 2004). However, BW effects can be attributed largely to increases in energy intake with BW (Weis *et al.,* 2004). Therefore, a simple (linear) relationship with energy intake may be used to routinely characterize TargetL/P in different pig genotypes, and based on measured or estimated L/P in pigs during the energy dependent phase of Pd at either two or more levels of energy intake, or two or more BW.

PHYSIOLOGICAL CONTROL OF GROWTH

Complex physiological systems are in place to determine the actual rates of Pd and Ld reflecting growth potential and environmental constraints, such as those imposed by available energy and nutrient intake. Extensive reviews have been written on the physiological control of energy and nutrient utilization by Waterlow (1986), Reeds *et al.* (1993), Ferré (1999), Grizard *et al.* (1999), Averous *et al.* (2003), Lawrence and Fowler (2002) and Scanes (2003). The impacts of fluctuations in energy and nutrient intake on key anabolic and catabolic hormones, hormone receptors and gene expression have been characterized. For example, in cattle (Hornick *et al.*, 2000) and pigs (Buonomo and Baile, 1991), feed intake restrictions results in lower plasma level of anabolic hormones, such as insulin like growth factor I (IGF-1), insulin, triiodothyronine (T3) and thyroxine (T4), while plasma levels of cortisol and growth hormone (GH) remained unchanged. When feed intake levels were subsequently increased, higher plasma levels of GH and reduced plasma levels of cortisol were observed (Yambayamba *et al.*, 1996; Hornick *et al.*, 2000). However, until the discovery of leptin, a clear link body composition, or L/P, and control of energy and nutrient partitioning and feed intake had not been established (Barb *et al.*, 1998; Houseknecht *et al.*, 1998; Barb *et al.*, 2001). At the University of Guelph, close relationships between plasma leptin levels and L/P during energy and nutrient intake restriction and after the energy and nutrient intake restriction was removed were observed (Martínez and de Lange, 2005), providing further evidence that there is a physiological control system in place linking nutritional history with energy and nutrient partitioning once a nutrition or feed intake restriction is removed. Leptin not only functions as an "adipostat" to signal the status of body energy stores to the brain, and perhaps other tissues, but also as a sensor of energy balance and energy metabolism (Houseknecht *et al.*, 1998; Martínez-Ramírez, 2005). Such observations support the application of mathematical relationships, to represent causal relationships, between L/P and utilization of available energy and nutrient intake for Pd and Ld.

Hypothesis

Based on the concepts described in the previous section and observations on the dynamics of CG following a period of amino acid intake restriction, it may be hypothesized that the extent and rate of CG is (a) constraint by PdMax, and (b) driven by TargetL/P that pigs try to achieve (Figure 1). These concepts imply that CG following a period of amino acid intake restriction occurs primarily during the energy-dependent phase of Pd and is unlikely to occur in growing pigs with a relatively low PdMax. In practical terms, this means that, at the end of the amino acid intake restriction period, body fatness (L/P) of pigs is higher than TargetL/P and, once the amino acid intake restriction period is removed, pigs will increase Pd and reduce Ld to achieve TargetL/P. These concepts may also apply to CG following a period of feed intake restriction (Quantitative nutrient intake restriction). However, in that case feeding level and diet composition effects on the size and chemical composition of the visceral organs – especially those that are involved in food processing – should be considered explicitly. These hypotheses will be tested against experimental observations in the next section.

Experimental Observations

QUALITATIVE NUTRIENT (AMINO ACID) INTAKE RESTRICTION

It has been suggested that the growth rate of piglets nursing on the sow without an additional source of energy and nutrients is below their potential (Braude and Newport, 1977; Lecce *et al.*, 1979; Harrell *et al.*, 1993; Pluske *et al.*, 1995). In accordance with Campbell and Dunkin (1982), sow's milk is deficient in amino acids, relative to energy, for maximum Pd. As a result, nursing piglets rapidly accumulate large body lipid stores, implying that at weaning, actual L/P is larger than TargetL/P. In a similar manner, and when applying typical phase feeding programs, pigs will or should be fed below their dietary amino acid requirements when a new diet is first introduced, causing at least a temporary reduction in growth and Pd as well as a temporary increase in Ld/Pd and L/P (Kyriazakis *et al.*, 1991; de Greef *et al.*, 1992; Whang *et al.*, 2003; Skiba and Fandrejewski, 1998; Martínez and de Lange, 2004, 2005). As mentioned earlier, the relative proportion of visceral organs mass to empty BW is normally not altered by a period of amino acid intake restriction, in comparison to control pigs that were not restricted in amino acid intake (Whang *et al.*, 2003; Martínez-Ramírez, 2005; Skiba, 2005). Theoretically and because of increased L/P, the maintenance energy requirements per kg of live BW or metabolic BW should be lower in pigs that are fed amino acid limiting diets (Birkett and de Lange, 2001), but this has not been established experimentally.

During the re-alimentation phase, when the amino acid intake restriction is removed, improvements in live BW gains or Pd have been observed in some groups of pigs (e.g. Kyriazakis *et al.*, 1991, de Greef *et al.*, 1992; Skiba and Fandrejewski, 1998; Whang *et al.*, 2003; MLC, 2004; Martínez and de Lange, 2005; Collins *et al.*, 2006), but not in others (e.g. Fergunson and Theeruth, 2002; Martínez and de Lange, 2004; O'Connell *et al.*, 2006; O'Doherty 2006). For example, in studies at the University of Guelph no CG in scale-fed castrates was observed, but full CG was apparent in scale-fed entire male pigs in terms of BW gain and L/P (Table 1) as well as in the relationship between P and time (Figure 2); Martínez-Ramírez, 2005; Martínez and de Lange, 2004, 2005). When improvements in growth rates have been observed during the re-alimentation phase, this has been associated with improvements in feed efficiency (e.g. Tullis *et al.*, 1986; Fabian *et al.*, 2004; Martínez-Ramírez, 2005). However, the (marginal) biological efficiency of using available amino acid intake for Pd is not improved during CG (Whang *et al.*, 2000a, 2003).

Entire male pigs have higher growth rates, better feed efficiency and higher lean tissue growth potentials, and thus PdMax, than castrates (Campbell *et al.*, 1983b; Whittemore, 1983; Campbell and Taverner, 1988). During the re-alimentation phase in the studies of Martínez and de Lange (2004, 2005), the growth rate was higher in entire male pigs, that shows complete CG, than in castrates that showed no CG (Table 1). Similarly, Robinson (1964) observed complete CG in gilts than in castrates. These observations strongly suggest that the extent of CG is determined by genotype and is higher in pigs with higher PdMax. It must be mentioned that several studies have failed to demonstrate that CG is influenced by gender (e.g. Campbell and Dunkin, 1983b; Kyriazakis *et al.,* 1991; Stamataris *et al.,* 1991; Critser *et al.,* 1995; Therkildsen *et al.,* 2002; 2004). For example, Kyriazakis *et al.*

Table 1. Growth performance and chemical body composition (ratio between whole body lipid and whole body protein, L/P) of scale-fed castrates and entire male pigs during (restriction phase) and after (re-alimentation phase) a period of amino acid intake restriction (Adapted from Martínez-Ramírez, 2005).

	Dietary treatment*		Probability of treatment effect
	Control	*Amino acid intake restriction*	
	Castrates		
Live body weight gain, g/d			
Restriction phase (15 to 35 kg BW)	556	410	<0.001
Re-alimentation phase (35 to 70 kg BW)	917	919	0.57
Overall (15 to 65 kg BW)	734	624	0.091
L/P			
End of restriction phase	0.65	1.20	0.005
End of re-alimentation phase	0.79	1.15	0.027
	Entire male pigs		
Live body weight gain, g/d			
Restriction phase (16 to 38 kg BW)	784	650	<0.001
Re-alimentation phase (38 to 54 kg BW)	1035	1149	0.028
Re-alimentation phase (38 to 111 kg BW)	1077	1170	0.002
Overall (16 to 111 kg BW)	990	995	0.79
L/P			
End of restriction phase (38 kg BW)	0.68	1.10	0.012
During re-alimentation phase (54 kg BW)	0.83	1.02	0.16
End of re-alimentation phase (111 kg BW)	1.15	1.14	0.86

* Pigs were scaled-fed relative to BW. During the restriction phase, amino acid intake was estimated to be 20% above requirements for body protein deposition for pig on the control treatment, and 40% (castrates) or 30% (entire male pigs) below requirements for pigs on the amino acid intake restriction treatment.

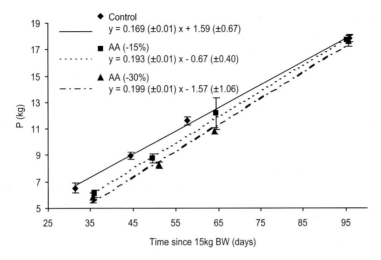

Figure 2. Relationship between whole body protein mass (P) and time during the re-alimentation phase (38 to 110 kg BW) in entire males pigs exposed to different levels of amino acid intake (Control, AA -15%, AA -30%) during the restriction phase (15 to 38 kg BW). Adapted from Martínez-Ramírez (2005).

(1991) observed no differences in CG between gilts and entire male pigs between 12 and 30 kg BW. This may be attributed to the small number of observations or the smaller difference in PdMax between gilts and entire male pigs, or between castrates and gilts, than between castrates and entire male pigs. Few studies have been conducted comparing CG in entire male pigs and castrates.

Based on sequential N-balance measurements in scale-fed entire male pigs following a period of amino acid intake restriction, Pd remained constant between 40 and 83 kg BW (Martínez-Ramírez, 2005; Figure 3) and approached the value for PdMax observed previously for this population of entire male pigs at higher BW (Weis *et al.*, 2004). Apparently, immediately after the amino acid intake restriction was removed, these entire male pigs were able to express PdMax, most likely because the need for Ld was reduced. These pigs were thus able to partition a larger portion of available energy intake towards Pd, as compared to the control pigs that were previously not exposed to an amino acid intake restriction. In contrast, Pd in scale-fed castrates, following a period of amino acid intake restriction up to 35 kg BW, was the same as Pd in control castrates that were previously not exposed to an amino acid intake restriction. For both groups of castrates Pd was independent of BW. Apparently, after 35 kg BW castrates on the control treatment were not within their energy dependent phase for Pd and Pd represented PdMax. Therefore, during the re-alimentation phase, Pd, and thus Ld, were not influenced by previous amino acid intake restriction in castrates and CG did not occur. These observations provide further evidence that Pd during a period of CG is constrained by PdMax and that PdMax is largely independent of BW until pigs start to mature. The latter was discussed earlier.

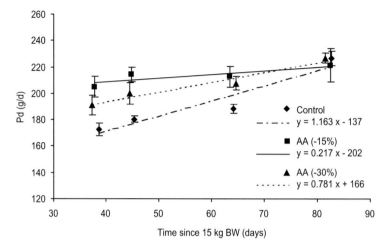

Figure 3. Relationship between whole body protein deposition (Pd; nitrogen balance) and days during the re-alimentation phase (38 to 110 kg BW) in entire males pigs exposed to different levels of amino acid (AA) intake (Control, AA -15%, AA -30%) during the restriction phase (15 to 38 kg BW). At the first three of four N-balance periods, values for Control were lower than those for the other two treatments (P<0.05); Values for AA -15% did not differ from those for AA -30% (P>0.10). Adapted from Martínez-Ramírez (2005).

In order to correct the nutrition induced increase in L/P, relative to TargetL/P, accumulated during the period of amino acid intake restriction, pigs are able to reduce Ld and Ld/Pd during the re-alimentation phase and when the amino acid intake restriction is removed (de Greef *et al.*, 1992; Skiba and Fandrejewski, 1998; Martínez and de Lange, 2005). Consequently, both ad libitum and scale-fed pigs are capable of directing more energy to Pd and achieve Pd that approach estimates of PdMax as soon as the amino acid restriction is removed. Higher growth rates, increased Pd, and reduced Ld/Pd can only be observed as long as pigs are fed non-limiting diets as observed by Whang *et al.* (2003) and Collins *et al.* (2006), and until TargetL/P is achieved (Martínez and de Lange, 2005; Figure 4).

In studies where pigs were fed ad libitum following a period of amino acid intake restriction, Wyllie *et al.* (1969), de Greef *et al.* (1992), Chiba *et al.* (2002) and Fabian *et al.* (2004) observed that average daily feed intake during the first part of the re-alimentation phase was reduced by 6, 10, 8% and 10%, respectively, apparently to reduce further Ld following a period of amino acid intake restriction. This effect may be attributable to the excessive fatness accumulated during the period of amino acid intake restriction and the negative impact of body fatness on apatite, mediated via leptin (Barb *et al.*, 1998; Houseknecht *et al.*, 1998). Since feed intake was controlled in the studies of Whang *et al.* (2003) and Martínez and de Lange (2004, 2005) CG was attributed fully to improvement in feed efficiency

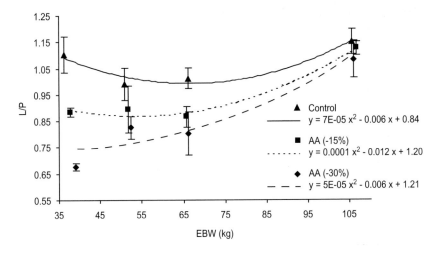

Figure 4. Relationship between body composition (whole body lipid to whole body protein ratio; L/P) and empty body weight (EBW) during the re-alimentation phase (38 to 110 kg BW) in entire males pigs exposed to different levels of amino acid (AA) intake (Control, AA -15%, AA -30%) during the restriction phase (15 to 38 kg BW). Adapted from Martínez-Ramírez (2005).

as a result of a change in the partitioning of retained energy between Pd and Ld, and not by feed intake mechanisms. This implies that, under ad libitum feeding conditions, pigs will more quickly achieve TargetL/P than under scale-feeding conditions.

At the end of the re-alimentation phase some experiments have shown complete CG (Fabian *et al.*, 2004; Martínez and de Lange, 2004, 2005; Collins *et al.*, 2006) and achieved a body composition that was similar to pigs that were previously not exposed to amino acid intake restriction (Figure 4). Moreover, carcass characteristics and weight of primal meat cuts were not influenced by previous amino acid intake restriction (Fabian *et al.*, 2004; Martínez and de Lange, 2005; O'Connell *et al.*, 2005, 2006). These observations clearly illustrate that CG is driven by a target body composition (TargetL/P; Figure 4) and not by constraints on composition of growth (Martínez-Ramírez, 2005). These mechanisms are consistent with the findings of Kyriazakis *et al.* (1991) and de Greef *et al.* (1992).

In the literature, there are five well conducted studies with young pigs or pigs with high PdMax that support current findings on CG in entire male pigs (Martínez-Ramírez, 2005). After a period of amino acid intake restriction, Kyriazakis *et al.* (1991), de Greef *et al.* (1992), Skiba and Fandrejewski (1998), Whang *et al.* (2003) and Collins *et al.*, (2006) observed CG and increased rates of Pd. Even when amino acid restriction was applied in young pigs (6.5 to 12 kg BW, Kyriazakis *et al.*, 1991; 4 to 8 weeks old, Collins *et al.*, 2006), CG and compensatory Pd was observed. Unfortunately, in these studies dynamics of compensatory Pd were not evaluated and pigs were slaughtered at low BW (Kyriazakis *et al.*, 1991; Skiba and

Fandrejewski, 1998; Whang *et al.*, 2003), which limited the extent of CG. However, in the study by Kyriazakis *et al.* (1991) and in pigs previously fed amino acid-limiting diets, average daily gains were rather constant during the re-alimentation phase, whereas average daily gain in the control pigs increased with BW and approached values for pigs showing CG. Given the close association between BW gain and Pd these observations are highly consistent with the current observations on entire male pigs in the study of Martínez-Ramírez (2005).

In summary, based on the literature and supported by previous findings in Guelph, it can be concluded that CG is more likely to occur in pigs with high lean tissue growth potentials, i.e. high PdMax. In fact, PdMax appears the main factor that determines the extent and duration of CG (Figure 4), while CG is driven by a target body composition which may be represented by constraints on the L to P ratio (TargetL/P; Figure 4).

QUANTITATIVE ENERGY AND NUTRIENT INTAKE RESTRICTION

During development towards maturity pigs may experience periods of feed intake restrictions, in particular during the immediate post-weaning period (Tokach *et al.*, 1992; Pluske *et al.,* 1995). Moreover, there has recently been some interest in a temporary restriction of feed intake in growing pigs, aimed at improving meat quality, in particular pork meat tenderness by inducing increased muscle protein turnover at the time of slaughter (Kristensen *et al.*, 2004; Therkildsen *et al.*, 2002, 2004).

Generally, during a period of feed or energy intake restriction, growth rate is reduced, while Ld, Ld/Pd and final L/P are lower as compared to non-restricted control pigs (Stamataris *et al.*, 1991; Bikker *et al.*, 1996a,b; Skiba and Fandrejewski, 1998; Weis *et al.*, 2004; Heyer and Lebret, 2007). Feed or energy intake restriction usually also reduce the size and metabolic activity of visceral organs, especially those that are involved in food processing (Koong *et al.*, 1982; Stamataris *et al.*, 1991; Bikker *et al.*, 1996a,b). This metabolic adaptation may suggest a reduction in maintenance requirements of these organs (Koong *et al.*, 1982; Noblet *et al.*, 1997). However, when energy intake restriction is induced by increasing the dietary fibre content (dilution effect), the size of visceral organs may be increased compared to control pigs (Pond and Mersmann, 1990; Raj, *et al.*, 2005; Skiba *et al.*, 2005, 2006). Thus, potential mechanisms for CG may vary with the manner in which quantitative energy and nutrient intake restriction is achieved.

During the first weeks following feed intake restriction, it is usual to observe increased live weight gains (up to 20%), improvements in feed efficiency (0 to 11%) and increased feed intakes (0 to 18%) (Nielsen, 1964; Campbell *et al.*, 1983b; Prince *et al.*, 1983; Valaja *et al.*, 1992; Oksbjerg *et al.*, 2002; Therkildsen *et al.*,

2004). Apart from the study by Robinson (1964), where gilts showed 7% higher rates of CG than castrates, the impact of pig genotype or gender on CG following a period of feed intake restriction has not been explored extensively or shown to be minimal (Campbell and Dunkin, 1983b; Stamataris *et al.*, 1991; Critser *et al.*, 1995; Therkildsen *et al.*, 2002; 2004).

CG following a period of feed intake restriction can largely be attributed to CG in visceral organs and gut fill, and especially to increases in protein mass and associated water mass in organs that are involved in food processing (Stamataris *et al.*, 1991; Bikker *et al.*, 1996a; Skiba and Fandrejewski, 1998). In well-controlled studies, Bikker *et al.* (1996b) and Skiba and Fandrejewski (1998) observed that during CG Pd was increased only in viscera when compared to control pigs (36.2 vs. 21.2 g/d and 21 vs. 17 g/d; P<0.01; respectively); in the carcass no compensatory Pd was observed (158 vs. 159 g/d and 109 vs. 105 g/d; P>0.10; respectively). It should be mentioned that, in studies where only whole animal performance was monitored, some compensatory Pd may have occurred in the carcass (e.g. Campbell *et al.*, 1983b, Donker *et al.* 1986; Critser *et al.* 1995; Therkildsen *et al.*, 2002, 2004). These observations stress the need to measure and explicitly represent Pd in visceral organs, and to apply the concept of PdMax to the carcass, as discussed earlier. These studies also suggest that PdMaxCarc may limit compensatory Pd following a period of feed intake restriction, explaining why no compensatory Pd was observed in some studies, while it has been observed in other studies. This concept, however, remains to be tested in well-controlled studies.

Observed increases in Ld and Ld/Pd in *ad libitum* fed pigs following a period of feed intake restriction (Stamataris *et al.*, 1991; Skiba and Fandrejewski, 1998) reflect the desire to achieve a TargetL/P that is consistent with increased daily energy intake. Even though these observed changes in Ld/Pd are in agreement with a TargetL/P which is increased with energy intake, the dynamics of Pd and Ld, and thus L/P, following a period of feed or energy intake restriction remain to be explored. Based on the concepts that were presented earlier, it may be speculated that a quick and sudden increase in energy intake during the energy-dependent phase of Pd in young growing pigs would lead to a rapid increase in Ld and zero or even negative Pd in the carcass until the new TargetL/P is achieved. The latter appears inconsistent with the live BW gains reported by Stamataris *et al.* (1991) immediately after the feed intake restriction is removed. Apparently, a mechanism is in place to facilitate a gradual transition to the new and increased TargetL/P after a period of feed or energy intake restriction in young growing pigs.

At the end of the re-alimentation phase, some experiments have shown partial or full compensation in body composition, i.e. pigs achieved the same carcass characteristics and weight of primal meat cuts when compared to pigs that were never fed restricted (Smith *et al.*, 1999; Therkildsen *et al.*, 2002; 2004; Oksbjerg *et al.*, 2002; Kristensen *et al.*, 2002; 2004). In most cases full compensation in body composition was achieved, even though no or incomplete CG was observed. The latter may be attributed to within-treatment variability in carcass characteristics and 'dilution' effect of BW gained after the feed intake restriction has been removed.

In summary, CG following a period of feed or energy intake restriction is usually incomplete and can be attributed largely to compensatory growth in visceral organs. The explicit representation of feeding level and diet composition effects on size and chemical composition of visceral organs is required for the prediction of the rate and extent of compensatory growth following a period of feed intake restriction. The dynamics of Ld and Pd during CG and following a period of feed intake restriction have not been well-characterized.

Conclusion and implications

In growing pigs, the extent and rate of compensatory growth (CG) varies with the type, degree, timing and duration of nutrient intake restriction, as well as genotype and energy and nutrient availability following the period of nutrient intake restriction. In case of CG induced by amino acid intake restriction (Qualitative nutrient intake restriction), the extent of CG appears constrained by the upper limit to body protein deposition (PdMax) and is driven by a target whole body lipid to whole body protein ratio (TargetL/P), implying that CG following a period of amino acid intake restriction occurs primarily during the energy dependent phase of body protein deposition (Pd) and is unlikely to occur in growing pigs with relatively low lean tissue growth potentials. These concepts may also apply to CG following periods of feed intake restriction (Quantitative nutrient intake restriction). However, in that case feeding level and diet composition effects on the size and chemical composition of the visceral organs – especially those involved in feed processing – should be considered explicitly. In most well-controlled studies CG following a period of food intake restriction can be attributed fully to CG in visceral organs. However, in other studies some CG may have been observed in the carcass following a period of feed intake restriction. The dynamics of voluntary feed intake during CG are not well understood, especially following a period of feed intake restriction, when pigs will attempt to increase both body lipid deposition, to achieve TargetL/P, and Pd, to reach a target body protein mass relative to the pigs' physiological age. In order to exploit CG commercially, populations of pigs need to be characterized in aspects of nutrient partitioning for growth. Dynamic and mechanistic pig growth models will be useful to exploit CG in commercial pork production.

Literature cited

Allden, W.G. (1970). The effects of nutritional deprivation on the. subsequent productivity of sheep and cattle. *Nutrition, Abstracts and. Reviews* **40**, 1167-1184.

Averous, J., Bruhat, A., Mordier, S. and Fafournoux, P. (2003). Recent advances in the understanding of amino regulation of gene expression. *Journal of Nutrition* **133**, 2040S-2045S.

Barb, C.R., Hausman, G.J. and Houseknecht, K.L. (2001). Biology of leptin in the pig. *Domestic Animal Endocrinology* **21**, 297-317.

Barb, C.R., Yan, X., Azain, M.J., Kraeling, R.R., Rampacek, G.B. and Ramsay, T.G. (1998). Recombinant porcine leptin reduces feed intake and stimulates growth hormone secretion in swine. *Domestic Animal Endocrinology* **15**, 77-86.

Baron, J., Klein, K.O., Colli, M.J., Yanovski, J.A., Novosad, J.A., Bacher, J.D. and Cutler, G.B. Jr. (1994). Catch-up growth after glucocorticoid excess: a mechanism intrinsic to the growth plate. *Endocrinology* **135**, 1367–1371.

Bikker, P. (1994). Protein and lipid accretion in body components of growing pigs. PhD. Thesis Department of Animal Nutrition Wageningen Agricultural University, Haagsteeg 4, 6708 PM Wageningen, The Netherlands.

Bikker, P., Vertegen, M.W., Kemp, B. and Bosch, M. (1996a). Performance and body composition of fattening gilts (45 - 85 kg) as affected by energy intake and nutrition in early life. I. Growth of the body and body components. *Journal of Animal Science* **74**, 795-805.

Bikker, P., Verstegen, M.W. and Campbell, R. G. (1996b). Performance and body composition of finishing gilts (45 to 85 kilograms) as affected by energy intake and nutrition in earlier life: II. Protein and lipid accretion in body components. *Journal of Animal Science* **74**, 806-817.

Black, J.L., Campbell, R.G., Williams, I.H., James, K.J. and Davies, G.T. (1986). Simulation of energy and amino acid utilization in the pig. *Research and Development in Agriculture* **3**, 121-145.

Bohman, V.R. (1955). Compensatory growth in beef cattle. The effect of hay maturity. *Journal of Animal Science* **14**, 249-255.

Buonomo, F.C. and Baile, C.A. (1991). Influence of nutritional deprivation on insulin-like growth factor 1, somatotropin and metabolic hormones in swine. *Journal of Animal Science* **69**, 755-760.

Campbell, R.G. and Dunkin, A.C. (1982). The effect of birth weight on the estimate milk intake, growth and body composition of sow-reared piglets. *Animal Production* **35**,193-197.

Campbell, R.G. and Dunkin, A.C. (1983a). The influence of nutrition early in life on growth and development of the pigs. I. The effects of protein nutrition to and subsequent to 6.5 kg on growth and development to 45 kg. *Animal Production* **36**, 415-423.

Campbell, R.G. and Dunkin, A.C. (1983b). The influence of nutrition early in life on growth and development of the pigs. II. Effects rearing method and feeding level on growth and development to 75 kg. *Animal Production* **36**, 425-434.

Campbell, R.G. and Taverner, M.R. (1988). Genotype and sex effects on the relationship between energy intake and protein deposition in growing pigs. *Journal of Animal Science* **66**, 676-686.

Campbell, R.G., Taverner, M.R. and Curic, D.M. (1983b). Effects of feeding level from 20 to 45 kg on the performance and carcass composition of pigs grown to 90 kg live weight. *Livestock Production Science* **10**, 265-272.

Campbell, R.G., Taverner, M.R. and Curic, D.M. (1983a). The influence of feeding level from 20 to 45 kg live weight on the performance and body composition of female and entire males. *Animal Production* **36**, 193-199.

Campbell, R.G., Taverner, M.R. and Curic, D.M. (1985). The influence of feeding level on the protein requirements of pigs between 20 and 45 kg live weight. *Animal Production* **40**, 489-496.

Chiba, L. (1994). Effects of dietary amino acid content between 20 and 50 kg and 50 and 100 kg live weight on the subsequent and overall performance of pigs. *Livestock Production Science* **39**, 213-221.

Chiba, L. (1995). Effects of nutritional history on the subsequent and overall growth performance and carcass traits of pigs. *Livestock Production Science* **41**, 151-161.

Chiba, L., Ivey, H., Cummins, K. and Gamble, B. (1999). Growth performance and carcass traits of pigs subjected to marginal dietary restrictions during the grower phase. *Journal of Animal Science* **77**, 1769-1776.

Chiba, L., Kuhlers, D., Frobish, L., Jungst , S., Huff-Lonergan, E., Lonergan, S. and Cummins, K. (2002). Effect of dietary restrictions on growth performance and carcass quality of pigs selected for lean growth efficiency. *Livestock Production Science* **74**, 93-102

Collins, C. L., Fu, S. X., Hinson, R., Leury, B. J., Tatham, B. G., Allee, G. L. and Dunshea, F. R. (2006). Lysine requirement of gilts following a protein restriction from 4 to 8 weeks of age. *Journal of Animal Science* **84** (Suppl. 1), 41 (Abstract).

Critser, D., Miller, P. and Lewis, A. (1995). The effects of dietary protein concentration on compensatory growth in barrows and gilts. *Journal of Animal Science* **73**, 3376-3383.

De Greef, K., Kemp, B. and Verstegen, M. (1992). Performance and body composition of fattening pigs of two strains during protein deficiency and subsequent realimentation. *Livestock Production Science* **30**, 141-153.

De Greef, K.H. (1992). Prediction of Production. Nutrition induced tissue partitioning in growing pigs. PhD Thesis. Department of Animal Nutrition Wageningen Agricultural University, Haagsteeg 4, 6708 PM Wageningen, The Netherlands.

de Lange, C.F.M., Birkett, S.H. and Morel, P.C.H. (2001). Protein, fat and bone tissue growth in swine. In: Lewis, A. and Southern, L. (Ed.) Swine Nutrition. Boca Raton, Florida, USA.

de Lange, C.F.M., Morel, P.C.H. and Birkett, S.H. (2003). Modeling chemical and physical body composition of the growing pig. *Journal of Animal Science* **81,** E159-165E.

Donker, R.A., denHartog, L.A., Brascamp, E.W., Merks, J.W.M., Noordewier, G.J. and Buiting, G.A.J. (1986). Restriction of feed intake to optimize overall performance and composition of pigs. *Livestock Production Science* **15**, 353-365.

Doyle, F. and Leeson, S. (1998). Compensatory growth in farm animals. Factors influencing response. Novus Nutrition Update 6 No. 01. Novus International Inc. St. Louis, Missouri.

Emmans, G.C., and Kyriazakis, I. (1997). Models of pig growth: problems and proposed solutions. *Livestock Production Science* **51**, 119-129.

Fabian, J., Chiba, L. I., Kuhlers, D. L., Frobish, K., Nadarajah, K. and McElhenney, W. H. (2003). Growth performance, dry matter and nitrogen digestibilities, serum profile, and carcass and meat quality of pigs with distinct genotypes. *Journal of Animal Science* **81,** 1142-1149.

Fabian, J., Chiba, L.I., Frobish, K., McElhenney, W., Kuhlers, D. and Nadarajah, K. (2004). Compensatory growth and nitrogen balance in grower-finisher pigs. *Journal of Animal Science* **82**, 2579-2587.

Fabian, J., Chiba, L.I, Kuhlers, D.L, Frobish, K., Nadarajah, K., Kerth, C., McElhenney, W. and Lewis, A. (2002). Degree of amino acid restriction during the grower phase and compensatory growth in pigs selected for lean growth efficiency. *Journal of Animal Science* **80**, 2610-2618.

Ferguson, N.S. and Gous, R.M. (1993). Evaluation of pig genotypes. 1. Theoretical aspects of measuring genetic parameters. *Animal Production* **56,** 233-243.

Ferguson, N.S. and Gous, R.M. (1997). The influence of heat production on the voluntary food intake in growing pigs given protein deficient diets. *Animal Science* **64**, 365-378.

Ferguson, N.S. and Theeruth, B.K. (2002). Protein and lipid deposition rates in growing pigs following a period of excess fattening. *South African Journal of Animal Science* **32**, 97-105.

Ferré, P. (1999). Regulation of gene expression by glucose. *Proceedings of the Nutrition Society*. **58**, 621-623.

Gill, B.P. (1998). Phase feeding: Effects on production efficiency and meat quality. Meat and Livestock Commission, Milton Keynes, UK.

Hogberg, M.G. and Zimmerman, D.R. (1978). Compensatory responses to dietary protein, length of starter period and strain of pig. *Journal of Animal Science* **47**, 893-899.

Hornick, J.L., van Eenaeme, C., Gérard, O., Dufrasne, I. and Istasse, L. (2000). Mechanisms of reduced and compensatory growth. *Domestic Animal Endocrinology* **19**, 121-132.

Hornick, J.L., van Eenaeme, C., Diez, M., Minet, V. and Istasse, L. (1998). Different periods of feed restriction before compensatory growth in Belgian Blue bulls: II. Plasma metabolites and hormones. *Journal of Animal Science* **76**, 260-271.

Houseknecht, K.L., Baile, C.A., Matteri, R.L. and Spurlock, M.E. (1998). The biology of leptin: A review. *Journal of Animal Science* **76**, 1405-1420.

Kristensen, L., Therkildsen, M., Aaslyng, M.D., Oksbjerg, N. and Ertbjerg, P. (2004). Compensatory growth improves meat tenderness in gilts but not in barrows. *Journal of Animal Science* **82**, 3617-3624.

Kristensen, L., Therkildsen, M., Riis, B., Sorensen, M.T., Oksbjerg, N., Purslow, P.P. and Ertbjerg, P. (2002). Dietary-induced changes of muscle growth rate in pigs: Effects on in vivo and post-mortem muscle proteolysis and meat quality. *Journal of Animal Science* **80**, 2862-2871.

Kyriazakis, I. and Emmans. G. (1992a). The effects of varying protein and energy intakes on the growth and body composition of pigs: 2. The effects of varying both energy and protein intake. *British Journal of Nutrition* **68**, 615-625.

Kyriazakis, I. and Emmans, G. (1992b). The growth of mammals following a period of nutritional limitation. *Journal of Theoretical Biology* **156,** 485-498.

Kyriazakis, I., Stamataris, C., Emmans, G. and Whittemore, C. (1991). The effects of food protein content on the performance of pigs previously given foods with low or moderate protein content. *Animal Production* **52**, 165-173.

Lawrence, T.L. and Flower, V.R. (2002). Growth of farm animals. CABI Publishing. Cab International. Wallingford Oxon OX10 8DE. UK.

Levin, N., Nelson, C., Gurney, A., Vadlen, R. and de Sauvage, F. (1996). Decreased food intake does not completely account for adiposity reduction after protein infusion. *Proceedings of the National Academy of Sciences of the United States of America* **93**, 1726-1730.

Lovatto, P.A., Sauvant, D. and van Milgen, J. (2000). Étude et modélisation du phénomène de crosissance compensatrice chez le porc. *Journées Recherche Procine en France* **32**, 241-246.

Martínez-Ramírez, H.R. (2005). Characterization of the dynamics of body protein deposition response following sudden changes in amino acid intake. M.Sc. Thesis. Department of Animal and Poultry Science, University of Guelph,

Guelph, Ontario, Canada.

Martínez, H.R., and de Lange, C.F.M. (2004). Body protein deposition response following sudden changes in ideal protein intake differs between pig types. *Journal of Animal Science* **82** (Suppl. 1), 420 (Abstract).

Martínez, H.R. and de Lange, C.F.M. (2005). Nutrition induced variation in body composition, compensatory growth, cortisol and leptin in growing pigs. *Journal of Animal Science* **82**(Suppl. 1), 214 (Abstracts).

Möhn, S. and de Lange, C.F.M. (1998). The effect of energy intake on body protein deposition in a defined population of gilts between 25 and 70 kg body weight. *Journal of Animal Science* **76**, 124-133.

Möhn, S., Gilles, A.M., Moughan, P.J. and de Lange, C.F.M. (2000). Influence of lysine and energy intakes on body protein deposition and lysine utilization in the growing pig. *Journal of Animal Science* **78**, 1510-1519.

Mosier, H.D. (1990). The determinants of catch-up growth. *Acta Paediatrica Scandinavia* (Suppl) **367**, 126-129.

Moughan, P.J. 1999. Protein metabolism in the pig. In: Kyriazakis, I. (Ed.). A Quantitative Biology of the Pig. CABI Publishing. CAB International. Wallingford, Oxon UK.

Moughan, P.J. and Verstegen, M.W.A. (1988). The modelling of growth in the pig. *Netherlands Journal of Agricultural Science* **36**, 145-166.

Moughan, P.J., Jacobson, L.H. and Morel, P.C.H. (2006). A genetic upper limit to whole-body protein deposition in a strain of growing pigs. *Journal of Animal Science* **84**, 3301-3309.

Nielsen, H.E. (1964). Effects on bacon pigs of differing levels of nutrition to 20 kg body weight. *Animal Production* **6**, 301-308.

Noblet, J., Bernier, J.F., Dubois, S., Le Cozler, Y. and van Milgen J. (1997). Effect of breed and body weight on components of heat production in growing pigs. In: K. McCracken, E.F. Unsworth, A.R. G. Wylie (Editors). Energy Metabolism of Farm Animals. Newcastle, Co. Down (Northern Ireland), pp. 225-228.

O'Donovan, P.B. (1984). Compensatory gain in cattle and sheep. *Nutrition, Abstracts and Reviews. Series B* **54**, 389-409.

O'Connell, M.K., Lynch, P.B. and O'Doherty, J.V. (2005). A comparison between feeding a single diet or phase feeding a series of diets, with either the same or reduced crude protein content, to growing finishing pigs. *Animal Science* **81**, 297-303.

O'Connell, M.K., Lynch, P.B. and O'Doherty, J.V. (2006). The effect of dietay lysine restriction during the grower phase and subsequent dietary lysine concentration during the re-alimentation phase on the performance, carcass characteristics and nitrogen balance of growing – finishing pigs. *Livestock Science* **101**, 169-179.

Oksbjerg, N., Sørensen, M. T. and Vestergaard, M. (2002). Compensatory growth and its effect on muscularity and technological meat quality in growing pigs. *Acta Agriculturæ Scandinavica, Section A, Animal Science* **52**, 85-90.

Osborne, T.B. and Mendel, L.B. (1916). Acceleration of growth after retardation. *American Journal of Physiology* **40**, 16-20.

Pitts, G. (1986). Cellular aspects of growth and catch-up growth in rats: A re-evaluation. *Growth* **50**, 419-436.

Pluske, J.R., Williams, I.H. and Aherne, F.X. (1995). Nutrition of the neonatal pig. In: The Neonatal pig. Development and Survival. (Ed) Varley, M.A. CAB International. Wallingford, UK.

Pond, W.G. and Mersmann, H.J. (1990). Differential compensatory growth in swine following control of feed intake by a high alfalfa diet fed ad libitum or by limited feed. *Journal of Animal Science* **68**, 352-362.

Pond, W.G., Yen, J.T. and Lindvall, R.N. (1980). Early protein deficiency: Effect on later growth and carcass composition of lean or obese swine. *Journal of Nutrition* **110**, 2506-2513.

Prince, T. J., Jungst, S. B. and Kuhlers, D. L. (1983). Compensatory responses to short-term feed restriction during the growing period. *Journal of Animal Science* **56**, 846-852.

Quiniou, N., Dourmand, J. and Nobblet, J. (1996). Effects of energy intake on the performance of different types of pigs from 45 to 100 kg body weight. I. Protein and lipid deposition. *Animal Science* **63**, 277-288.

Quiniou, N., Nobblet, J., van Milgen., J. and Dourmand, J. (1995). Effect of energy intake on performance, nutrient and tissue gain and protein and energy utilization in growing boars. *Animal Science* **61**, 133-143.

Raj, St., Skiba, G, Weremko, D., Fandrewski, H. (2005). Growth of the gastrointestinal tract of pigs during realimentation following a high-fibre diet. *Journal of Animal and Feed Sciences* **14**, 675-684.

Reeds, P. Burrin, D. Fiorotto, M., Mersmann, H. and Pond, W. (1993). Growth regulation with particular reference to the pig. In: Hollis, G. (Ed). Growth of the pig. CAB International, Wallingford, UK.

Reynolds, A.M. and O'Doherty, J.V. (2006). The effect of amino acid restriction during the grower phase on the compensatory growth, carcass composition and nitrogen utilization in grower – finishing pigs. *Livestock Science* **104**, 112-120.

Robinson, D. (1964). The plane of nutrition and compensatory growth in pigs. *Animal Production* **6**: 227-236.

Scanes, C.G. (2003). Hormones and growth. In: Scanes, C.G. (Ed.) Biology of growth of domestics animals. Iowa State Press. Iowa, USA.

Schinckel, A.P. (1999). Describing the pig. In: Kyriazakis (Ed.). A quantitative biology of the pig. CABI Publishing. CAB International, Wallingford, UK.

Schinckel. P. and de Lange, C.F.M. (1996). Characterization of growth parameters needed as inputs for pig growth models. *Journal of Animal Science* **74**, 2021-2036.

Skiba, G. (2005). Physiological aspects of compensatory growth in pigs. *Journal of Animal and Feed Sciences* **14** (Suppl. 1), 191-203.

Skiba, G. and Fandrejewski, H. (1998). Energy utilization in re-alimentated pigs in relation to initial body composition. In: McCracken, K., Unsworth, E.F., and Wylie, A.R.G. (Ed.). Energy Metabolism of farm animals. CAB International, Wallingford, UK, pp 229-232.

Skiba, G, Raj, St., Weremko, D., Fandrewski, H. (2005). Growth of the gastrointestinal tract in weaning pigs as affected by crude fibre content in the diet. *Journal of Animal and Feed Sciences* **15**, 403-415.

Skiba, G, Raj, St., Weremko, D., Fandrewski, H. (2006a). The compensatory response of pigs previously fed a diet with an increased fibre content. 2. Chemical and body components and composition of daily gain. *Journal of Animal and Feed Sciences* **15**, 403-415.

Skiba, G, Raj, St., Weremko, D., Fandrewski, H. (2006a). The compensatory response of pigs previously fed a diet with an increased fibre content. 2. Growth rate and voluntary feed intake. *Journal of Animal and Feed Sciences* **15**, 393-402.

Smith, J.W. II, Tokach, M.D., O'Quinn, P.R., Nelssen, J.L., Goodband, R.D. (1999). Effects of dietary energy density and lysine:calorie ratio on growth performance and carcass characteristics of growing-finishing pigs. *Journal of Animal Science* **77**, 3007-3015.

Stamataris, C., Kyriazakis, I. and Emmans, G. (1991). The performance and body composition of young pigs following a period of growth retardation by food restriction. *Animal Production* **53**, 373-381.

Tanner, J.M. (1963). Regulation of growth size in mammals. *Nature* **4896,** 825-850.

Therkildsen, M., Riis, B.M., Karlsson, A., Kristensen, L., Ertbjerg, P., Purslow, P.P., Aaslyng, M.A. and Oksbjerg, N. (2002). Compensatory growth response in pigs, muscle protein turn-over and meat texture: Effects of restriction/ re-alimentation period. *Animal Science* **75**, 367-377.

Therkildsen, M., Vestergaard, M., Busk, H., Jensen, M.T., Riis, B., Karlsson, H.A., Kristensen, L., Ertbjerg, P. and Oksbjerg, N. (2004). Compensatory growth in slaughter pigs-in vitro muscle protein turnover at slaughter, circulation IGF-I, performance and carcass quality. *Livestock Production Science* **88**, 63-75.

Tokach, M.D.; Goodband, R.D.; Nelssen, J.L. and Kats, L.J. (1992). Influence of weaning weight and growth during the first week post weaning on subsequent pig performance. Swine Day. Kansas State University.

Valaja, J., Alaviuhkola, T., Suomi, K. and Immonen, I. (1992). Compensatory growth after feed restriction during the rearing period in pigs. *Agricultural and Food Science in Finland* **1**, 15–20.

Waterlow, J.C. (1986). Metabolic adaptation to low intakes of energy and protein. *Annual Review of Nutrition* **6**, 495-526.

Waters, H.J. (1908). The capacity of animals to grow under adverse conditions. *Proceedings of the Society for the Promotion of Agricultural Science*, NY. **29**, 71-96.

Weis, R.N., Birkett, S.H., Morel, P.C.H. and de Lange, C.F.M. (2004). Effects of energy intake and body weight on physical and chemical body composition in growing entire male pigs. *Journal of Animal Science* **82**, 109-121.

Wilson, P. and Osbourn, D. (1960). Compensatory growth after under-nutrition in mammals and birds. *Biological Reviews* **35**, 324-363.

Whang, K., Donovan, S. and Easter, R. (2000a). Effect of protein deprivation on subsequent efficiency of dietary protein utilization in finish pigs. *Asian-Australasian Journal of Animal Science* **13**, 659-665.

Whang, K., McKeith, F., Kim, S. and Easter, R. (2000b). Effect of starter feeding program on growth performance and gains of body components from weaning to market weight in swine. *Journal of Animal Science* **78**, 2885-2895.

Whang, K., Kim, S., Donovan, S. McKeith, F. and Easter, R. (2003). Effects of protein deprivation on subsequent growth performance, gain of body components, and protein requirements in growing pigs. *Journal of Animal Science* **81**, 705-716.

Whittemore, C.T., and Fawcett, R.H. (1976). Theoretical aspects of a flexible model to simulate protein and lipid growth in pigs. *Animal Production* **22**, 87-96.

Whittemore, C. T., Tullis, J.B. and Hastie, S.W. (1978). Efficiency of use of nitrogen from dried microbial cells after a period of N deprivation in growing pigs. *British Journal of Nutrition* **39**, 193-200.

Wyllie, D., Speer, V.C., Ewan, R.C. and Hays, V.W. (1969). Effects of starter protein level on performance and body composition of pigs. *Journal of Animal Science* **29**, 433-438.

Yambayamba, E.S., Price, M.A., and Foxcroft, G.R. (1996). Hormonal status, metabolic changes, and restring metabolic rate in beef heifers undergoing compensatory growth. *Journal of Animal Science* **74**, 57-69.

Zubair, A. K. (1994). Compensatory growth in the broiler chicken. Ph.D. Thesis. Department of Animal and Poultry Science, University of Guelph, Guelph, Ontario, Canada.

LIST OF PARTICIPANTS

The forty-first University of Nottingham Feed Conference was organised by the following committee:

MR N.J. CHANDLER (*National Renderers Association*)
DR Z. DAVIES (*Defra*)
MR M. HAZZLEDINE (*Premier Nutrition*)
MR W. MORRIS (*BOCM PAULS Lt*d)
DR D. PARKER (*Novus International*)
MR M. ROGERS (*Volac International*)
DR R. TEN DOESCHATE (*ABNA Ltd*)
DR M.A. VARLEY (*Provimi Ltd*)

DR J.M. BRAMELD
PROF P.J. BUTTERY
DR P.C. GARNSWORTHY (*Secretary*)
DR J.N. HUXLEY
DR T. PARR   *University of Nottingham*
DR A.M. SALTER
DR K.D. SINCLAIR
PROF R. WEBB
DR J. WISEMAN (*Chairman*)

The conference was held at the University of Nottingham Sutton Bonington Campus, 4-6 September 2007. The following persons registered for the meeting.

Aikman, Dr P	University of Reading, Dept of Agriculture, Earley Gate, P O Box 237, Reading RG6 6AR, UK
Anderson, Dr R	Merlin Veterinary Group, Edinburgh Rd, Kelso TD5 7EN, UK
Bain, Mr M	Vistavet, 211 Castle Rd, Randalstown, Co Antrim BT41 2EB, UK
Bakke, Mr M J	Custom Dairy Performance Inc, P O Box 99, Clovis, CA 93613-0099, USA
Bartram, Dr C	Southern Valley Feeds, Huntworth Mill, Bridgewater TA6 6LQ, UK
Beever, Prof D	Keenan Rumans, Ryecroft Munday Dean, Marlow, Bucks SL7 3BU, UK
Bird, Mr N	Farm Energy & Control Services Ltd, Pingewood Business Estate, Pingewood, Reading, Berks RG30 3UR, UK
Blake, Dr J	Dietcheck Ltd, Highfield, Little London, Andover SP11 6JE, UK
Brameld, Dr J M	University of Nottingham, Sutton Bonington Campus, Loughborough LE12 5RD, UK
Castillejos, Dr L	Diamond V Europe, P O Box 14, Marum 9363, The Netherlands
Chew, Mr R	Pfizer Ltd, Ramsgate Rd, Sandwich CT13 9NJ, UK
Chuffart, Mr M	DSM Nutritional Products SA, Rue de la Combe 15, Gland 1196, Switzerland
Contreras, Mr D	University of Nottingham, Sutton Bonington Campus, Loughborough, Leics LE12 5RD, UK
Dart, Miss A	Woodhayes House, Clyst Hydon, Cullompton EX 15 2NT, UK

353

Davies, Mr T	KITE, 18 Greenway, Ashbourne, Derbyshire DE6 1EF, UK
Davies, Dr Z	DEFRA, Area 4B, Nobel House, 17 Smith Square, London SW1P 3JR, UK
De Jong, Miss L	CCL BV, Postbus 107, Veghel 5460 AC, The Netherlands
de Lang, Dr K	University of Guelph, Dept of Animal & Poultry Science, Guelph N1G 2W1, Canada
Dinamani, Dr R	Tetragib Chemie Pvt Ltd, IS-40, KHB Industrial Area, Yelahanka New Town, Bangalore 560064, India
Doppenberg, Dr J	Schothorst Feed Research, Box 533, Lelystad 8200 AM, The Netherlands
Downey, Mr N	SCA Nutec, SCA Mill, Dalton, Thirsk, N Yorks YO7 3HE, UK
Drackley, Dr J	University of Illinois, 1207 West Gregory Drive, Urbana, Illinois 61801, USA
Edwards, Prof S	Newcastle University, School of Agriculture, Food & Rural Development, King George V1 Building, Newcastle Upon Tyne NE1 7RU, UK
Flint, Prof A P F	University of Nottingham, Sutton Bonington Campus, Loughborough LE12 5RD, UK
Fordyce, Mr J	Country Wide Farms, Suite 2, Grateley Business Park, Cholderton Road, Grateley, Hants SP11 9SH, UK
Fowers, Miss R	Frank Wright Ltd, Blenheim House, Blenheim Rd, Ashbourne, Derbyshire DE6 1HA, UK
Fullarton, Mr P	Forum Bioscience, 41-51 Brighton Rd, Redhill, Surrey RH1 6YS, UK
Galbraith, Dr H	University of Aberdeen, 23 St Machar, Aberdeen AB24 3RY, UK
Garnsworthy, Dr P C	University of Nottingham, Sutton Bonington Campus, Loughborough, Leics LE12 5RD, UK
Gill, Dr P	MLC, P O Box 44, Winterhill House, Milton Keynes MK5 8AJ, UK
Golds, Mrs S P	University of Nottingham, Sutton Bonington Campus, Loughborough LE12 5RD, UK
Gould, Mrs M	Volac International Ltd, Volac House, Orwell, Royston SG8 5QX, UK
Graham, Dr H	AB Vista, 3 Woodstock Court, Marlborough Business Park, Marlborough SN8 4AN, UK
Graham, Mr M R	CMD Agribusiness and AS Associates, Tremywawr, Brezdden Ave, Arddleen, Llanymynech SY22 6SP, UK
Green, Mrs K	Fishmeal Information Network, 1010 Regus House, Cambourne Bus Park, Cambourne CB23 6DP, UK
Green, Prof M	University of Nottingham, Sutton Bonington Campus, Loughborough, Leics LE12 5RD, UK
Gregson, Miss E	University of Nottingham, Sutton Bonington Campus, Loughborough, Leics LE12 5RD, UK
Hall, Miss C	BOCM Pauls, First Avenue, Royal Portbury Dock, Portbury, Bristol BS20 7XS, UK

Hamid, Mr N A	University of Nottingham, Sutton Bonoington Campus, Loughborough, Leics LE12 5RD, UK
Hazzledine, Mr M	Premier Nutrition, The Levels, Rugeley WS15 1RD, UK
Hooley, Mrs E	University of Nottingham, Sutton Bonington Campus, Loughborough LE12 5RD, UK
Hough, Mr T	NWF Agriculture Ltd, Wardle, Nantwich, Cheshire CW5 6AQ, UK
Husband, Mr J	University of Nottingham, EBVC, 68 Arthur St, Penrith, Cumbria CA11 7TX, UK
Huxley, Dr J N	University of Nottingham, Sutton Bonington Campus, Loughborough, Leics LE12 5RD, UK
Ingham, Mr Roger	Kemira Growhow UK Ltd, Ince, Chester CH2 4LB, UK
Irwin, Mr R	United Feeds Ltd, 8 Northern Rd, Belfast BT3 9AL, UK
Isaac, Mr P	Mole Valley Farmers, Huntworth Mill, Bridgewater TA6 6LQ, UK
Jacklin, Mr D	Consultant, 10 Station Close, Ridingmill, Northumberland NE44 6HF, UK
Jagger, Dr S	ABN, Oundle Road, Peterborough PE2 9PW, UK
Jones, Mr H	Roquette UK Ltd, Sallow Rd, Corby NN17 5JX, UK
Keeling, Mrs S	Nottingham University Press, Manor Farm, Church Lane, Thrumpton, Notts NG11 0AX, UK
Kirkland, Dr R	Volac International Ltd, Volac Houe, Orwell, Royston SG8 5QX, UK
Lee, Miss E	University of Nottingham, Sutton Bonington Campus, Loughborough, Leics LE12 5RD, UK
Lomax, Prof M	University of Nottingham, Sutton Bonington Campus, Loughborough, Leics LE12 5RD, UK
Lucey, Mr P	Dairygold Co-op Ltd, Lambardstown, Co Cork , Ireland
Ludger, Miss A K	Nutreco SRC, Boxmeerseweg 30, Sint Anthonis 5845 ET, The Netherlands
Mafo, Mr A	Hi Peak Feeds Ltd, Hi Peak Feeds Mill, Sheffield Rd, Kilamarsh S21 1ED, UK
McClelland, Mr D J	Norvite, Wardhouse, Insch, Aberdeen AB52 6YD, UK
McIlmoyle, Dr D	Rumenco, Stretton House, Derby Rd, Burton-on-Trent, Derbyshire DE13 0DW, UK
Meeusen, Ir A	Kemin Europe N V, Toekomstlaan 42, Industriezane Wolfstee, Herentals 2200, Belgium
Morris, Mr W	BOCM Pauls Ltd, First Ave, Royal Portbury Dock, Portbury, Bristol BS20 9XS, UK
Mounsey, Mr A	Pentlands Publishing Ltd, Station Rd, Great Longstone, Bakewell DE45 1TS, UK
Nettleton, Dr P	Moredun Research Institute, Pentlands Science Park, Penicuik EH26 0PZ, UK
Overend, Dr M	Forum Bioscience, 41-51 Brighton Rd, Redhill, Surrey RH1 6YS, UK

Packington, Mr A	DSM Nutritional Products (UK) Ltd, Delves Road, Heanor DE75 7GG, UK
Parker, Dr D	Novus Europe, 200 Avenue Marcel Thiry, Building D, Brussels B-1200, Belgium
Parr, Dr T	University of Nottingham, Sutton Bonington Campus, Loughborough LE12 5RD, UK
Pass, Mr R	Diageo, Oerlil House, Carsebridge Rd,, Alloa, Clackmannanshire FK10 3LT, UK
Pine, Mr P	Premier Nutrition, The Levels, Rugeley WS15 1RD, UK
Rapp, Dr C	Zinpro Animal Nutrition, Gerard Doustraat 4A, Boxmeer 5831CC, The Netherlands
Remmer, Mr R J Retford	Optivite International Ltd, Drayton Court, Manton Wood Bus Pk, Rd, Worksop, Notts S80 2RS, UK
Richards, Dr S	SCA Nutec, SCA Mill, Dalton Airfield, Dalton, Thirsk, N Yorks YO7 3HE, UK
Robinson, Miss M J	John Thompson and Sons, 35-39 York Rd, Belfast BT15 3GW, UK
Roger, Mr P	Veterinary Consultant Services, Victoria Cottage, Reath, Nr Richmond, N Yorks DL11 6SZ, UK
Rogers, Mr M	Volac International Ltd, Volac House, Orwell, Royston SG8 5QX, UK
Rose, Mr D	CBA Technical, Lansil Industrial Estate, Lansil Rd, Lancaster LA1 3QY, UK
Royle, Mr N	United Feeds, 8 Northern Rd, Belfast BT3 9AL, UK
Rudd, Mr G	AIC - Agricultural Industries Confederations, Confederation House, East of England Showground, Peterborough PE2 6XE, UK
Rundle, Ms E	Pilgrims Veterinary Centre, 5-7 Castle Street, Cranbourne BH21 5PZ, UK
Salter, Prof A	University of Nottingham, Sutton Bonington Campus, Loughborough LE12 5RD, UK
Santos, Prof J	University of California, Davis, VMTRC, 18830 Rd 112, Tulare CA 93274, USA
Seppala, Miss S	Raisio Feed Ltd, P O Box 101, Raisio 21201, Finland
Sinclair, Dr K D	University of Nottingham, Sutton Bonington Campus, Loughborough LE12 5RD, UK
Sissons, Mr J	ABN, ABN House, Oundle Rd, Woodston, Peterborough PE2 9PW, UK
Starkl, Dr V	Biomin GmbH, Industriestrasse 21, A-3130 Herzogenburg , Austria
Sterten, Mr H	Felleskjopet Forutvikling, N-7005 Trondeim, Trondeim 7005, Norway
Sudekum, Dr K H	University of Bonn, Endenicher Allee 15, Bonn 53115, Germany
Sundrum, Prof A	University of Kassel, Novdbahnhof str 7, Witzenhausen 37273, Germany
Taylor, Mr M J	Calibre Control, 5 Asher Court, Lyncastle Way, Appleton, Warrington, Cheshire WA4 4ST, UK
van Kempem, Dr T	Provimi Ltd, Lenneke Marelaan 2, St Stevens Woluwe 1932, Belgium

Varley, Dr M	Provimi Ltd, Eastern Ave, Lichfield, Staffs WS13 7SE, UK
Vecqueray, Mr R J	EBVC, 68 Arthur St, Penrith CA11 7TX, UK
Wallace, Dr R J	Rowett Research Institute, Bucksburn, Aberdeen AB21 9SB, UK
Ward, Ms M	Ermine Farms Ltd, Waddingham Grange, Kirton Rd, Waddingham, Gainsborough, Lincs DN21 4TB, UK
Webb, Mrs R	Nottingham University Press, Manor Farm, Church Lane, Thrumpton, Notts NG11 OAX, UK
Webb, Prof R	University of Nottingham, Sutton Bonington Campus, Loughborough LE12 5RD, UK
Whitehead, Mr J	Wyreside Products, Lune Bank, School Lane, Pilling, Preston, Lancs PR3 6AA, UK
Whitney, Miss H	BQP, 1Stradbroke Business Centre, New St, Stradbroke, Suffolk IP21 5JJ, UK
Wilde, Mr D	Alltech UK Ltd, Ryhall Raod, Stamford PE9 1TZ, UK
Wilkinson, Dr M	University of Nottingham, Sutton Bonington Campus, Loughborough, Leics LE12 5RD, UK
Williams, Dr A	Cranfield University, Natural Resource Management Centre, Building 42a, Cranfield, Beds MK43 OAL, UK
Wiltbank, Prof M	University of Wisconsin, Dept of Dairy Science & Endocrinology, 1675 Observatory Drive, Madison W15 3706, USA
Wiseman, Prof J	University of Nottingham, Sutton Bonington Campus, Loughborough LE12 5RD, UK
Wonnacott, Miss K	University of Nottingham, Sutton Bonington Campus, Loughborough, Leics LE12 5RD, UK

INDEX

Moulton
College

NORTHAMPTONSHIRE

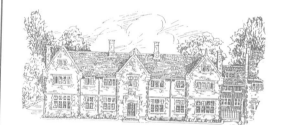